The Toxic Truth About Fruits and Vegetables

Plant Poisons, Mineral Traps, Metabolic Burdens, and the Hidden Chemistry of "Healthy" Foods

First Edition: April 2026
ISBN: 978-1-966035-08-4
Published by Elite Nutrition Research
EliteNutritionResearch.com

ELITE

NUTRITION RESEARCH

Elite Nutrition Research is a science-driven health and education company dedicated to understanding and optimizing human physiology at its most fundamental level. Our work is built on an architecture-first approach—examining how nutrients interact with cellular systems, membranes, energy production, and signaling pathways to shape overall health and performance. Rather than following trends, we focus on first principles, combining biochemical insight, formulation precision, and practical application to create both advanced nutritional products and in-depth educational systems.

Through our books, courses, and formulations, Elite Nutrition Research aims to give individuals direct access to the mechanisms that govern their biology empowering them to think clearly, act intentionally, and build lasting health from the inside out.

To explore our full system of products, courses, and research, visit:
www.elitenutritionresearch.com

Table of Contents

Introduction. The Body Does Not Eat Nutrition Labels 7

Part I - The Plant Is Not Passive 19

Chapter 1 - Plant Tissue Is Defensive Tissue 21

Chapter 2 - What Digestion Has to Do to a Plant 33

Chapter 3 - Poison, Burden, Irritant, and Blocker 45

Part II - The Gut Event 57

Chapter 4 - The Gut as the First Site of Loss 59

Chapter 5 - Fiber, Bulk, and the Problem of False Virtue 71

Chapter 6 - FODMAPs and the Fermentation Burden 83

Chapter 7 - Lectins and the Problem of Chemical Contact 95

Chapter 8 - Protease Inhibitors and Poor Protein Yield 105

Chapter 9 - Tannins, Polyphenols, and the Cost of Astringency 115

Chapter 10 - Saponins and Detergent-Like Plant Chemistry 127

Part III - Mineral Theft and Nutritional Loss 137

Chapter 11 - Oxalates: Mineral Traps and Urinary Burden 139

Chapter 12 - Phytates: Mineral Locking 153

Chapter 13 - When a Food Tests Dense but Nourishes Poorly 165

Part IV - Direct Plant Toxins in Common Foods 175

Chapter 14 - Glycoalkaloids in Potatoes and Nightshades 177

Chapter 15 - Cyanogenic Glycosides 187

Chapter 16 - Cucurbitacins: 199

Chapter 17 - Other Natural Plant Toxins Worth Understanding 209

Part V - Endocrine and Metabolic Interference 221

Chapter 18 - Goitrogens and the Thyroid 223

Chapter 19 - Drug and Hormone Handling 237

Chapter 20 - Liver Workload and Chemical Clearance 247

Part VI - The Kidney, Urine, and the Organ of Consequence 259

Chapter 21 - The Kidney as a Filter of Failed Food Logic 261

Chapter 22 - Crystal Burden, Irritation, and Stone Vulnerability 271

Chapter 23 - Sensitive Hosts and High-Risk Physiology..........................281
Part VII - Fruit Is Not Exempt..291
Chapter 24 - The Chemical Problem with Fruit..293
Chapter 25 - Sugar Delivery, Fructose Load, and Intestinal Overrun.....303
Chapter 26 - Fruit Acids, Polyols, Seeds, and Peel Chemistry.................313
Chapter 27 - Fruits with Special Risks...325
Part VIII - Preparation, Dose, and Exposure Pattern...............................335
Chapter 28 - Why Preparation Changes the Biological Event.................337
Chapter 29 - Dose Makes the Burden Visible..351
Chapter 30 - Illusion of Safety by Rotation..363
Part IX - How to Judge a Food Correctly...375
Chapter 31 - A Better Standard Than "Contains Nutrients"...................377
Chapter 32 - How to Think About Fruits and Vegetables.......................385
Chapter 33 - The Foods Most Likely to Burden the Body.......................395
Conclusion...411

Introduction

The Body Does Not Eat Nutrition Labels

The modern conversation about fruits and vegetables usually begins after the most important part has already been erased. The plant arrives in public language as a category, a color, a serving, a source of vitamins, fiber, antioxidants, or phytochemicals. It does not arrive as a defended tissue. It does not arrive as a leaf built around oxalate crystals, a seed built around mineral-binding storage compounds, a tuber carrying glycoalkaloids near the peel, or a fruit carrying sugars, acids, polyols, seeds, skins, and enzyme-active molecules inside one structure. The chemistry gets flattened before digestion even begins. A food is praised for what laboratory analysis can extract from it, while the body is left to deal with the actual structure that reaches the mouth, the stomach, the intestinal lumen, and the absorptive membrane. That is the first failure. The conversation treats the nutrient list as the food itself, when the nutrient list is only a partial inventory of what can be measured after the tissue has already been destroyed in the lab.

The body does not eat that laboratory printout. It eats physical plant matter that has to be torn apart, acidified, enzymatically cleaved, mixed with bile, exposed to microbes, and held in solution long enough for usable compounds to reach the intestinal surface. A calcium number on paper says nothing by itself about whether calcium remains available in the gut once oxalate is released from the same leaf. An iron number says little about actual iron entry into the body if phytate, tannins, or competing fibers are holding that mineral in the lumen and carrying it toward the toilet. A carbohydrate number says little about tolerance if the sugars are paired with polyols or fermentable carbohydrates that stay unabsorbed, pull water into the bowel, and then feed gas production in the colon. The shallow conversation keeps asking what the plant contains. Digestion is asking a different question. What survives the plant matrix. What stays soluble. What gets trapped. What crosses. What has to be cleared.

This flattening also hides the fact that plant compounds do different kinds of damage or interference in different compartments. Some problems stay in the gut, where they irritate the mucosa, slow protein breakdown, alter transit, or increase fermentation pressure. Some move into the blood and become renal work, hepatic work, endocrine interference, or drug metabolism problems. Oxalate is a clean example because the burden shifts location as the sequence moves forward. In the gut it can bind calcium and reduce mineral value from the meal. After absorption it becomes a urinary solute that the kidney must filter and excrete, and under the wrong conditions it contributes to crystal formation. Grapefruit makes the same point through a different route. The fruit is still discussed as produce, but its furanocoumarins can inhibit intestinal cytochrome P450 3A4, one of the enzyme systems that helps break down many drugs during first-pass metabolism. The chemistry does not care about the produce aisle. It acts where it lands. The modern conversation stays shallow because it keeps grouping unlike biological events under one moralized food category and calling that nutrition.

The same shallowness shows up in the way preparation, dose, and frequency are treated as afterthoughts. A raw spinach smoothie every morning is not the same exposure as occasional cooked spinach beside a mixed meal. An undercooked bean is not the same object as a properly soaked and thoroughly boiled bean. A peeled and pressure-cooked plant food is not the same intestinal problem as the raw, intact, daily version. Yet public nutrition language often speaks as if the category settles the matter. Fruit. Vegetable. Whole food. Plant-based. Those words do not describe what digestion is actually handling. They do not describe whether a compound is heat-labile, meaning it breaks down with sufficient heat, water-soluble, meaning it can leach into cooking water, or mechanically protected inside skins, seed coats, and fibrous cell walls. They do not describe whether a burden is occasional and trivial or chronic enough to become part of the intestine's daily workload, the thyroid's iodine problem, or the kidney's filtration burden.

A chemically serious conversation has to start lower and closer to the tissue. What kind of plant structure is this. What defensive compounds are concentrated there. What does chewing rupture. What does acid release. What do pancreatic enzymes fail to break. What gets bound before absorption. What reaches the brush border, the enzyme-rich surface of the small intestine that finishes digestion and helps move nutrients into the body. What crosses into portal blood on the way to the liver. What leaves through urine because the body cannot use it. Once those questions are asked, the public language around fruits and vegetables starts looking thin and ceremonial. The food may keep the reputation. The gut, liver, thyroid, and kidney still have to handle the chemistry.

The Gap Between Nutrient Charts and Biological Reality

A nutrient chart is a chemical inventory taken after the food has been reduced to analyzable matter. It tells you what can be detected in the sample. It does not tell you what the mouth can break open, what stomach acid can release, what pancreatic enzymes can separate, what remains trapped inside plant cell walls, what precipitates in the intestinal lumen, or what the absorptive surface can actually move into the body. This is the first distortion. The chart makes the food look like an open container of nutrients waiting for pickup. The body meets a structure instead. Leaf tissue, seed tissue, tuber tissue, fruit tissue. Fiber scaffolds. crystal deposits. storage compounds. enzyme inhibitors. binding agents. acids. sugars. bitter molecules. Defense chemistry is still part of the food when it enters the mouth. The chart does not show the conflict inside the meal. It only lists what was present when the laboratory finished dismantling what digestion may not dismantle nearly as well.

This is why two foods can carry similar numbers on paper and produce very different biological returns. A plant can test high in calcium while delivering far less usable calcium once oxalate is released into the same intestinal contents and binds it. A seed can test rich in zinc or iron while phytate, the phosphorus storage compound in many seeds and legumes, holds those minerals in complexes that human digestion cannot break efficiently. A protein value can look respectable while protease inhibitors, compounds that block protein-digesting enzymes such as trypsin and chymotrypsin, reduce how much amino acid actually becomes available for absorption. The chart records gross content. The body lives on liberated content, retained content, and tolerated content. Those are not the same numbers.

The gap widens further at the intestinal surface. Nutrients do not enter the body because they exist in the bowl. They have to reach the brush border, the enzyme-rich surface of the small intestine, in a form that remains soluble and transportable. Soluble means dissolved and available to move through the watery environment of the gut. Transportable means small enough and chemically suitable for intestinal cells to carry or admit across the membrane. Many things go wrong before that point. Minerals can bind other compounds and become unavailable. Carbohydrates can remain poorly absorbed, pull water into the bowel, and then pass into the colon where bacteria ferment them into gas. Proteins can remain partially digested and continue downstream as larger fragments. Polyphenols and tannins can bind proteins and minerals. Fiber can hold material inside a bulk matrix long enough to change the speed and quality of contact. The nutrient chart sees a list. The intestine sees a traffic problem.

Even absorption is not the end of the story. Once a compound crosses into blood, the question shifts from availability to handling. Can the liver use it, transform it, store it, or neutralize it. Can the kidney clear it without concentrating it into a crystal risk. Can the thyroid function normally in the presence of compounds that interfere with iodine handling. A food can look generous at the level of content and still create a poor net return once burden is counted. Oxalate illustrates the whole sequence clearly. In the gut it can lower mineral availability. In the blood it becomes a compound the body must carry. In the kidney it becomes a filtration burden. In the urine it can contribute to calcium oxalate crystallization if concentration rises high enough. The chart only showed that the leaf contained calcium, magnesium, potassium, and vitamin C. The kidney sees the rest of the story.

The chart also ignores preparation, which means it ignores the chemistry of change. Boiling can lower soluble oxalate because some of it leaves the tissue and enters the cooking water. Proper heat can denature lectins and protease inhibitors, which means it changes their shape enough to reduce their biological activity. Fermentation and sprouting can lower phytate by activating phytase, the enzyme that breaks phytic acid down. Peeling can remove compounds concentrated near the outer tissue. Juicing can strip away some structural resistance while concentrating sugar delivery and shrinking the amount of chewing, gastric slowing, and bulk that once moderated the exposure. A chart that treats raw and cooked values as simple variations of the same food misses the central point. Preparation changes what digestion is dealing with.

This is why the public argument so often feels persuasive and thin at the same time. It points to measurable nutrients and assumes the biological case is closed. But the body does not run on nutrient presence. It runs on digestive release, chemical availability, membrane transport, tissue tolerance, and clearance cost. The number on the page is the beginning of the question, not the answer. A food earns its place only after the gut has broken it down, the intestine has absorbed what remains usable, the tissues have taken what they need, and the organs of clearance have finished with what the body could not use. Until that full sequence is accounted for, the chart is describing composition. It is not yet describing nourishment.

Why "Contains Vitamins" Is Not the Same as "Nourishes the Body"

A food can contain vitamins and still nourish poorly because containment is a laboratory fact, while nourishment is a physiological result. The vitamin has to survive the structure it is packaged in, survive preparation, survive the digestive sequence, remain chemically available in the intestinal contents, reach the absorptive surface, cross into the body, and then enter tissues that can actually use it. That is a much narrower path than nutrition language usually admits. A leaf, fruit, seed, or root is not a loose pile of vitamins waiting for pickup. It is organized tissue. Cell walls hold compounds in place. fibers slow release. acids shift pH. polyphenols bind proteins and minerals. oxalate can change the mineral environment of the meal. enzyme inhibitors can reduce digestion upstream. The vitamin may be present in the sample and still be carried through a meal that delivers less usable nourishment than the label implies.

The body also does not use all vitamin forms equally. Plant foods often contain precursors, unstable forms, or compounds that require additional conversion before they become useful inside human tissue. Beta-carotene is a clear example. It is not vitamin A itself. It is a carotenoid precursor that the intestinal lining and liver must convert into retinol, the active vitamin A form used in vision, immune signaling, epithelial maintenance, and many other functions. That conversion is variable. It depends on digestion, fat presence, bile release, enzyme activity, genetics, thyroid status, and overall nutritional state. A chart may count beta-carotene generously and then let the public language drift into "high in vitamin A." The body is dealing with a conversion problem, not a direct vitamin delivery. The same inflation happens whenever a chart treats precursor presence as if it were identical to active tissue availability.

Even when the vitamin itself is present, access is still conditional. Fat-soluble vitamins such as vitamin K, vitamin E, and carotenoids need proper fat digestion to move well through the intestine. They do not float freely into the body on reputation alone. They need emulsification, which means bile has to break dietary fat into tiny droplets, and they need micelles, small lipid transport particles that carry fat-soluble compounds across the watery environment of the intestinal lumen. The lumen is the inside space of the intestine where digestion and absorption are happening. If bile flow is weak, fat intake is too low, pancreatic output is poor, or the plant matrix resists release, the vitamin can remain in the bowel and leave in stool. Water-soluble vitamins face a different problem. They may be more chemically mobile, but they are also vulnerable to heat, oxidation, storage loss, and washout into cooking water. Presence in raw tissue and delivery after cooking, chewing, acid exposure, intestinal transport, and host use are not the same biological fact.

Nourishment also depends on what the rest of the food is doing while the vitamin is present. A plant can deliver some vitamin C and still burden the intestine with fermentable carbohydrates that pull water into the bowel and feed rapid gas production in the colon. A green can carry folate and vitamin K while also carrying enough oxalate to reduce the mineral value of the meal and increase urinary oxalate load later. A legume can bring B vitamins and minerals while still requiring the intestine to work around lectins, phytate, tannins, and protease inhibitors. The body does not experience each vitamin in isolation. It experiences the whole tissue at once. Release, binding, fermentation, irritation, transit speed, absorption, and clearance are happening in the same meal. A food is not nourishing because a beneficial molecule is somewhere inside it. A food is nourishing when the total digestive outcome leaves the body with more usable material than burden.

That is the real gap between nutrient praise and biological result. "Contains vitamins" describes composition. "Nourishes the body" describes net return after digestion, absorption, conversion, retention, and tissue cost. The distinction matters because the intestine is not grading the food for good intentions. It is breaking down structures, sorting soluble from insoluble material, transporting what can cross, and pushing the rest downstream. The liver then has to handle what enters portal blood, the blood vessel system that carries absorbed compounds from the intestine to the liver first. The kidney later has to clear what the body cannot use. A food can test dense and still underperform. The vitamin can be there from the start and still arrive in tissues thinly, inconsistently, or with enough attached burden that the body pays heavily for what little it gets.

The Central Framework of the Book

The book rests on a simple correction. Food is not judged by its reputation, its category, or its nutrient label. It is judged by what happens when living tissue meets human physiology. That means the analysis has to begin with structure. A leaf is not a vitamin list. A seed is not a mineral list. A fruit is not a sugar list. Each is a built piece of biology with its own storage strategy, water content, fibers, crystalline deposits, acids, pigments, enzyme inhibitors, protective skins, seed coatings, and defensive compounds. The body does not receive nutrients in abstraction. It receives matter arranged in a form that has to be broken down, held in solution, moved across a membrane, and then either used or cleared. The framework of this book follows that sequence because that is the sequence the body is forced to follow.

The first question is food structure. What kind of tissue is this. Is it a leaf built for mineral handling and environmental exposure, a seed built to protect stored energy and phosphorus, a tuber built for storage beneath the ground, or a fruit built to surround and protect reproductive tissue while attracting consumption at the right stage of ripeness. Structure determines the chemistry that comes with the food and the physical resistance digestion will face. Tough cell walls, fibrous scaffolds, seed coats, oxalate crystals, starch granules, lectins, phytate, tannins, glycoalkaloids, acids, and sugars are not side details. They are part of the food itself. If the tissue is chemically defended or physically resistant, that matters before any nutrient discussion begins.

The second question is digestive liberation. A nutrient has no value to the body while it is still locked inside intact plant structure or still bound inside a complex the intestine cannot use. Chewing fractures tissue. Stomach acid denatures proteins, meaning it unfolds them and makes them easier for enzymes to attack. Pancreatic enzymes cleave carbohydrates, fats, and proteins into smaller units. Bile emulsifies fat, which means it breaks larger fat masses into tiny droplets that can move through the watery environment of the small intestine. But digestion does not liberate everything equally. Some nutrients stay trapped. Some are released only partially. Some are released into a lumen, the hollow interior of the gut, that is already crowded with compounds ready to bind them, precipitate them, ferment them, or carry them away. The question is never whether the food contains the nutrient. The question is whether digestion can free it cleanly enough for the body to gain access.

That leads directly to binding and inhibition. This is where many plant foods lose the nutritional argument while still keeping the nutritional reputation. Oxalate can bind calcium in the gut and reduce the amount of calcium that remains available for absorption. Phytate can sequester zinc, iron, calcium, and magnesium inside complexes human digestion handles poorly. Tannins can bind proteins and minerals. Protease inhibitors can block enzymes such as trypsin and chymotrypsin, which are supposed to break dietary protein into absorbable amino acids. Lectins can survive weak preparation and make aggressive contact with the intestinal surface. None of that shows up honestly when the food is reduced to a praise phrase like rich in minerals or full of nutrients. The meal is not a nutrient parade. It is a competitive chemical environment. Some compounds are trying to cross into the body. Others are trapping them before they get there.

Absorption is the next checkpoint, and it is narrower than people think. A nutrient has to remain soluble, meaning dissolved and mobile in intestinal fluid, or packaged appropriately for transport. It has to reach the brush border, the enzyme-rich surface of the small intestine where final digestion and uptake occur. It then has to cross into the intestinal cell or pass between cells under conditions the body can tolerate. Fat-soluble compounds need proper bile handling and micelle formation, which means they must be incorporated into tiny lipid transport particles that can move through intestinal fluid. Minerals need the right chemical environment to stay available. Sugars and amino acids depend on transport systems that can saturate, compete, or fail under stress. A food can contain useful compounds and still deliver very little because the intestinal surface never receives them in a form it can move into the blood.

Once something crosses, the story is still not over. The body now has to handle what entered. This is the organ burden phase, and it is where shallow nutrition language usually stops paying attention. The liver has to process compounds arriving from the intestine through portal blood, the venous system that carries absorbed material from the gut to the liver first. The thyroid has to keep functioning in the presence of compounds that interfere with iodine handling or hormone formation. The kidney has to filter and excrete compounds the body cannot use. Oxalate shows the whole sequence clearly. In the gut it can reduce mineral availability. After absorption it becomes part of blood transport. In the kidney it becomes filtration work. In concentrated urine it can contribute to calcium oxalate crystal formation. A food that looks generous on paper can still leave behind a trail of digestive friction, endocrine interference, hepatic processing demand, or urinary burden. The body counts that cost whether the label does or not.

The final question is net biological result. After the tissue has been broken down, after some compounds have been released and others bound, after some have crossed and others have been excreted, after the organs have spent energy sorting use from waste, what is the body left with. More usable nourishment than burden, or more burden than return. That is the standard of this book. Not what the food promised. Not what the chart listed. Not what the public reputation says it should have done. The real judgment comes after the digestive sequence is over and the organs have finished paying for the meal.

How This Book Will Judge Foods

This book will not judge a food by category, public reputation, or the number of favorable compounds that appear on a nutrient chart. It will judge the food the way the body judges it. The first question is digestibility. What does the stomach have to denature, what do pancreatic enzymes have to cleave, what does bile have to emulsify, what remains locked inside fibrous plant structure, and what reaches the small intestine only half-processed. A food that resists breakdown is already lowering its own value. If protein remains poorly cleaved, if minerals remain embedded in a plant matrix, if carbohydrate arrives in the bowel faster than the intestine can handle it, the meal is already moving in the wrong direction before absorption even begins. The body is not fed by what enters the mouth. It is fed by what digestion can actually dismantle.

The next question is bioavailability, which means the fraction of a nutrient that remains chemically available, reaches the absorptive surface, crosses into the body, and becomes usable inside tissue. This is where a large part of nutrition rhetoric falls apart. A leaf may contain calcium, but if that same leaf releases oxalate into the intestinal contents, the calcium number on paper is no longer telling the truth about what the meal will deliver. A seed may contain zinc and iron, but if phytate holds those minerals in complexes human digestion handles poorly, the intestine sees less than the chart promised. A vegetable may carry carotenoids, but if fat digestion is weak and bile release is poor, those fat-soluble compounds move poorly through the lumen, the interior space of the intestine where digestion and absorption are happening, and less reaches the brush border, the enzyme-rich surface where final uptake occurs. This book will keep asking the same hard question. How much of what the food contains survives the whole trip into the body in a usable form.

Then comes toxic load. This does not mean every plant food is an acute poison. It means the food may carry compounds that irritate, inhibit, interfere, or force clearance. A kidney bean that is undercooked carries lectin activity that can injure the digestive sequence quickly and violently. A green potato carries glycoalkaloids that are still acting as plant defense molecules when the person eats it. Cassava can carry cyanogenic glycosides that release cyanide if the tissue is handled badly. Bitter squash can announce abnormal cucurbitacin burden through taste before the gut pays for it with vomiting and pain. Even when the compound does not produce obvious poisoning, it may still create a lower-grade chemical problem. A high-oxalate green, a phytate-heavy seed, a tannin-rich plant tissue, or a high-FODMAP fruit may push the intestine, blood, liver, thyroid, or kidney into unnecessary work. This book will count that work. A food does not become innocent because the burden falls short of emergency.

Excretion burden is where the argument becomes harder to evade. Once a compound crosses into blood, the organs of handling inherit the problem. The liver has to transform what arrives through portal blood, the venous system that carries absorbed material from the intestine to the liver first. The kidney has to filter what the body cannot use and concentrate it into urine without allowing it to precipitate, meaning fall out of solution into crystals. Oxalate again shows the whole sequence with unusual clarity. Inside the gut it can reduce mineral value from the meal. After absorption it becomes part of the circulating load. At the kidney it becomes filtration work. In urine it can become crystal pressure if concentration rises high enough. The same food can therefore fail twice. It can nourish poorly on the way in and burden the urinary tract on the way out. That is not a side issue. That is part of the food's actual biological cost.

Dose and frequency decide whether a burden remains occasional or becomes structural. A single exposure and a staple exposure are not the same physiological event. A handful of cooked greens once in a while is not the same intestinal sequence as a daily raw smoothie made from oxalate-rich leaves. A properly prepared bean eaten intermittently is not the same as repeated reliance on legumes as a protein foundation while the intestine is still dealing with lectins, protease inhibitors, phytate, and fermentation load. Repetition changes the tissue consequence because the same binding, irritation, osmotic pull, fermentation pressure, endocrine interference, or urinary load keeps returning to the same surfaces and organs. The bowel is asked to tolerate it again. The thyroid is asked to compensate again. The kidney is asked to clear it again. This book will judge foods not only by what they can do once, but by what they do when they become part of the daily pattern.

Host vulnerability is the final filter because the same food is not the same biological decision in every body. A person with intact fat digestion does not handle oxalate the same way as a person with fat malabsorption, where unabsorbed fat binds calcium in the gut and leaves more oxalate free for absorption. A person with robust iodine status and a resilient thyroid does not face crucifer exposure the same way as a person already running close to insufficiency. A person with a calm bowel does not experience fermentable fruit and vegetable carbohydrates the same way as a person with visceral hypersensitivity, altered motility, or chronic bloating. Reduced kidney function changes the risk attached to compounds that require urinary clearance. Medication use changes the risk attached to fruits such as grapefruit that interfere with intestinal enzyme systems. This book will not pretend that one verdict fits every physiology. It will keep the host in view because the body receiving the food is part of the food's meaning.

These six standards work together. A food has to be digestible enough to break down, bioavailable enough to deliver what it contains, low enough in toxic load to avoid imposing needless chemical stress, light enough in excretion burden that the organs of clearance are not forced to pay heavily for it, moderate enough in dose and frequency that the burden does not become daily tissue workload, and compatible enough with the host that the meal does not exceed the body's handling capacity. That is how this book will judge foods. Not by label content. Not by moral status. By what the body can extract, what the body has to fight through, and what the organs are left carrying after the meal is over.

Part I

The Plant Is Not Passive

Chapter 1

Plant Tissue Is Defensive Tissue

A plant is fixed in place. It cannot bite, run, hide, or heal a damaged structure the way an animal can. Its leaves sit exposed to insects, fungi, drought, sunlight, bruising, and repeated contact from anything that wants to chew, pierce, rot, infect, or consume it. So the plant manages contact with chemistry. The chemistry is not decorative. It is built into the tissue. Bitter compounds discourage eating. Enzyme inhibitors interfere with digestion in the eater. Lectins bind surfaces. Tannins bind proteins. Oxalate can stiffen or protect tissue while also storing or handling calcium in a form the plant can tolerate. Glucosinolates sit in crucifer tissue until damage brings them into contact with the enzymes that convert them into sharper compounds. Cyanogenic glycosides remain stable until plant cells are broken and the chemistry is allowed to proceed toward cyanide release. This is how a rooted organism controls the terms of contact. It does not need a nervous system to make a leaf difficult, a seed resistant, a peel irritating, or a tuber chemically costly.

That chemical logic changes with the tissue because the job changes with the tissue. A leaf is thin, exposed, and metabolically active. It is built to capture light, move water, exchange gases, and keep its living surface intact despite constant environmental contact. Its defenses often concentrate around the outer tissue, the vacuole, which is the fluid-filled compartment inside plant cells where many compounds are stored, or in crystalline deposits that can physically and chemically change the experience of eating it. A seed has a different problem. It is a compact storage structure that holds phosphorus, minerals, starch, fat, or protein for the next growth cycle. Its task is not to be easy to digest. Its task is to remain intact long enough to protect that stored material. That is why seeds so often carry phytate, lectins, tannins, protease inhibitors, and tough outer coats. A tuber stores energy underground and still has to resist rot, insect damage, and overconsumption. A fruit can be soft and attractive when ripe, but even there the sugars are not the whole story. The skin, the seeds, the acids, the peel oils, and the ripening chemistry all shape how that tissue is handled by animals, microbes, and the environment.

This means plant chemistry is organized around controlling access. The plant does not have to make itself absolutely inedible. It only has to make feeding less favorable, less efficient, less comfortable, or more selective. A protease inhibitor does not need to kill the eater. It only needs to interfere with proteases, the enzymes that break protein into absorbable amino acids, so that digestion becomes less successful. A lectin does not need to destroy the intestine outright. It only needs to survive enough of the digestive sequence to reach the gut surface and make unwanted contact there. Phytate does not need to act like a poison in the emergency-room sense. It only needs to hold zinc, iron, calcium, or magnesium tightly enough that the mineral leaves the body with the plant residue instead of entering the blood. Oxalate does not need to behave like a venom. It only needs to alter the mineral environment of the meal and, if absorbed, add to the kidney's filtration burden later. The plant's chemistry often works by shaving away value from the eater while preserving value inside the tissue.

The important point is that these compounds are part of the food before cooking, before chewing, before digestion, and before any nutrient analysis is turned into a health claim. Public language tends to isolate the favorable compound and detach it from the tissue that carries it. Kale becomes vitamin K and folate. Spinach becomes iron and calcium. Almonds become magnesium. Beans become fiber and plant protein. That is a laboratory and marketing simplification. The actual food arrives as structured tissue carrying both nutrients and resistance. When the leaf is fractured, the seed is soaked, the bean is undercooked, the potato greens, or the fruit is concentrated into juice, the human digestive tract does not receive a vitamin slogan. It receives a packet of plant architecture with its defensive chemistry still attached. The mouth begins tearing cells apart. Acids begin changing protein structure. Enzymes begin cleaving starch, fat, and protein. At the same time, oxalate is being released, phytate is still holding minerals, lectins may still be active, tannins may still be binding proteins, and fermentable carbohydrates may still be moving toward bacterial fermentation. The nutrients and the obstacles enter the intestine together.

This is why the first question in this book is not whether a fruit or vegetable contains something beneficial. The first question is what kind of plant tissue it is and what that tissue is trying to hold, protect, deter, or survive. Once that is understood, the rest of the sequence becomes easier to see. Digestion is not meeting an innocent container of vitamins. It is meeting defended biological material. Some of that defense will be dismantled by heat, soaking, fermentation, peeling, boiling, or proper cooking. Some of it will remain active enough to reduce mineral uptake, slow protein digestion, irritate the mucosa, increase fermentation, interfere with iodine handling, or add solute load to the urine. The chemistry begins in the plant. The cost is paid in the eater.

Leaves, Seeds, Roots, Tubers, Skins, and Fruits as Different Defensive Structures

Plants do not defend every tissue the same way because the tissues are doing different jobs. A leaf is a live exposed surface. It has to hold water, exchange gases, capture light, and stay intact while insects chew it, fungi land on it, and weather keeps abrading it. That exposure changes the chemistry. Leaves often carry bitter compounds, oxalate, glucosinolates, nitrates, tannins, and other molecules that make feeding less rewarding or less safe. The defenses do not have to make the leaf absolutely uneatable. They only have to increase friction. A thin green tissue that looks delicate to the eye can still arrive in the gut carrying a mineral-binding burden, a thyroid burden, or a fermentation problem once its cells are broken open. Spinach and beet greens make the point clearly. The leaf can test rich in minerals while the same tissue releases enough oxalate to lower the mineral value of the meal and increase urinary oxalate load later. A crucifer leaf can look clean and harmless while still carrying glucosinolate chemistry that becomes more biologically relevant when the tissue is cut, chewed, and digested.

Seeds are built with a harder attitude because they are packages of stored value. They hold phosphorus, minerals, protein, starch, and fat for the next growth cycle. The plant has no interest in making that storage easy for another organism to digest. So seeds are often wrapped in coats, fibers, tannins, lectins, and storage chemistry that resists access. Phytate is central here because it stores phosphorus for the seed while also binding zinc, iron, calcium, and magnesium in the eater's intestine. Protease inhibitors matter for the same reason. A seed rich in protein still has reason to interfere with the eater's proteases, the enzymes that are supposed to break protein into absorbable amino acids. The seed is trying to preserve concentrated nutrition through time, pressure, moisture shifts, microbial exposure, and predation. Nuts, legumes, grains, and many pseudograins all carry some version of this logic. Their public reputation usually tracks their nutrient density. Their biological behavior is shaped just as much by the compounds that protect that density from being surrendered easily.

Roots and tubers live underground, which changes the threat pattern but does not remove it. A root has to move water and minerals while staying chemically tolerable to the plant itself and resistant enough to organisms in the soil. A tuber stores energy, usually as starch, and has to survive damage, microbial invasion, and opportunistic feeding while buried in a wet, microbe-rich environment. That is why underground tissues so often mix stored carbohydrate with protective chemistry. Potatoes are the common example because their glycoalkaloids, especially near the peel and in greened or sprouting tissue, remain part of the food when people eat them. The starch gives the potato its comforting identity. The glycoalkaloids remind you that it is still a defended storage organ. Cassava carries the same principle through a different chemistry. It stores carbohydrate, but its cyanogenic glycosides also mean the tissue may release cyanide if processing is inadequate. A storage organ can look like a simple energy food and still require soaking, peeling, fermenting, boiling, or careful selection before it stops behaving like a defended plant structure.

Skins, peels, and outer layers deserve special attention because they sit at the boundary between plant tissue and the external world. They are the first contact zone for insects, molds, abrasion, ultraviolet light, and bruising. That boundary role often concentrates waxes, phenolics, bitter compounds, pigments, volatile oils, and other chemically active substances. Sometimes those outer compounds are mild. Sometimes they are the most reactive part of the food. Citrus peel oils, potato peel glycoalkaloids, fruit skin tannins, and many bitter or irritating outer layers all fit this pattern. The outer tissue is not there to make the plant easy to digest. It is there to slow water loss, resist invasion, and control how other organisms interact with what lies beneath. When a peel is removed, the biological sequence changes. When it is kept, juiced, blended, or ground, the intestine receives more of the boundary chemistry along with the inner tissue. The difference between peeled and unpeeled is not cosmetic. It is a change in chemical exposure.

Fruit is often treated as the exception because sweetness makes the tissue seem cooperative, but fruit is not a surrender of defense. It is a controlled package built around seed protection and timed consumption. The flesh may become attractive when ripe, but the seeds still need protection, the skin still regulates contact, and the chemistry of the fruit still shapes how it is handled in the mouth and gut. Acids, sugars, polyols, tannins, salicylates, furanocoumarins, and seed compounds can all matter depending on the fruit. Grapefruit shows that fruit chemistry can reach beyond digestion and alter intestinal drug metabolism. Apple, pear, and stone fruit show that a sweet reputation does nothing to prevent fructose and polyol burden from overwhelming a sensitive intestine. Apricot kernels and other pits remind you that reproductive tissue remains chemically defended even when the surrounding flesh is edible. The fruit offers access under specific terms. It does not abandon control.

Once these tissues are seen as different defensive structures, the nutritional argument changes. You stop asking whether plants contain useful compounds and start asking what kind of plant part is entering the meal, what that part was built to protect, and what chemistry is likely to be released when digestion starts breaking it down. A leaf is not a seed with green color. A tuber is not a fruit without sweetness. A peel is not just a wrapper. Each tissue brings its own form of resistance, and each form of resistance changes the digestive sequence in its own way. That is why one plant burdens the thyroid, another binds minerals, another interferes with protein digestion, another irritates the gut, and another raises urinary crystal pressure. The structure tells you where the trouble is likely to begin.

Why Sweetness, Color, or Reputation Do Not Erase Plant Defense Chemistry

Sweetness changes behavior. It does not change tissue history. A fruit becomes sweet because its chemistry shifts during ripening, starch can be converted into simpler sugars, acids can fall, volatile aroma compounds can rise, pigments can intensify, and the flesh becomes more attractive to whatever will carry the seed away. That attractive phase often gets treated as proof that the food is now nutritionally innocent. It is not. The sweet flesh is still wrapped around reproductive tissue, still carrying acids, polyphenols, salicylates, polyols, enzymes, peel compounds, seed compounds, and sugars that must be absorbed or fermented. The sweetness is a signal to the eater. It is not a cancellation of the rest of the chemistry. A ripe fruit can still overload fructose handling if the dose is high enough. It can still bring poorly absorbed polyols into the bowel. It can still expose the intestine to peel chemistry and the liver to compounds that have to be transformed or cleared. The sweet taste makes the exposure easier to welcome. It does not make the exposure biologically simple.

Color creates the same kind of false simplification. A deep green leaf, a dark berry, a bright orange root, or a richly pigmented peel is usually taken as evidence of nutritional virtue. What it actually proves is that the plant made pigments. Those pigments may carry antioxidant activity in a laboratory assay, but the tissue carrying them still has to be chewed, acidified, broken down by enzymes, and moved through a gut where other compounds in the same plant can bind minerals, irritate surfaces, change motility, or alter absorption. A bright green leaf can still release oxalate. A crucifer with a strong nutritional reputation can still bring glucosinolate chemistry that becomes more relevant once the tissue is cut and chewed. A vividly colored fruit can still deliver enough fructose, acid, or polyol burden to create gas, distension, and unstable bowel movement in a sensitive intestine. Pigment is not a verdict. It is one visible part of a much larger chemical structure.

Reputation is even weaker than sweetness and color because it is built outside the body entirely. A food becomes wholesome in public language long before the intestine has shown whether it can handle it well. Spinach carries the reputation of iron and calcium while its oxalate content can lower mineral availability in the same meal. Beans carry the reputation of fiber and plant protein while lectins, phytate, protease inhibitors, and fermentable carbohydrates can all change the digestive return. Grapefruit carries the reputation of fresh fruit while its furanocoumarins can inhibit intestinal cytochrome P450 3A4, usually shortened to CYP3A4, one of the enzyme systems that breaks down many drugs during first-pass metabolism in the gut wall. The chemistry keeps working whether the reputation is clean or not. Public approval does not enter the stomach. Molecules do.

This is why plant foods are so often misjudged. People keep isolating the favorable feature and letting it stand in for the whole tissue. Sweetness becomes natural energy. Color becomes antioxidant value. Fiber becomes digestive virtue. Vitamin content becomes nourishment. The full sequence is rarely followed. What else is released when the cells break. What binds calcium, zinc, or iron before those minerals reach the absorptive surface. What survives cooking. What is reduced by boiling and what is not. What reaches the brush border, the enzyme-rich surface of the small intestine, in a soluble form and what stays tied up in the intestinal contents. What enters portal blood, the blood flowing from the intestine to the liver first, as something useful and what enters as something that will simply add handling work. The shallow reading stops at the plant's image. The physiological reading keeps going until the organs are done with it.

Plants also benefit from being judged by the part of their chemistry that attracts rather than the part that defends. Sweet fruit flesh can recruit an eater while the seed remains chemically protected. A colorful peel can signal ripeness while still holding tannins, waxes, acids, or aromatic defense compounds near the surface. A leaf can look fresh, crisp, and harmless while still changing the mineral environment of the meal the moment its cells are ruptured. The attractive trait and the defensive trait often occupy the same tissue at the same time. That is not a contradiction from the plant's side. It is strategy. The plant does not need to choose between appeal and resistance. It can use both.

So the book will not let sweetness, color, or reputation settle the question. Those are surface cues. The body works underneath them. It meets the actual tissue, releases the actual compounds, absorbs only what remains available, and clears what it cannot use. If a food arrives with sugar and fragrance, the intestine still has to sort out the acids, polyols, peel compounds, seeds, and fermentation load. If a vegetable arrives with a nutrient-dense reputation, the same meal may still bind minerals, slow protein digestion, irritate the mucosa, or add urinary burden later. The plant keeps its image. The body still has to survive the chemistry.

The Difference Between a Food Being Edible and a Food Being Low-Burden

Edible is a very low standard. It means the body can survive the encounter, at least in the short term. It does not mean the food breaks down easily, yields nutrients efficiently, leaves the intestinal surface undisturbed, spares the liver unnecessary work, or exits through the kidney without adding to urinary burden. A food can be edible because its toxins are below the level of acute poisoning, because cooking has reduced part of the defense chemistry, or because the body can absorb enough usable material to offset some of the cost. That still leaves a large middle ground where the meal is tolerated yet biologically expensive. The gut can keep moving. The person can remain alive. The food can still be imposing friction at every stage from digestion to excretion.

Low-burden is a different judgment. It asks how much resistance the food brings with it and how much work the body has to do to extract value from it. Does the tissue open easily under chewing, acid, enzymes, and bile. Do the proteins cleave cleanly into absorbable amino acids. Do the minerals remain soluble in the intestinal contents, or do oxalate, phytate, and tannins trap them before they reach the absorptive surface. Do the carbohydrates absorb in the small intestine, or do they pass downstream, pull water into the bowel, and feed fermentation in the colon. Does the fat carry fat-soluble vitamins into micelles, the tiny lipid transport particles that move through intestinal fluid, or is the whole sequence weak and wasteful. A low-burden food is one that gives the body access without attaching a large penalty to the process.

This distinction matters because many defended plant foods stay on the right side of edibility while remaining far from low-burden. A bowl of spinach is edible. That does not mean it is a light mineral food once oxalate is released into the meal and begins binding calcium. Beans are edible after proper preparation. That does not mean they become frictionless once lectins, protease inhibitors, phytate, and fermentable carbohydrates are counted. A potato is edible. A greened or sprouting potato is still carrying glycoalkaloids near the peel that the stomach and intestine have to absorb or clear. Grapefruit is edible. Its furanocoumarins can still inhibit intestinal cytochrome P450 3A4, usually shortened to CYP3A4, and alter drug handling in the gut wall. The word edible hides these differences because it treats survival as if it were the same thing as nutritional cooperation.

The body itself keeps the categories separate. In the gut, a food can be tolerated while still causing incomplete digestion, mineral loss, bloating, cramping, altered transit, or repeated mucosal contact with irritating compounds. The mucosa is the living lining of the intestine, the tissue that has to absorb nutrients while maintaining a barrier against unwanted material. Beyond the gut, the same food can still create downstream work. The liver has to transform absorbed compounds arriving through portal blood, the blood vessel system that carries material from the intestine to the liver first. The kidney has to filter compounds the body cannot use and concentrate them into urine without allowing them to precipitate into crystals. Edible means the body managed. Low-burden means the body did not have to spend much to manage.

That is why this book will not praise a food merely because people can eat it without collapsing. The useful question is what the food costs relative to what it returns. Does it deliver nourishment with little interference, or does it arrive carrying enough binding, inhibition, irritation, fermentation pressure, endocrine interference, or excretion load that the body pays heavily for modest return. A food can be edible for years and still keep the intestine under daily strain, keep minerals from entering efficiently, keep the thyroid compensating, or keep the kidney clearing compounds that should never have been a staple burden in the first place. Edibility keeps the food on the plate. Low burden is what earns it a place in the diet.

Why the Human Body Must Negotiate with Plant Chemistry Before It Can Gain Value from Plant Tissue

The human body does not receive plant nutrients in a free state. It receives them inside living structures that were built for the plant's needs first. A leaf is built to hold water, move minerals, capture light, and survive repeated exposure. A seed is built to preserve concentrated energy, phosphorus, and reproductive potential through time and damage. A root or tuber is built to store material underground without surrendering it easily to microbes or animals. That architecture matters because the nutrient is packaged inside fibers, cell walls, storage vacuoles, crystalline deposits, protein matrices, starch granules, oils, acids, and defense compounds that are all entering the mouth together. The body has to break the structure open before it can even approach the nutrient. Chewing fractures tissue. Stomach acid denatures proteins, meaning it unfolds them and makes them easier for enzymes to attack. Pancreatic enzymes cleave carbohydrate, fat, and protein into smaller units. Bile breaks dietary fat into fine droplets so fat-soluble compounds can move through intestinal fluid. But this dismantling is never happening in a neutral environment. The same ruptured tissue that releases vitamins, minerals, sugars, or amino acids may also release oxalate, phytate, tannins, lectins, protease inhibitors, salicylates, glucosinolates, or fermentable carbohydrates. The nutrient and the obstacle are often liberated in the same moment.

That is why plant eating is always a negotiation rather than a simple transfer of nutrition. The body is not just extracting useful compounds. It is separating them from the chemistry that limits access. Oxalate can bind calcium before calcium reaches the absorptive surface. Phytate can sequester zinc, iron, calcium, and magnesium inside complexes the intestine handles poorly. Tannins can bind proteins and minerals. Protease inhibitors can block enzymes such as trypsin and chymotrypsin, which are supposed to reduce dietary protein into absorbable amino acids. Fermentable carbohydrates can remain poorly absorbed in the small intestine, draw water into the bowel, and then pass into the colon where bacteria convert them into gas and organic acids. Even when a favorable compound is present, its path into the body is crowded. It has to remain soluble, meaning dissolved and mobile in intestinal fluid. It has to survive contact with binding agents. It has to reach the brush border, the enzyme-rich surface of the small intestine where final digestion and uptake occur. It then has to cross into the intestinal cell or pass between cells under conditions the body can tolerate. A plant may contain the nutrient. The body still has to win access to it.

The negotiation continues after absorption because entry into blood is not the same thing as useful delivery. Once a plant compound crosses the intestinal wall, the liver has to handle it first through portal blood, the venous system that carries absorbed material from the intestine to the liver. Some compounds are stored, some are transformed, some are neutralized, and some simply add to the organ's workload. The kidney later inherits what the body cannot use or must keep within safe concentration limits. Oxalate shows the full argument with unusual clarity. In the gut it can lower mineral value from the meal by binding calcium. After absorption it becomes part of the circulating load. At the kidney it becomes filtration work. In concentrated urine it can contribute to calcium oxalate crystal formation. Grapefruit makes the same point through a different mechanism. Its furanocoumarins can inhibit intestinal cytochrome P450 3A4, usually shortened to CYP3A4, one of the enzyme systems that helps metabolize many drugs in the gut wall. The fruit is edible. The chemistry still changes what the body has to do. Plant value is therefore never just a matter of what entered the mouth. It is a matter of what the intestine could absorb cleanly and what the organs could handle without paying too much for it.

This is why the public habit of reducing fruits and vegetables to nutrient content misses the most important part of the physiology. A plant tissue becomes valuable to the body only after the body has broken it down, defended itself from the parts that interfere, absorbed what remains usable, and cleared what it could not use. The negotiation is built into the meal. Some foods require only light negotiation because their structure opens easily and their chemical resistance is modest. Others arrive with harder terms. They bind, block, ferment, irritate, resist cleavage, alter mineral traffic, or add excretion burden later. The body can still survive those foods. It may even get some value from them. But survival is not the same thing as efficient nourishment. Plant tissue pays out only after the chemistry has been worked through. Until then, the intestine is not receiving a health food. It is dealing with a defended biological structure that has to be overcome before it can become useful.

Chapter 2

What Digestion Has to Do to a Plant

The first problem plant tissue presents is physical, not nutritional. Before the intestine can absorb anything, the food has to be fractured. Plant cells are built with cellulose-rich walls, pectin, hemicellulose, fibrous scaffolds, water compartments, starch granules, oils, pigments, acids, and storage bodies that keep the tissue organized and intact. Digestion has to undo that organization. In the mouth, the teeth begin the first act of force. They shear leaves, crush fruits, rupture skins, crack softer seed structures, and reduce larger pieces into smaller particles that can be swallowed. That sounds simple until the plant's architecture is kept in view. Chewing is not just making food smaller. It is breaking cell walls, exposing vacuoles, which are the fluid-filled storage compartments inside plant cells, releasing acids, sugars, minerals, oxalate, and polyphenols into saliva, and increasing surface area so later digestive steps can reach more of the tissue. A leaf that stays poorly chewed stays more structurally intact. A seed swallowed with its shell largely unbroken may pass with much of its stored material still protected. The plant begins the meal as organized tissue. Mastication, the formal term for chewing, is the first attempt to turn that tissue into digestible matter.

Saliva starts chemical work, but its mechanical role is just as important. It wets the plant fragments, binds them into a bolus, the soft mass prepared for swallowing, and begins starch digestion through salivary amylase, an enzyme that starts cleaving starch into smaller carbohydrate units. That action is limited and short-lived, but it matters because many plant foods arrive with starch packed into granules inside cells that must first be opened. If chewing is weak, the enzyme has less access. If the tissue is tough, stringy, or swallowed too quickly, more intact plant structure leaves the mouth than people realize. The mouth is already sorting foods by how much force they demand. Crisp fruit flesh usually ruptures easily. Fibrous greens require repeated shearing. Nuts and seeds challenge the teeth more directly. Raw root vegetables resist fracture more than cooked ones because heat softens structure and changes how water and starch are held inside the plant. A cooked carrot and a raw carrot are not the same mechanical problem. The same is true all across the plant world. Cooking often does not improve a food because it adds virtue. It improves it because it partially dismantles the tissue before the eater has to.

The stomach takes over where chewing leaves off, but the stomach cannot do the whole job by chemistry alone. Its muscular wall churns the meal, folds it, compresses it, and repeatedly drives it against itself to reduce particle size further. This is especially important for plant foods because the stomach is often working on material that still contains intact cell clusters, fibrous strands, seed fragments, skins, and ungelatinized or only partly accessible starch. Gastric acid lowers pH, which means it makes the stomach contents strongly acidic. That acid denatures proteins by unfolding them, activates pepsin, the major protein-digesting enzyme in the stomach, and helps loosen some food structures. But stomach acid does not digest cellulose. It does not dissolve every plant barrier. It does not liberate minerals cleanly from every plant matrix. The stomach is mixing, softening, unfolding, and grinding. It is not performing a miracle. If the meal arrives as raw fibrous matter with defensive compounds still embedded in the tissue, the stomach can only prepare that material for the next stage. It cannot erase the plant's structure on its own.

This is where particle size starts to matter in a serious way. The stomach does not empty large, resistant fragments efficiently. It meters partly processed food through the pylorus, the muscular exit valve at the bottom of the stomach, into the small intestine in a controlled stream. Smaller particles move forward more easily. Larger or tougher particles stay behind for more churning. That means poor chewing increases downstream work. It also means plant foods that retain coarse structure can slow gastric processing while still escaping in a form that is only partly opened. Raw greens blended into a smoothie and raw greens chewed in a salad may create different mechanical sequences, but neither sequence guarantees full liberation of nutrients. Blending reduces particle size aggressively, yet it can also deliver a large plant load quickly, with less chewing, less oral signaling, and less pacing. The stomach then receives a different kind of workload: finer particles, yes, but often in larger volume and with the same oxalate, polyphenol, fiber, acids, and fermentable compounds still present. Mechanical reduction helps. It does not settle the question of whether the plant will nourish well.

The stomach also separates what can be softened from what remains structurally stubborn. Soft fruit flesh may collapse quickly. Cooked tubers may disperse once heat has swollen and gelatinized starch, meaning the starch granules have absorbed water and lost their native tight packing. Bean skins, seed fragments, nut particles, and raw fibrous stems are different. They often persist longer, carrying with them nutrients that remain partly enclosed and defense compounds that remain attached to the same particles. This is one reason plant foods can test dense while yielding less than expected. The digestive tract is not analyzing the food after complete destruction in a laboratory mill. It is handling a moving mass of fragments that vary in size, softness, permeability, and chemical content. Some fragments open early. Some keep their contents to themselves until much later. Some never surrender much at all before they leave the body.

So the mouth and stomach are doing more than preparing food for absorption. They are determining whether plant tissue will become accessible at all. Teeth fracture the structure. Saliva wets and begins starch cleavage. The stomach acidifies, denatures, churns, and sorts by particle size. Every one of those steps is a negotiation with plant architecture. If the tissue breaks well, later digestion has a chance. If it stays resistant, the rest of the digestive tract inherits a more difficult problem. The intestine can only absorb what the upper digestive tract has made reachable. When the first mechanical steps underperform, the plant keeps more of its structure, and with it, more control over what the body actually gets.

Acid, Enzymes, Bile, and Microbial Fermentation as Stages of Plant Handling

Once the mouth and stomach have reduced plant tissue to smaller fragments, the digestive sequence shifts from force to chemistry. The stomach acidifies the meal first. Hydrochloric acid lowers pH, which means it turns the stomach contents sharply acidic, unfolds many proteins, loosens some food structure, and prepares the mass for enzymatic attack. That acid environment matters because it changes what later enzymes can reach and how tightly parts of the meal remain assembled. But acid has limits. It can denature plant proteins and soften some tissue. It cannot digest cellulose, the structural carbohydrate that reinforces plant cell walls. It cannot dissolve every crystal, unlock every mineral, or neutralize every defense compound. A plant does not become nutritionally available just because it has entered acid. The stomach is preparing the material, not finishing the work. It is breaking protein shape, reducing microbial load, mixing the particles into chyme, the semi-fluid mass that leaves the stomach, and sending that mass forward in controlled pulses. Plant handling is now underway, but much of the architecture is still intact.

The small intestine receives that acidic chyme and immediately has to correct the environment. Pancreatic bicarbonate, an alkaline secretion that neutralizes acid, raises the pH so digestive enzymes can function. Pancreatic amylase continues starch digestion. Proteases such as trypsin and chymotrypsin cleave proteins into smaller peptides, which are short chains of amino acids. Lipase attacks fats. Brush border enzymes at the intestinal surface finish much of the last carbohydrate and peptide work before absorption. This is where plant structure starts separating into usable and unusable fractions. If starch granules were softened by cooking, enzymes gain better access. If proteins are tied up inside dense seed structure or protected by protease inhibitors, enzyme action becomes less efficient. If minerals were released from the tissue but immediately met oxalate or phytate, the intestine may now be full of nutrient numbers on paper and very little freely absorbable mineral in reality. Enzymes do not work in abstraction. They work inside a crowded chemical mixture where plant compounds can block, trap, or slow access to the very nutrients that made the food look impressive in the first place.

Bile enters the sequence when fat and fat-soluble compounds need handling. Bile is made in the liver, stored in the gallbladder, and released into the small intestine to emulsify fat, which means it breaks larger fat masses into much smaller droplets. That matters because the lumen, the hollow interior of the intestine where digestion is taking place, is water-based. Fat does not move well through that environment on its own. Bile salts help build micelles, tiny transport assemblies that carry fatty acids, cholesterol, carotenoids, and fat-soluble vitamins through intestinal fluid toward the absorptive surface. This is one reason plant nutrition is often overstated. A vegetable may contain carotenoids or vitamin K, but those compounds do not move efficiently into the body unless they are released from the plant structure, exposed to adequate fat handling, and carried properly through the lumen. Low-fat meals, weak bile release, poor pancreatic function, or plant matrices that resist breakdown all lower that transfer. The nutrient is still present in the sample. The intestine is still dealing with a transport problem.

Not everything is digested in the small intestine, and that remainder becomes the substrate for microbial fermentation in the colon. Fermentation is not digestion by human enzymes. It is digestion by microbes. Fibers, resistant starches, oligosaccharides, polyols, and other poorly absorbed carbohydrates arrive in the large bowel and are metabolized by bacteria into gases and short-chain fatty acids, which are small fatty acids such as acetate, propionate, and butyrate produced during fermentation. In the right amount and in the right host, this can be tolerated or even useful. In the wrong amount, or in a bowel already prone to visceral hypersensitivity, altered motility, or unstable microbial balance, fermentation becomes mechanical stress. Gas expands the lumen. Water shifts into the bowel. Distension stretches the wall. Transit changes. Pain, urgency, pressure, and bloating follow. This is why a plant food can be praised for fiber and still destabilize digestion. The chemistry that escaped small-intestinal absorption does not disappear. It simply changes hands and becomes bacterial work.

These stages are continuous, and the same plant can create problems at more than one point in the sequence. Acid may denature its proteins but leave its fibers standing. Pancreatic enzymes may reach some starch but lose efficiency against inhibitors in seeds and legumes. Bile may help carry fat-soluble compounds while oxalate or phytate is simultaneously lowering mineral availability elsewhere in the same meal. Microbial fermentation may salvage some residual carbohydrate while also producing enough gas and osmotic pressure to turn the colon into a symptom generator. That is why the body cannot judge a plant by nutrient content alone. It has to process the tissue stage by stage. Acid prepares it. Enzymes dismantle what they can. Bile escorts what can move through fat pathways. Microbes finish what escaped upstream digestion. Only after that sequence is over can the plant be judged by its real yield. Until then, the food is still negotiating.

Cell Walls, Fibers, Seed Coats, and Crystalline Deposits as Barriers to Access

Plant tissue does not give its contents up freely. The nutrients are inside structures that were built to hold shape, resist collapse, control water, protect storage material, and survive damage. Cell walls are the first barrier. Unlike animal cells, plant cells are wrapped in a rigid outer wall made largely from cellulose, hemicellulose, and pectin. Cellulose is a structural carbohydrate that human digestive enzymes do not break down. Hemicellulose and pectin add further strength, spacing, and gel behavior to the tissue. This means the body is not simply digesting nutrients. It is trying to reach nutrients that are still enclosed inside microscopic compartments. Chewing can rupture some of those walls. Cooking can soften some of them. Acid can help loosen the arrangement. But many walls remain partly intact long enough to delay or reduce access to what sits inside. A nutrient trapped inside an unbroken or only partly broken plant cell is present in the food and absent from the body at the same time.

Fiber adds another layer of difficulty because it is not one thing and it does not behave one way. Insoluble fiber tends to hold structure, resist dissolution, and preserve bulk. Soluble fiber absorbs water, swells, and can form viscous material, meaning a thicker gel-like mass that slows movement of digestive contents. Both can interfere with access, though by different routes. Insoluble fiber can physically shield cell contents from enzymes and keep plant particles structurally stubborn farther down the tract. Soluble fiber can slow diffusion, which means it can slow the movement of digestive enzymes toward their targets and the movement of liberated nutrients back toward the intestinal surface. That does not make fiber imaginary or inert. It makes it mechanical. The same plant structure that helps the plant stand upright or retain water can also keep digestive chemistry from reaching stored starch, protein, fat, or micronutrients efficiently. A nutrient chart measures content after complete destruction of the tissue. The intestine works on partially dismantled matter moving through fluid, time, pressure, and chemical competition.

Seed coats make the problem harder because seeds are built to preserve value, not surrender it. The seed coat is a protective shell around a concentrated storage package of phosphorus, minerals, fat, protein, or starch. It reduces water penetration, slows microbial damage, and protects the embryo until conditions favor growth. In food terms, that means it often delays or limits digestive access. Inside that coat, the chemistry becomes even less cooperative. Phytate stores phosphorus for the future plant while binding minerals in the eater's intestine. Tannins can bind proteins. Protease inhibitors can interfere with the enzymes that are supposed to cleave protein into absorbable amino acids. Even when chewing breaks a seed or when grinding turns it into flour, the seed's stored material is still arriving with its protective chemistry attached. This is why seeds, legumes, nuts, and grains so often require soaking, cooking, fermenting, sprouting, grinding, or prolonged processing before they stop behaving like guarded biological packages. The storage value is real. The resistance to release is real too.

Crystalline deposits show the same principle in a more visible form. Some plants store calcium as calcium oxalate crystals. These are mineral structures formed when oxalate binds calcium inside the plant tissue. They help the plant manage calcium, deter feeding, and maintain internal balance. In the eater, they change the whole mineral story of the meal. The crystal itself is not a free gift of calcium. It is calcium already locked to oxalate. Some oxalate remains insoluble, meaning it stays bound and poorly absorbed. Some is present in more soluble forms that can dissolve more readily in the intestinal contents, bind additional calcium from the meal, or become available for absorption. That is why a high-oxalate leaf can test mineral-dense while delivering less usable mineral than expected and later contributing to urinary oxalate burden if some of that oxalate is absorbed. The crystal is a storage and defense solution for the plant. It becomes a nutritional and renal problem for the eater.

When these barriers are kept in view, plant digestion stops looking like a simple act of extraction. The body is not opening a package of ready nutrients. It is grinding through walls it cannot digest, moving enzymes through swollen fiber, trying to penetrate seed defenses, and dealing with minerals already tied up in crystal or binding chemistry. Some plant foods yield enough despite those barriers. Some yield very little for the amount of digestive effort and tissue burden they impose. That difference is one of the central questions of the book. A nutrient inside a plant is only a possibility. The barrier in front of it is the first part of the real story.

Why Liberation of Nutrients Is Not Guaranteed by Presence on Paper

A nutrient chart records presence after the food has been dismantled by laboratory methods. The body does not receive the food in that state. It receives a structured tissue that still has to be fractured, acidified, cleaved by enzymes, mixed with bile, and held in a soluble state long enough for usable compounds to reach the absorptive surface. That difference is where much of modern nutrition language goes wrong. A mineral can be present inside a leaf and still remain unavailable once that leaf releases oxalate into the same intestinal contents. A seed can contain zinc, iron, calcium, and magnesium while phytate keeps those minerals tied up in complexes the intestine handles poorly. A vegetable can contain carotenoids while weak fat digestion, low bile release, or incomplete tissue breakdown prevents those compounds from moving efficiently through the watery contents of the small intestine. The number on paper describes composition. Liberation describes whether digestion can actually free that compound from the structure that is holding it.

Plant structure is the first reason liberation fails. Nutrients are enclosed inside cells, storage bodies, protein matrices, starch granules, oil droplets, and vacuoles, the fluid-filled compartments inside plant cells that often hold acids, pigments, minerals, and defense compounds. Those compartments are wrapped in cell walls the body does not digest well. Chewing breaks some of them. Cooking softens some of them. Acid and enzymes loosen more. But none of that guarantees full release. A plant particle can move through the stomach and small intestine still partly intact, still holding material that a nutrient database counted confidently. That is one reason finely milled, fermented, soaked, cooked, raw, chewed, and blended versions of the same plant do not behave the same way in the gut. The tissue structure changes, and with it the degree of access. Presence in the plant and liberation during digestion are separate questions.

Even when the nutrient is physically released, chemistry can still stop it from becoming available. The intestinal lumen, the hollow interior of the gut where digestion is happening, is not an empty tube waiting to collect nutrients. It is a crowded chemical mixture. Minerals compete with one another. Acids change solubility. Fibers swell and alter movement. Tannins bind proteins and minerals. Oxalate binds calcium. Phytate sequesters several minerals at once. Protease inhibitors reduce the efficiency of protein digestion by interfering with enzymes such as trypsin and chymotrypsin. A nutrient can therefore be liberated from the plant cell and still fail to reach the brush border, the enzyme-rich absorptive surface of the small intestine, in a usable form. Release is only the first hurdle. Remaining soluble, unbound, and transportable is the next one.

The form of the nutrient matters as much as the fact of its presence. Beta-carotene is not retinol. It is a precursor that has to be converted into active vitamin A. Non-heme iron in plants is not handled like heme iron from animal tissue. Calcium locked in calcium oxalate crystals is not equivalent to freely available calcium in the intestinal contents. Folate in a food and folate retained after storage, preparation, gastric exposure, and intestinal transport are not the same quantity. A chart often collapses these distinctions because it is built to record detectable compounds, not to follow the full physiological sequence into tissue use. The body cannot live on detection. It lives on conversion, transport, uptake, storage, and retained function. A nutrient that exists only as a technical entry in a database has not yet nourished anyone.

This is why the book keeps returning to net biological result instead of label content. A food earns nutritional value only after digestion has opened the structure, enzymes have reduced the contents into usable units, binding chemistry has failed to trap them, the intestine has absorbed them, and the organs have handled the rest without paying too much for the meal. Until that sequence is complete, presence on paper is only a possibility. The nutrient may be there. The body still has to get to it.

The Idea of Net Yield Versus Label Content

Label content is a static description of what can be measured inside a food sample. Net yield is the biological remainder after the body has finished wrestling with that food. Those are not the same thing. A chart can tell you that a leaf contains calcium, magnesium, folate, vitamin K, carotenoids, and vitamin C. It cannot tell you how much of that calcium stays available once oxalate is released into the intestinal contents, how much of those carotenoids are actually liberated from the plant structure and carried through the small intestine in micelles, the tiny lipid transport particles that move fat-soluble compounds through intestinal fluid, or how much of the rest is carried out in stool because the tissue resisted breakdown. The label is an inventory. Net yield is an outcome. The first is easy to print. The second has to be paid for in digestion.

That payment begins with tissue structure and ends only after absorption and clearance. The food has to be chewed into fragments small enough for acid and enzymes to reach. Cell walls have to be broken. Starch granules have to be opened. Proteins have to be denatured, which means unfolded so enzymes can attack them, and then cleaved into smaller pieces. Minerals have to remain soluble in the lumen, the interior space of the gut where digestion is taking place, instead of becoming trapped in complexes with oxalate, phytate, or tannins. Fat-soluble compounds have to be released from the plant tissue, emulsified with bile, and carried to the brush border, the enzyme-rich absorptive surface of the small intestine. If any of those steps underperform, the label content stays in the food or in the waste stream. The number was real. The delivery was poor.

This is why a food can look dense and still undernourish. Spinach is the easy example because the contradiction is built into the same leaf. The calcium is present. The oxalate is also present. Once the tissue is broken down, the oxalate changes the mineral environment of the meal by binding calcium and lowering the amount that remains available for absorption. Seeds and legumes do the same kind of damage through different chemistry. Their phosphorus storage compound, phytate, can hold zinc, iron, calcium, and magnesium tightly enough that human digestion gains less of those minerals than the label suggests. A bean can also carry protease inhibitors that interfere with trypsin and chymotrypsin, the pancreatic enzymes that are supposed to reduce protein into absorbable amino acids. The food keeps the number. The intestine loses part of the return.

Net yield also has to subtract burden. A food is not giving the body its full value if the same meal adds significant digestive friction, fermentation pressure, thyroid interference, hepatic work, or urinary solute load. A high-oxalate green can lower mineral yield in the gut and then become kidney work later if some oxalate is absorbed and excreted in urine. A high-FODMAP fruit or vegetable can deliver some vitamins while also leaving enough poorly absorbed carbohydrate in the bowel to pull in water, feed bacterial fermentation, and produce gas, bloating, pain, and unstable transit. Grapefruit can be fresh, fragrant, and rich in vitamin C while still carrying furanocoumarins that inhibit intestinal cytochrome P450 3A4, usually shortened to CYP3A4, an enzyme system involved in first-pass drug metabolism in the gut wall. The body does not judge the food by what it gave in one column and ignore what it cost in another. Net yield includes both sides.

That is the standard this book will use. A food is not impressive because a chart can list favorable compounds inside it. It becomes valuable only when digestion can release those compounds, the intestinal contents can keep them available, the absorptive surface can move them into the body, the tissues can use them, and the organs of clearance are not left carrying an avoidable burden afterward. Label content tells you what the plant contains when the laboratory destroys it completely. Net yield tells you what the human body is actually left with after the plant has been chewed, acidified, enzymatically reduced, absorbed where possible, and excreted where necessary. The gap between those two numbers is where most of the nutritional deception lives.

Chapter 3

Poison, Burden, Irritant, and Blocker

The word poison is usually reserved for the dramatic event. A person eats something, symptoms arrive quickly, and the connection is hard to miss. Vomiting, diarrhea, abdominal pain, neurologic change, collapse. That model is real, but it is narrow. It captures the plant compound that injures fast and visibly. It misses the larger field of foods that do not produce a crisis and still impose repeated biological cost. A kidney bean that still carries active lectin can produce an acute gastrointestinal reaction because the dose is high enough and the chemistry is direct enough to disrupt the digestive sequence quickly. A greened potato carrying excess glycoalkaloids can produce nausea, abdominal distress, and neurologic symptoms because the compound itself is overtly toxic at sufficient intake. Those are poison problems in the ordinary sense. The body is overwhelmed in a short window. The reaction announces itself. Chronic metabolic burden is different. The food does not have to produce an emergency. It only has to keep stealing mineral access, keep slowing digestion, keep increasing fermentation pressure, keep interfering with thyroid chemistry, or keep adding compounds the liver and kidney must clear day after day.

That difference begins with the way the compound behaves in the tissue and in the body. An acute poison usually has enough direct chemical force to damage quickly once it is released, absorbed, or brought into contact with the gut surface. The timescale is short because the mechanism is strong. The compound binds, injures, inhibits, or destabilizes fast enough that the body shows obvious distress before compensation can smooth the problem out. Chronic burden works through smaller repeated failures. Oxalate does not need to produce collapse to matter. It only needs to bind calcium in the intestinal contents, reduce mineral availability from the meal, and in some people cross into blood in enough quantity that the kidney must keep filtering and excreting it. Phytate does not need to poison the eater in the emergency-room sense. It only needs to hold zinc, iron, calcium, or magnesium tightly enough that the intestine absorbs less over months and years. A high-FODMAP plant food does not need to contain a classical toxin. It only needs to leave enough poorly absorbed carbohydrate in the small intestine and colon to keep drawing water into the bowel and feeding rapid fermentation. One problem is explosive. The other is cumulative. Both are real. They are not the same biological event.

The body also experiences these categories in different compartments. Acute poisoning is often easiest to see because the gut becomes the stage first. The mucosa, the living lining of the intestine, gets hit hard enough that nausea, cramping, vomiting, secretory diarrhea, or pain follow rapidly. In other cases the absorbed compound reaches the nervous system, liver, or circulation fast enough to produce broader symptoms. Chronic burden is usually distributed. Part of the cost may stay in the gut as incomplete digestion, bloating, irritation, altered transit, or repeated chemical contact with the same absorptive surface. Another part may show up only after absorption. The liver has to transform compounds arriving through portal blood, the venous system carrying absorbed material from the intestine to the liver first. The thyroid may have to keep functioning in the presence of compounds that interfere with iodine handling. The kidney may have to keep filtering a load that adds nothing to tissue nourishment. Because that burden is spread across time and organs, people often misread it as normal eating, minor sensitivity, aging, or bad luck. The chemistry is quieter, not weaker.

Irritant and blocker are useful words because they describe two major ways burden operates without requiring a classical poison. An irritant is a compound or tissue feature that increases friction at the mucosal surface, changes motility, pulls water into the bowel, increases gas pressure, or otherwise makes contact with the digestive tract more costly. The food may be technically edible and still keep the gut under strain. A blocker works by interfering with access rather than by announcing distress. It binds minerals, inhibits proteases, which are the enzymes that digest protein, alters transport, or changes the chemical environment enough that nutrients remain in the lumen instead of crossing into the body. Many plant foods combine both roles. A legume can carry fermentable carbohydrate that increases luminal pressure while also carrying phytate and protease inhibitors that reduce nutrient return. A leafy plant can deliver vitamins on paper while simultaneously changing the mineral chemistry of the meal. Once these categories are separated, the argument becomes cleaner. A food does not have to poison acutely to underperform chronically. It can irritate. It can block. It can burden. That is enough to matter.

This distinction changes how foods should be judged. The ordinary question asks whether the food is poisonous, as if the absence of acute toxicity settles the matter. The physiological question asks what the food keeps forcing the body to do. Does the digestive tract keep losing minerals to binding chemistry. Does the intestine keep dealing with fermentable residues, unstable transit, or repeated mucosal contact. Does the thyroid keep compensating. Does the kidney keep clearing compounds that never should have become a staple urinary load. An acute poison is easy to condemn because the damage is concentrated and visible. Chronic metabolic burden hides inside normal eating because the injury is spread out and paid in installments. That does not make it trivial. It makes it easier to miss until the cost has become part of the body's daily workload.

Direct Toxins Versus Compounds That Bind Minerals or Inhibit Enzymes

A direct toxin harms by acting on tissue fast enough and strongly enough that the damage can be recognized as poisoning. The compound itself is the main problem. Once enough of it is released, absorbed, or brought into contact with the gut, the body starts losing control of the situation. Cyanogenic glycosides in poorly processed cassava can release cyanide, which blocks cytochrome c oxidase, an enzyme inside mitochondria that allows cells to use oxygen to make energy. Glycoalkaloids in stressed or greened potatoes can disrupt cell membranes and interfere with acetylcholinesterase, the enzyme that normally breaks down the neurotransmitter acetylcholine after a nerve signal. Lectin-rich undercooked kidney beans can make aggressive contact with the intestinal lining and trigger abrupt nausea, vomiting, and diarrhea. In each of those cases, the food is not merely reducing nutritional return. It is delivering a compound that can injure quickly enough to force an obvious reaction. The body is no longer negotiating over efficiency. It is trying to contain damage.

Mineral binders work differently. They do not have to create a dramatic toxic episode because their damage is subtractive rather than explosive. The compound enters the gut and changes what the meal can yield. Oxalate is the cleanest example because it can bind calcium in the intestinal contents and reduce the amount of calcium that remains soluble and available for absorption. Phytate does the same kind of work across a wider mineral range. It can hold zinc, iron, calcium, and magnesium inside complexes that human digestion handles poorly. The person may feel nothing dramatic after the meal. No crisis announces the loss. But the mineral never reaches the brush border, the absorptive surface of the small intestine, in the form the body needs. This is why a food can test rich in minerals and still nourish thinly. The nutrient is present inside the plant. The binder changes whether it ever becomes part of the body.

Enzyme inhibitors create another kind of hidden loss. Digestion depends on enzymes cleaving larger food structures into smaller absorbable units. Proteases such as trypsin and chymotrypsin break protein into peptides and amino acids. Amylases reduce starch into smaller carbohydrate fragments. Lipases split fat into fatty acids and monoglycerides, which are partial fat breakdown products small enough to move toward absorption. When a plant compound inhibits one of these systems, the nutrient can remain in the bowel as unfinished material. Protease inhibitors in legumes and seeds are the clearest example. The food may contain substantial protein, but if the intestine cannot reduce that protein efficiently, the amino acid return falls. The chart keeps the number. The body receives less of the material that number was supposed to promise. This is not poisoning in the ordinary sense. It is digestive sabotage.

The difference matters because these compounds injure by different routes and produce different kinds of evidence. A direct toxin often announces itself through fast gut distress, neurologic symptoms, or systemic instability. A mineral binder may produce no clear symptom at the time of eating while steadily lowering mineral entry across repeated meals. An enzyme inhibitor may show up as bloating, heaviness, incomplete digestion, or chronically poor protein yield rather than obvious toxicity. One category attacks sharply. The others degrade the value of the meal and increase physiological cost without creating a scene. But the quieter mechanism should not be mistaken for a harmless one. Repeated mineral loss, repeated incomplete protein digestion, and repeated chemical friction at the intestinal surface can change the body just as surely as a stronger toxin changes it more suddenly.

Many plant foods combine these categories. A legume may carry lectin activity, protease inhibitors, phytate, and fermentable carbohydrate in the same tissue. A leafy plant may bring useful vitamins while also releasing oxalate that changes the mineral chemistry of the meal. A tuber may deliver starch while still carrying direct toxic potential near the peel if stress chemistry has risen. That is why foods cannot be judged by asking whether they are poisonous in the narrowest sense. The better question is what kind of chemical opposition the tissue creates. Does it injure directly. Does it bind. Does it inhibit. Does it keep the nutrient from reaching blood. A food can fail the body through more than one mechanism at the same time, and many defended plant tissues do exactly that.

Gut Irritation Versus Endocrine Interference Versus Renal Burden

Plant chemistry does not injure the body in only one place, and one reason the modern conversation stays confused is that it keeps collapsing very different kinds of burden into one vague category of sensitivity. The gut, the endocrine system, and the kidney are not experiencing the same problem even when the meal is the same. Gut irritation begins at the point of contact. The intestinal lining, or mucosa, is the living surface that has to absorb nutrients while holding the boundary between the body and everything still inside the bowel. When a plant arrives carrying poorly digested carbohydrate, lectins, abrasive fiber, tannins, saponins, acids, or other chemically active compounds, the first cost may be local. Water shifts into the lumen, the hollow interior of the gut. Gas expands from fermentation. Transit changes. The bowel wall stretches. Protein digestion becomes less complete. The person feels pressure, bloating, pain, urgency, heaviness, or irregularity. This is a contact burden. The chemistry is acting where the food still physically is.

Endocrine interference is a different event because the problem is no longer mechanical contact with the gut surface. The problem is disruption of signaling chemistry the body depends on to regulate growth, metabolic pace, temperature, stress response, and substrate use. The thyroid is the clearest example in this book. Thyroid hormone production depends on iodine delivery into thyroid tissue, oxidation of that iodine, and its incorporation into tyrosine residues on thyroglobulin, the large storage protein from which thyroid hormones are made. Some plant compounds interfere with that sequence. Goitrogenic compounds from cruciferous vegetables, especially when iodine status is weak or intake is repetitive and poorly balanced, can reduce iodine handling or otherwise increase the gland's workload. The plant is no longer just irritating a mucosal surface. It is altering a gland's ability to maintain hormone output. That shift matters because endocrine burden often hides better than gut burden. The bowel complains quickly. The thyroid compensates quietly until it cannot keep pace as easily.

Renal burden begins after absorption. The kidney only inherits what entered the blood and remained part of the circulating load long enough to require filtration. This is why oxalate is such a strong model compound. In the gut, oxalate can already be a nutritional problem because it binds calcium and lowers the usable mineral yield of the meal. If some oxalate remains soluble, crosses the intestinal wall, and enters the bloodstream, the burden moves downstream. Now the kidney has to filter it, concentrate it into urine, and keep it dissolved well enough that it does not precipitate into crystals. Precipitate means to fall out of solution and form a solid. In this context it means the urine can no longer keep calcium and oxalate dissolved together, and crystal formation begins. That is not a gut symptom and it is not an endocrine problem. It is an excretory problem created by a compound the body cannot use and must remove.

The same food can therefore impose different categories of burden in sequence. A high-oxalate leaf can first reduce calcium availability in the intestine, then add oxalate to the blood, then increase urinary crystal pressure later. A legume can first irritate digestion through fermentation and incomplete protein breakdown, then lower mineral absorption through phytate, and then leave the tissues undernourished despite respectable nutrient numbers on paper. A crucifer-heavy pattern in a person with poor iodine status may cause little obvious gut distress while still increasing thyroid strain over time. The mistake is to talk as if all adverse food effects belong to one basket. They do not. The gut pays in contact, distension, motility disruption, and incomplete digestion. The endocrine system pays in compensatory signaling and altered hormone handling. The kidney pays in filtration and excretion of compounds that never should have become part of the daily urinary workload.

This distinction also changes how symptoms should be interpreted. Gas, bloating, cramping, reflux, irregular bowel movement, and post-meal heaviness point first toward digestive friction, incomplete breakdown, osmotic load, fermentation pressure, or mucosal irritation. Cold intolerance, slowing, fatigue, altered hair or skin texture, and other thyroid-pattern symptoms point toward a different physiological lane entirely, one involving hormone production and signaling rather than simple bowel tolerance. Flank pain, urinary irritation, crystals, or stone formation point toward a clearance problem, where the meal has already passed through digestion and entered the kidney's domain. The food may be the same. The burden is not. A serious nutritional framework has to separate these pathways because the body does. Otherwise every plant problem gets mislabeled as a vague sensitivity when the real issue may be local irritation in one person, gland interference in another, and urinary burden in a third.

That is why foods have to be judged by where the cost lands. Some foods mainly irritate. Some mainly interfere. Some mainly burden excretion. Many defended plant foods do more than one. The intestine absorbs only part of the meal. The rest of the body inherits the consequences.

Why a Food Can Be Nonlethal and Still Biologically Expensive

A food does not have to kill quickly to cost the body dearly. Lethality is a crude threshold. It tells you when the chemistry overwhelmed the organism fast enough to force collapse, obvious poisoning, or emergency symptoms. Most foods that burden people never reach that threshold. They stay below it and keep charging smaller tolls instead. The intestine loses mineral access. Protein digestion becomes less complete. Fermentation pressure rises. The thyroid compensates harder. The liver processes compounds that brought little return. The kidney filters and concentrates solutes the body cannot use. None of that has to look dramatic after a single meal. The body can survive the encounter and still come away with less nourishment, more work, and more tissue friction than the food's reputation would suggest.

This is the category modern nutrition language misses most easily because it is trained to look for deficiency on one side and poisoning on the other, as if everything important happens only at the extremes. Real physiology spends most of its time in the middle. A high-oxalate leaf may not poison the person, but it can still lower calcium availability in the intestinal contents and then send absorbed oxalate to the kidney for excretion later. A phytate-rich seed may not trigger obvious symptoms at the table, but it can still keep zinc, iron, calcium, and magnesium tied up in complexes that the small intestine handles poorly. A legume can be edible and still arrive carrying protease inhibitors that reduce protein cleavage, fermentable carbohydrate that expands the bowel with gas and water, and lectin activity that was reduced by cooking but not erased by the label. The food can be tolerated in the ordinary sense and still perform badly when judged by what it yielded versus what it cost.

The body feels that cost in stages. First comes digestive expense. More chewing, more gastric work, more enzyme demand, more time spent trying to break apart structure that resists dismantling. Then comes absorptive expense. Nutrients have to remain soluble, reach the brush border, the enzyme-rich surface of the small intestine, and cross into the body before binding chemistry or poor digestion carries them farther downstream. Then comes handling expense. Compounds that do cross into portal blood, the venous blood moving from the intestine to the liver first, have to be sorted. Useful material is stored, transformed, or sent onward. Useless or disruptive material is modified, filtered, concentrated, and excreted. A food can therefore fail in more than one place. It can underdeliver in the gut and overburden the organs afterward. That is a bad trade even when nobody calls it toxicity.

This is also why repetition matters more than people think. A single meal can remain trivial because the body has room to compensate. Daily exposure is different. The same binding chemistry keeps recurring in the same intestinal lumen. The same fermentable residues keep reaching the same colon. The same goitrogenic pressure keeps asking the thyroid to work around interference. The same urinary solute keeps returning to the kidney. A single exposure and a staple exposure are not the same physiological event. The first may leave no obvious trace. The second can become part of the tissue's normal workload. At that point the food is no longer just edible. It is part of the body's maintenance problem.

That is the standard this book will use when it calls a food biologically expensive. The claim is not that the food is instantly deadly. The claim is that the body has to spend too much to get too little. Digestion strains, absorption narrows, useful yield falls, clearance burden rises, and the organs keep paying for a food that looked better on paper than it behaved in tissue. Nonlethal only means the chemistry stayed below the level of immediate collapse. It says nothing about whether the meal was cooperative, efficient, or worth repeating.

Reframing "Healthy Plant Foods" as Variable Exposures Rather Than Moral Objects

The phrase healthy plant foods usually enters the conversation as a verdict before the biology has even begun. The food is assigned a moral status, then everything else gets organized around protecting that status. If symptoms appear, the dose was too low, the preparation was wrong, the microbiome needs time, the person is unusually sensitive, or the rest of the diet must be the real problem. What almost never happens is a clean return to the tissue itself. What kind of plant part was eaten. What compounds did that tissue release when it was cut, chewed, blended, cooked, or juiced. What did those compounds do in the lumen, the hollow interior of the gut where digestion is taking place. What reached the absorptive surface in a soluble form and what stayed bound, fermented, or irritating. The moral frame blocks those questions because once a food is treated as virtuous by category, its chemistry is no longer being judged as chemistry. It is being defended as identity.

A variable exposure frame is harder and more honest. It begins by assuming that a fruit, leaf, seed, tuber, peel, or legume is not a stable moral object. It is an exposure with a specific dose, a specific structure, a specific preparation method, a specific frequency, and a specific host receiving it. A cooked carrot is one exposure. A large daily spinach smoothie is another. A peeled boiled potato is one exposure. A greened potato with stressed peel chemistry is another. A few well-cooked lentils beside a mixed meal are one exposure. A heavy legume-based diet eaten daily by a person already dealing with bloating, poor protein digestion, and mineral insufficiency is another. The plant category does not settle the matter because the body does not absorb categories. It handles actual compounds in actual amounts delivered inside actual tissues.

This changes the standard of judgment. Instead of asking whether the food belongs to the healthy side of a cultural divide, the book asks what kind of load the exposure creates. Does the plant release oxalate that changes the mineral environment of the meal. Does it bring phytate that holds zinc, iron, calcium, or magnesium in complexes the intestine handles poorly. Does it carry fermentable carbohydrate that stays in the bowel long enough to pull in water and feed gas production. Does it contain glucosinolate breakdown products that matter more in a person with weak iodine status. Does it create a kidney burden later because the body absorbed what it could not use and now has to clear it in urine. Those are exposure questions. They are measurable in physiology, not in public virtue. A food can have an admirable reputation and still perform badly when judged by digestive yield, endocrine cost, or urinary consequence.

The variable exposure frame also makes room for preparation and repetition, which the moral frame usually flattens. Boiling changes soluble oxalate exposure because some oxalate leaves the tissue and enters the cooking water. Proper heat reduces lectin activity and denatures protease inhibitors, which means it changes their shape enough to reduce their interference with digestion. Fermentation and sprouting can lower phytate. Peeling can reduce contact with compounds concentrated near the outer tissue. None of those steps magically turns a defended plant into a free gift. But they do change the chemistry the body receives. Frequency changes it further. A single exposure and a staple exposure are not the same physiological event. A small burden can remain trivial when it is rare. The same burden can become part of the intestine's daily workload when it is repeated as a foundation food. Once that is understood, the question is no longer whether the food is good or bad. The question is what repeated contact with that specific food, in that form, is doing to that specific body.

Host vulnerability becomes clearer as well when the moral language is removed. A person with strong bile flow, robust enzyme output, intact mineral status, good kidney function, and a calm bowel can often absorb or tolerate a plant exposure that destabilizes someone else. A person with fat malabsorption may absorb more oxalate because unabsorbed fat binds calcium in the gut and leaves more oxalate free to cross into the body. A person with thyroid fragility and low iodine reserves is not handling crucifer-heavy intake on the same terms as someone whose iodine status is strong. A person with visceral hypersensitivity or unstable motility is not meeting onions, apples, beans, and polyol-rich fruits as the same digestive experience as someone with a quiet intestine. The food did not become morally worse in one body and morally better in another. The exposure met a different physiology and produced a different result.

That is the frame this book will use from start to finish. Fruits and vegetables will not be treated as saints, villains, or symbols of discipline. They will be treated as chemical exposures with structure, dose, frequency, preparation state, and tissue consequence. Some exposures will be low burden and modestly useful. Some will be tolerable only in limited forms. Some will be poor staples because they bind, inhibit, irritate, interfere, or burden excretion more than they nourish. The category healthy plant foods hides those differences by turning food into a moral object. Physiology does the opposite. It breaks the food apart and tallies the cost.

Part II

The Gut Event

Chapter 4

The Gut as the First Site of Loss

The first real loss from a plant-heavy meal often happens before a single nutrient has entered the body. It happens in the intestinal lumen, the hollow interior space of the small intestine where food, acid-neutralizing secretions, bile, pancreatic enzymes, minerals, sugars, peptides, fibers, and plant defense compounds all mix together in suspension. Public nutrition language usually skips this space because it is not flattering. The food still looks virtuous on paper. The intestine is already sorting through conflict. Minerals are being released and bound in the same moment. Proteins are being exposed to digestive enzymes while plant inhibitors are still present in the same mixture. Carbohydrates are being reduced into smaller units while some fractions remain resistant, osmotically active, or ready for later fermentation. The lumen is not a passive tube carrying nutrients toward absorption. It is the first contested environment where the meal either becomes more available to the body or starts losing value before the absorptive surface ever sees it.

This is where plant chemistry begins to subtract. A leaf releases calcium and oxalate into the same fluid. A seed-derived food releases minerals and phytate into the same fluid. A legume sends protein, starch, protease inhibitors, lectins, and fermentable carbohydrate into the same fluid. Those compounds do not wait politely for the intestine to absorb the good parts first. They meet each other immediately. Oxalate can bind calcium. Phytate can hold zinc, iron, calcium, and magnesium in complexes that stay poorly available. Tannins can bind proteins and minerals. Protease inhibitors can slow the cleavage of dietary protein into smaller fragments the intestine can actually transport. The lumen therefore decides much of the meal's fate before absorption begins. A nutrient can be present in the bowl, released from the tissue, and still lost functionally because the chemistry of the lumen changed around it.

The lumen also determines how much of the meal stays dissolved, mobile, and reachable. That matters because a nutrient has to remain soluble, meaning dissolved in intestinal fluid, if it is going to move efficiently toward the brush border, the enzyme-rich surface of the small intestine where final digestion and uptake occur. Once a mineral precipitates, meaning it falls out of solution into a less mobile form, or becomes trapped in a larger complex, it is no longer behaving like a freely absorbable nutrient. Once a fat-soluble compound fails to enter micelles, the tiny bile-based transport particles that move lipids through the watery contents of the intestine, it is less likely to reach the membrane that has to take it into the body. Once proteins remain only partly digested because enzyme access was poor or inhibitors were present, the intestine is left with bulkier fragments and less efficient amino acid delivery. This is why nutrient content and nutrient availability part company so early. The lumen is already downgrading the meal while the food still carries a wholesome reputation outside the body.

Carbohydrates create another kind of battle in the same space. Some sugars and starch fragments absorb efficiently if the plant structure has been broken down well and the transport systems at the intestinal surface are not overloaded. Others do not. Fructose in excess of absorptive capacity, polyols, and fermentable oligosaccharides can remain in the lumen long enough to keep water there by osmotic effect, meaning they pull water into the bowel simply because dissolved particles attract it. That extra fluid can speed transit, loosen stool, and increase the volume the bowel has to manage. If those carbohydrates then pass into the colon, bacteria ferment them into gas and short-chain fatty acids. The symptom may be felt later as bloating, cramping, distension, or urgency, but the first failure began upstream when the lumen held onto material that the small intestine could not clear cleanly. The food may still be edible. The gut has already started losing control of the sequence.

This is why the lumen deserves to be treated as the first battleground rather than a neutral passageway. It is where the plant's structure has been broken open enough to release its contents but not yet resolved enough to deliver them cleanly into the body. Every weakness in the meal shows up here first. Binding chemistry shows up here. Incomplete protein digestion shows up here. Failed mineral release shows up here. Poor fat handling shows up here. Osmotic drag and the beginnings of fermentative burden show up here. By the time symptoms appear, or by the time the kidney has to clear what the gut allowed across, the first losses have already happened in this interior chemical field. The meal does not become nourishing because its nutrients entered the intestine. It becomes nourishing only if the lumen stops being a place of conflict and starts becoming a place of transfer.

Binding, Precipitation, Enzyme Inhibition, Osmotic Drag, and Microbial Fermentation

Once plant tissue has been broken open in the gut, the meal stops being a simple collection of nutrients and becomes a chemical traffic problem. Binding is one of the first ways value is lost. A mineral is released from the plant, enters the intestinal fluid, and then meets a compound that holds it tightly enough to keep it from reaching the absorptive surface. Oxalate does this with calcium. Phytate can do it with zinc, iron, calcium, and magnesium. Tannins can bind both proteins and minerals. The nutrient has not disappeared, but it has changed status. It is no longer moving freely in solution toward uptake. It is being held inside a complex that the small intestine handles poorly. That is why the lumen, the hollow interior of the intestine, is the first site of nutritional failure. The food may still contain what the label promised. The chemistry of the meal is already cutting the body off from part of it.

Precipitation is the next loss, and it is closely related to binding. To precipitate means to fall out of solution and become less mobile. In the gut, that matters because dissolved compounds can move through intestinal fluid toward the brush border, the enzyme-rich surface of the small intestine where final digestion and absorption occur. Once a mineral or other compound precipitates, it is behaving less like a freely available nutrient and more like sediment carried downstream. The meal may still look chemically rich if analyzed after complete destruction in a laboratory. The intestine is not performing that kind of destruction. It is working with a fluid mixture where pH, mineral ratios, bile activity, acids, fibers, and plant-derived binding compounds are all changing what stays dissolved and what does not. Availability is not determined only by what was released from the tissue. It is determined by what remains soluble long enough to be absorbed.

Enzyme inhibition creates a different kind of loss because now the food is interfering with the machinery that is supposed to dismantle it. Proteases such as trypsin and chymotrypsin reduce protein into smaller fragments and amino acids the intestine can absorb. Amylases reduce starch into smaller carbohydrates. Lipases break fat into absorbable components. When a plant carries protease inhibitors, the problem is not that protein is absent. The problem is that protein stays larger, less accessible, and less absorbable because the enzyme meant to cleave it has been blocked. The same logic applies across digestion. The intestine is not merely receiving nutrients. It is trying to reduce structure into transportable units. If the enzyme system is slowed, the meal remains bulkier, less finished, and more likely to continue downstream as partially digested material. A respectable protein number on paper means very little if the gut is still struggling to cut that protein into usable form.

Osmotic drag begins when poorly absorbed carbohydrates remain in the intestinal lumen and hold water there. Osmosis is the movement of water toward an area with more dissolved particles. In practical terms, if fructose, polyols, or fermentable oligosaccharides remain in the bowel because absorption is incomplete, they pull fluid into that space. The result is a thinner, heavier, more distended intestinal load. Transit can speed up. Stool can loosen. The gut wall stretches. The person feels pressure before bacteria have even started much of the secondary work. That secondary work is microbial fermentation. Fermentation means gut microbes break down carbohydrates the human small intestine did not absorb. In the colon, bacteria act on those leftovers and produce gas and short-chain fatty acids, small fats such as acetate, propionate, and butyrate. In a stable bowel and at a tolerable dose, that may be manageable. In a sensitive bowel, or when the plant load is too high, gas expands the lumen, pressure rises against the bowel wall, and the meal becomes pain, bloating, urgency, and altered transit. The food can still be called healthy outside the body. Inside the gut it has become water retention, gas production, and mechanical stress.

These are not separate academic concepts. They are overlapping ways a meal loses value before the body ever gets to count the nutrients as its own. Binding traps. Precipitation immobilizes. Enzyme inhibition slows dismantling. Osmotic drag pulls water into the bowel. Microbial fermentation converts unabsorbed residue into gas and pressure. A single plant food can trigger more than one of these losses at once. That is why the intestine is the first battleground and the first place where a nutritious-looking meal can start failing. The body does not live on what the food contained at the start. It lives on what remained accessible after the lumen finished sorting out what would cross and what would continue downstream as burden.

How Symptoms Begin Before Absorption

People often imagine that a food has to enter the bloodstream before it can do anything meaningful to the body. The gut makes that impossible. Symptoms can begin while the meal is still sitting in the lumen, the hollow interior of the intestine where digestion is unfolding in fluid, before a nutrient, toxin, or irritant has crossed into circulation. The bowel is not an inert pipe waiting to deliver material onward. It is a muscular, secretory, sensory organ with a living mucosal surface, dense nerve supply, immune surveillance, and constant exposure to pressure, stretch, acidity, osmotic load, and chemical contact. That means the body can begin reacting while the food is still outside the body in the strict sense, still inside the intestinal tube, still part of the gut contents rather than part of the bloodstream. If the lumen fills with poorly absorbed sugars, polyols, acids, fermentable residues, abrasive particles, or enzyme-resistant fragments, the intestine can start signaling distress immediately. Bloating, pressure, cramping, urgency, nausea, reflux, and altered motility do not require absorption first. They require contact, stretch, fluid shift, and failed handling inside the digestive tract.

Osmotic drag is one of the fastest ways this begins. If a meal leaves a high concentration of poorly absorbed particles in the small intestine, water moves into that space to dilute them. Osmosis is simply the movement of water toward the area with more dissolved material. The bowel now has more fluid to manage, more distension, and often faster transit. The person may feel heaviness, sloshing, cramping, or sudden bowel urgency before any meaningful downstream nutrient benefit has occurred. Fructose that exceeds absorptive capacity, sugar alcohols such as sorbitol, and other fermentable carbohydrates can all create this kind of luminal overload. The same sequence happens with some plant fibers and incompletely digested residues that hold water and expand bulk. The symptom is not mysterious. The bowel wall is being stretched by fluid and volume that should not still be there.

Mechanical and chemical irritation can begin just as early. A meal that arrives with partially digested protein, fibrous fragments, acids, lectin activity, tannin contact, or other irritating chemistry can increase friction along the mucosal surface. The mucosa is the living lining of the intestine, the tissue that has to absorb nutrients while protecting the body from unnecessary intrusion. That lining is sensitive to repeated contact with compounds that bind proteins, alter permeability, change secretion, or simply keep scraping past in poorly reduced form. A food does not need to contain a classical poison to create this kind of stress. It only has to keep the intestine working against difficult material. The bowel can respond by changing motility, increasing secretion, tightening in some segments while relaxing in others, and sending sensory signals upward that the person experiences as discomfort, nausea, or pain. The symptom begins in the handling problem itself.

Fermentation adds a second wave. When carbohydrates escape absorption in the small intestine and reach the colon, bacteria begin digesting what human enzymes left behind. That bacterial digestion produces gases and short-chain fatty acids, which are small fats made by microbial metabolism. Gas expands the lumen further. Distension increases. In a bowel with visceral hypersensitivity, meaning a nervous system that reacts strongly to normal or modest stretching, even ordinary amounts of gas can become pain, pressure, and bloating. The person often blames the symptom on something abstract like inflammation or poor gut health. The more immediate truth is simpler. The food left too much unfinished material in the bowel, microbes acted on it, and the intestine was forced to carry the pressure.

This is why symptoms can begin before absorption and why that fact matters so much to the way foods should be judged. A meal can fail while still inside the gut. It can draw in water, slow enzyme access, bind minerals, hold nutrients in bulky complexes, increase fluid volume, accelerate transit, and generate gas pressure before the bloodstream has gained anything from it. The food may still contain vitamins, minerals, carbohydrates, or phytonutrients on paper. The intestine is already showing whether the body is likely to benefit from the exposure or merely endure it. By the time something useful reaches blood, the first verdict has often already been delivered by the bowel wall, the fluid balance of the lumen, and the pressure building inside the tube.

Why Bloating, Gas, Pain, Diarrhea, Constipation, and Food Aversion Are Not Random

These symptoms are usually treated as loose complaints, as if the bowel simply decides to be difficult after certain meals for reasons nobody can trace. The intestine is not acting randomly. It is reacting to load, pressure, chemistry, and failed handling. Bloating begins when material remains in the gut that should have been broken down, absorbed, or moved forward cleanly without excess fluid or gas. Gas begins when bacteria ferment carbohydrates the small intestine did not absorb. Pain begins when the bowel wall stretches, spasms, or is forced into repeated contact with irritating compounds and poorly reduced food residue. Diarrhea begins when unabsorbed particles keep water in the lumen, the hollow interior of the bowel, or when secretion and motility rise in response to chemical irritation. Constipation can begin from the opposite pattern, where poorly digestible bulk, slowed transit, dehydration of stool, altered motility, or protective slowing keeps contents sitting too long. Food aversion follows when the nervous system learns the sequence. The body starts treating the food as a problem before the mind has finished naming it. None of this is mysterious. The symptoms are outputs from a digestive system that has been forced into the wrong kind of work.

Bloating and gas are usually the easiest examples because the mechanics are so direct. If a meal leaves too much fructose, polyol, resistant starch, fiber, or fermentable oligosaccharide in the bowel, the intestine has to carry that material forward while water and bacteria react to it.

Osmotic particles hold fluid in the intestinal contents. Bacteria ferment what escapes absorption and release gases such as hydrogen, methane, and carbon dioxide. The lumen expands. The bowel wall stretches. In a resilient gut, that may remain tolerable. In a sensitive gut, or after a sufficiently large plant load, the expansion becomes pressure, fullness, visible distension, belching, lower abdominal tightness, and the strange sensation that the meal is still physically occupying the gut long after it should have cleared. The symptom is not random discomfort. It is retained substrate becoming retained volume and then retained pressure.

Pain follows the same sequence but adds a stronger sensory response. The bowel wall is supplied with nerves that register stretch, chemical irritation, and changes in motility. When the intestine is forced to push against distending gas, excess fluid, incompletely digested residue, or chemically active compounds, the muscular wall begins changing its contraction pattern. Some segments tighten. Some stall. Some push too quickly. That altered motility can create cramping, gripping, or aching pain because the gut is no longer moving contents in a smooth coordinated way. Lectin-rich undercooked legumes, heavily fermentable meals, abrasive or poorly reduced plant matter, and meals that repeatedly irritate the mucosa, the living intestinal lining, can all contribute to this kind of pattern. The person feels pain and often assumes the meal must have triggered a vague intolerance. The physiology is more exact. The intestine was forced into abnormal pressure and contraction because the meal created more residue, more fluid, more chemical friction, or more bacterial activity than the system could manage comfortably.

Diarrhea and constipation look like opposites, but both can come from failed handling of the same food category under different conditions. Diarrhea often appears when poorly absorbed carbohydrates and other osmotic particles keep water in the bowel and speed transit. The intestine is trying to move an unstable load out. Secretion may rise. Time for absorption falls. Stool stays loose. Constipation can happen when bulky, resistant, slowly moving residue remains in the gut long enough for more water to be withdrawn, leaving harder stool behind. It can also happen when repeated irritation or fermentation changes motility in a way that produces stalling rather than acceleration. Methane is one factor that can slow transit in some people because methane-producing gut microbes are associated with slower bowel movement patterns. The same plant-heavy pattern can therefore produce diarrhea in one person and constipation in another depending on water shifts, microbial activity, motility pattern, nervous system sensitivity, and how much of the meal remained unfinished inside the bowel. The symptom differs. The common thread is that the gut was not handling the meal cleanly.

Food aversion is often the most intelligent symptom of the group. When a meal repeatedly leads to pressure, nausea, pain, urgency, reflux, or prolonged heaviness, the nervous system starts building avoidance around that food. This is not weakness or irrationality. It is pattern recognition. The stomach slows before an expected problem meal. The smell or taste becomes unpleasant. Appetite drops. The mouth resists chewing. The person may say the body does not want it. That is often exactly right. The body is learning that a certain tissue, in a certain dose, prepared a certain way, reliably leads to digestive friction. The aversion can appear before the person understands the mechanism, but the mechanism is still there. Symptoms are not random reactions scattered across meals without cause. They are the gut's record of what happened when digestion failed to reduce the load, absorption failed to clear it, and the bowel was left to manage the remainder as pressure, fluid, spasm, and distress.

The Gut as a Site Where Plant Chemistry Can Reduce Nourishment Before Blood Ever Sees the Meal

The bloodstream is not the first place a meal succeeds or fails. The first sorting happens in the gut, while the food is still outside the body in the strict physiological sense, still inside the tube of the digestive tract rather than inside tissue or circulation. That matters because a plant can begin losing nutritional value long before a vitamin, mineral, sugar, fatty acid, or amino acid crosses the intestinal wall. The gut does not simply receive nutrients and pass them inward. It tears structure apart, exposes compounds that were separated inside the plant, mixes them into a fluid environment, and forces them into contact with acid, bile, enzymes, minerals, fibers, and microbes. In that space, a favorable nutrient and an unfavorable plant compound are often released together. The leaf does not release calcium alone. It may release oxalate with it. The seed does not release minerals alone. It may release phytate with them. The legume does not release protein alone. It may release protease inhibitors and fermentable carbohydrate at the same time. The intestine is therefore not the place where nutrition merely begins. It is the place where the first losses are imposed.

Those losses happen by mechanism, not by abstraction. A mineral can be released from the plant matrix and then bound before absorption. Oxalate can tie up calcium. Phytate can hold zinc, iron, calcium, and magnesium in complexes that remain poorly available to the absorptive surface. Tannins can bind proteins and minerals and make them less usable. Protease inhibitors can interfere with trypsin and chymotrypsin, the pancreatic enzymes that are supposed to cut larger food proteins into absorbable amino acids. Poorly absorbed carbohydrates can remain in the lumen, the hollow interior of the intestine where digestion is happening, and pull water into the bowel by osmotic force before microbes ferment what remains downstream. A nutrient chart does not show this stage honestly because the chart is describing what was present in the food sample. The gut is deciding what remains soluble, what stays mobile, what reaches the brush border, the enzyme-rich surface of the small intestine, and what is already being diverted toward waste. A food can look dense on paper and begin thinning out in value the moment digestion opens it.

This is also where the difference between gross content and usable yield becomes real. Gross content is what the food carried into the mouth. Usable yield is what survives chewing, acid exposure, enzyme cleavage, bile handling, binding chemistry, precipitation, and luminal transport. Precipitation means a compound falls out of solution and becomes less mobile in intestinal fluid. Once that happens, access narrows further. The body does not absorb potential. It absorbs what remains reachable. A carotenoid in a vegetable has to be released from plant structure, incorporated into micelles, the tiny bile-based transport particles that move fats and fat-soluble compounds through intestinal fluid, and brought to the absorptive membrane. A mineral has to stay free long enough to be transported. A protein has to be cut small enough to cross. If the gut keeps losing compounds to binding, failed liberation, incomplete cleavage, poor micelle formation, or unstable transit, then nourishment has already been reduced before the liver, blood, kidney, muscle, or thyroid ever has a chance to use anything.

That is why the gut has to be treated as the first site of nutritional subtraction. The body is not waiting passively for nutrients to arrive in blood. It is fighting for access while the meal is still in the intestinal contents. Some foods cooperate with that process and give up their value with relatively little friction. Others arrive carrying their own interference. They release nutrients and obstacles in the same act. They ask the intestine to separate what can nourish from what will bind, inhibit, irritate, ferment, or continue downstream as burden. By the time something useful enters circulation, the first accounting has already been done. If the gut had to surrender minerals, tolerate incomplete digestion, carry excess water, manage fermentation pressure, or push partially usable material toward excretion, then the meal was already losing value before blood ever saw it.

Chapter 5

Fiber, Bulk, and the Problem of False Virtue

Fiber is the part of plant structure human digestive enzymes do not fully dismantle. That definition is already more useful than most nutrition language because it keeps the material visible. Fiber is not a moral property. It is not a cleansing force. It is not a magical regulator drifting through the bowel doing good by reputation. It is physical plant matter with specific structural behavior in water, acid, enzymes, and gut movement. Much of it comes from cell walls and supporting architecture. Cellulose forms rigid structural strands. Hemicellulose helps organize the wall around those strands. Pectin forms gel-like networks that hold water and influence the texture of fruits and vegetables. Lignin, though not a carbohydrate, adds further rigidity in tougher plant tissues. These materials help a plant stand upright, resist collapse, control water movement, and protect what is stored inside. When a person eats the plant, those same materials become part of the digestive workload because the body must sort nutrients out from a structure it does not fully digest.

That is why fiber is better understood as mechanics before it is discussed as nutrition. Insoluble fiber tends to keep shape, resist dissolution, and preserve bulk. Soluble fiber tends to absorb water, swell, and form more viscous material, meaning a thicker slower-moving gel within intestinal contents. Both change what digestion has to work through. Insoluble fiber can keep plant fragments coarse and physically separate nutrients from enzymes. Soluble fiber can slow diffusion, which means it can slow the movement of digestive enzymes toward food particles and the movement of liberated nutrients back toward the absorptive surface. Neither form is automatically good or bad in the abstract. The question is what that physical behavior does in a given meal and in a given intestine. A swollen gel can modestly slow sugar entry in one context and create heaviness, delayed emptying, and trapped material in another. Coarse bulk can increase stool mass in one person and increase abrasion, pressure, or incomplete digestion in another. The physics comes first. The health claim comes later, if it survives contact with the actual bowel.

Fiber also changes the meal before the colon ever sees it. In the stomach and small intestine, it alters particle dispersion, fluid retention, and the speed at which food components meet acid, bile, and enzymes. A fibrous plant matrix can keep starch granules enclosed longer, keep proteins less exposed, and hold minerals inside a structural mesh while binding compounds such as oxalate and phytate are being released from the same tissue. That means fiber is not just something that arrives in the colon to feed microbes. It is part of the upstream problem of access. A plant can test rich in minerals, carotenoids, or folate while the same structure slows liberation and transport of those compounds through the lumen, the hollow interior of the intestine where digestion is unfolding. The public conversation usually treats fiber as if it enters after the nutrient has already been secured. In reality it often sits in the middle of the negotiation, changing how much of the meal becomes absorbable at all.

Once fiber passes into the colon, the question shifts from structural interference to microbial handling. Some fibers and resistant carbohydrates become bacterial substrate. Microbes ferment them into gases and short-chain fatty acids, which are small fats such as acetate, propionate, and butyrate made during bacterial digestion. That outcome is often simplified into a universal good, but the bowel does not experience it so neatly. Fermentation means volume, gas, osmotic change, and mechanical stretch before it means any theoretical benefit. In a stable bowel, some of that may be tolerated. In a bowel already prone to bloating, slowed transit, rapid transit, or visceral hypersensitivity, meaning heightened nerve response to stretch and pressure, the same fiber load can become distension, pain, reflux, urgency, or constipation depending on how the gut handles pressure and water. Fiber is therefore not merely a nutrient category. It is structural residue with hydraulic and fermentative consequences.

So when this book asks what fiber physically is, the answer is not roughage, digestive support, or plant goodness. Fiber is plant architecture the human gut cannot fully reduce with its own enzymes. It holds water, preserves structure, slows access, alters viscosity, changes transit, feeds bacteria, and changes where the meal imposes its work. Sometimes that work is modest and well tolerated. Sometimes it becomes a major part of why a meal yields less nourishment than its label suggests. The word fiber sounds nutritional. The material behaves mechanically.

Soluble Versus Insoluble Fractions

The division between soluble and insoluble fiber matters because these fractions create different mechanical problems in the gut. Soluble means the fiber dissolves or disperses into water strongly enough to form a thicker, more viscous intestinal mixture. Viscous means it increases thickness and slows movement within the fluid contents of the bowel. Insoluble means the fiber does not dissolve well in water and tends to hold its structural identity as bulk, fragments, or coarse plant residue. Both are usually praised under the same word, as if fiber were a single beneficial substance moving through the body with a single function. The intestine does not experience them that way. One changes the fluid mechanics of digestion by swelling, trapping water, and slowing diffusion. The other changes the physical structure of the intestinal contents by preserving bulk, friction, and particulate load. The name stays the same. The digestive burden does not.

Soluble fiber is often treated as the gentler or smarter form because it can form gels and slow the movement of nutrients toward absorption. That description is not false, but it is incomplete. A gel is not an abstract virtue. It is a physical barrier. When soluble fiber swells in water, it thickens the contents of the stomach and small intestine, slows gastric emptying in some contexts, and slows the movement of digestive enzymes toward food particles and the movement of liberated nutrients back toward the absorptive surface. That can flatten glucose entry after a meal, but the same property can also create heaviness, prolonged fullness, delayed clearance, and a longer period of contact between the bowel and whatever else is trapped in that swollen matrix. Minerals, sugars, peptides, bile acids, plant acids, polyphenols, and fermentable residues are all moving through the same thickened mass. If the host handles that load poorly, the result can be bloating, pressure, incomplete meal clearance, or a slow drag through the upper gut rather than some tidy therapeutic effect. Once soluble fiber reaches the colon, bacterial fermentation can intensify quickly because many soluble fractions are more fermentable than coarse structural residues. The same swelling that looked useful upstream can become gas, luminal expansion, and unstable transit downstream.

Insoluble fiber behaves more like retained plant scaffolding. It tends to resist dissolution, keep its shape longer, and travel as physical residue. Cellulose-rich vegetable matter, bran-like fragments, seed hull material, and fibrous stems are common examples. This kind of material can increase stool bulk simply because more undigested matter is moving through the tract, but that should not be confused with improved nourishment or improved digestion. Bulk is not the same thing as successful extraction. Insoluble fiber can shield starch from enzymes, keep cell contents partly enclosed, and carry nutrients outward still trapped in the plant matrix. It can also create friction. In a bowel with strong motility and good hydration, that friction may be tolerated. In a bowel that is inflamed, slowed, narrowed, or already reacting poorly to pressure, the same coarse residue can become abrasion, distension, incomplete evacuation, or the strange pattern where the person feels full of material and undernourished at the same time. The bowel is moving mass. That does not mean the meal was handled well.

Most real foods contain both soluble and insoluble fractions, which is one reason simplified fiber language misleads people so badly. An apple is not soluble fiber in isolation. Oats are not beta-glucan in isolation. Greens are not cellulose in isolation. The plant arrives as mixed architecture. Some parts swell. Some parts resist. Some parts ferment quickly. Some parts hold their structure longer. The ratio changes with ripeness, cooking, grinding, juicing, drying, and processing.

Heating can soften pectin-rich tissues and alter how much water a plant fraction holds. Milling can reduce particle size and change how quickly microbes reach it. Juicing can remove much of the coarse fraction while concentrating sugar delivery and leaving a different burden behind. The gut is not handling a label claim. It is handling a physical blend of swelling material, coarse residue, trapped nutrients, bacterial substrate, and whatever plant defense chemistry came attached to the same tissue.

That is why soluble and insoluble fractions should be judged by what they force the digestive tract to do, not by whether a nutrition article assigned one a better public image. Does the soluble fraction thicken the intestinal contents enough to delay clearance, trap material, and increase fermentation burden later. Does the insoluble fraction preserve so much structure that nutrients remain physically enclosed and the bowel is left pushing bulk rather than absorbing value. Does the combination increase stool only because more undigested plant matter is being carried out. These are the real questions. Soluble and insoluble are not moral categories. They are different structural behaviors of plant residue inside water, enzymes, bile, and bowel motion. One swells and slows. One resists and bulks. Both can help under the right conditions. Both can become part of the digestive problem when the meal asks more of the gut than the gut can turn into useful return.

Water Holding, Swelling, Friction, and Fermentation

Fiber changes the bowel first through physics. Before it becomes a talking point about health, it becomes mass inside water. Some plant fractions hold water aggressively and expand. Others stay coarse, resist dissolution, and move through the gut as structural residue. That combination changes the shape and behavior of the intestinal contents. Water holding means the meal remains bulkier and wetter for longer. Swelling means the same amount of plant matter now occupies more space inside the lumen, the hollow interior of the bowel where digestion and transport are taking place. That increased volume changes pressure against the gut wall, changes how quickly contents move, and changes how easily enzymes, bile, and liberated nutrients can circulate through the meal. A swollen fiber mass is not an abstract benefit. It is a physical load the intestine has to push, mix, and clear.

That load can become friction. Friction in the gut is not only scraping in the crude sense, though coarse insoluble material can do some of that. It is also the repeated mechanical difficulty created when bulky plant residue slows smooth movement, holds contents in contact with the mucosa, the living intestinal lining, and forces the muscular wall to work harder to move material that remains structurally stubborn. A soft well-reduced meal and a gut full of swollen fibrous residue are not the same mechanical problem. One moves as digestible slurry. The other can move as retained bulk, thickened gel, coarse fragments, or some unstable mix of all three. That difference matters because a bowel already prone to pressure, cramping, incomplete evacuation, reflux, or bloating often does poorly when the meal keeps increasing physical workload without increasing nutritional return to the same degree. The stool may become larger. That does not prove the meal nourished well. It may simply prove that more undigested plant structure survived the trip.

Fermentation adds a second layer of pressure after the physical one. Once fiber and resistant carbohydrates pass into the colon, bacteria begin breaking down what human enzymes did not finish. That bacterial digestion produces gases and short-chain fatty acids, which are small fats made by microbial metabolism. In a bowel with good tolerance and modest substrate load, that may remain manageable. In a bowel already under strain, fermentation turns retained plant matter into expansion. Gas increases luminal pressure. Water shifts continue. The wall stretches. Transit may accelerate or stall depending on motility pattern and microbial composition. The person feels bloating, distension, cramping, urgency, heaviness, or constipation, not because the bowel is reacting mysteriously, but because water holding and swelling upstream became fermentation and pressure downstream. The same plant structure that looked wholesome on the plate can become retained bulk first and bacterial substrate second.

This is why water holding, swelling, friction, and fermentation have to be judged together. They are not separate virtues sprinkled across the digestive tract. They are linked stages of a physical burden. Plant residue holds water. Water expands volume. Volume increases pressure and slows or distorts movement. Retained material reaches the colon and becomes microbial fuel. Microbial breakdown produces gas and further distension. If the nutritional yield from that plant matter is modest while the mechanical and fermentative workload is high, the food is doing more to occupy the bowel than to nourish the body. The language of bulk makes that sound virtuous. The intestine still has to live inside the mechanics.

Why "Adds Bulk" Is Not Automatically Beneficial

Bulk is a physical description, not a nutritional verdict. It tells you that more material is occupying space in the bowel. It does not tell you whether that material was well digested, whether nutrients were efficiently liberated, whether minerals stayed available, whether the meal cleared smoothly, or whether the intestine had to tolerate excess pressure, retained water, and fermentation to get there. A larger stool can come from better hydration and better motility in one setting. It can also come from the far less flattering fact that more plant structure survived digestion and left the body as residue. The public language around fiber often treats bulk as if it were proof of digestive success. That reverses the order of the physiology. The first question is what the body extracted. Only then can stool volume mean anything.

A food that adds bulk may be doing so because its cell walls resisted breakdown, its fibers held water, its coarse fragments stayed intact, and its nutrients remained partly enclosed while the bowel pushed the residue onward. That is not automatically a gain. It may mean the intestine handled a larger physical load while recovering less nourishment from it. Insoluble plant residue can enlarge stool simply by remaining present. Soluble fractions can swell, trap water, thicken the intestinal contents, and increase volume before much of that material ever reaches the colon. The bowel then has to mix, propel, and clear a larger mass. In some people that produces what gets called regularity. In others it produces pressure, heaviness, incomplete evacuation, reflux, or the peculiar combination of abdominal fullness and poor nutritional return. The stool may be impressive. The meal may still have underperformed.

Bulk can also hide the fact that the intestine is solving the wrong problem. The goal of digestion is not to produce the largest output. The goal is to reduce food into absorbable material, move that material into the body, and carry away what remains with as little friction as possible. If a meal increases stool volume mainly because it leaves behind swollen fiber, resistant plant particles, trapped water, and bacterial byproducts, then the bowel is managing residue, not displaying success. Fermentation makes this harder to see because it can create the appearance of activity. The person feels movement, hears gas, sees output, and assumes the system is working. But microbial fermentation often means the small intestine failed to clear the meal cleanly upstream. The colon inherited excess substrate, bacteria consumed it, gas and short-chain fatty acids were produced, and the stool changed shape and volume afterward. The bowel moved more. That does not mean the body gained more.

There is also a cost to carrying bulk that health language tends to ignore. More bulk means more distension. More distension means more stretch on the bowel wall. More retained water and more fiber swelling mean more luminal pressure, meaning more pressure inside the hollow interior of the gut. In a calm robust intestine, some of that may remain tolerable. In a bowel prone to bloating, visceral hypersensitivity, slowed transit, rapid transit, or pelvic outlet dysfunction, it can become part of the problem itself. The colon has to push harder. The contents may stall in one segment and rush through another. The person can alternate between constipation and urgency while still being told the fiber is helping because it adds bulk. The bowel is not grading the meal by public doctrine. It is reacting to the mechanics in real time.

That is why bulk has to be demoted from virtue to observation. It may be useful in some settings, but it proves very little by itself. A larger stool does not tell you whether the food nourished well, whether the gut absorbed efficiently, or whether the intestine had to endure unnecessary structural load to get there. It may reflect improved bowel movement in one person. It may reflect failed extraction and increased residue in another. The body is not fed by volume leaving the colon. It is fed by what left the lumen and entered tissue. If a food adds bulk while lowering digestibility, trapping nutrients, increasing pressure, and feeding fermentation, then the bowel is carrying more material precisely because the meal delivered less of itself to the body.

When Bulk Becomes Irritation, Slowed Digestion, Nutrient Trapping, or Symptom Generation

Bulk stops being useful when the intestine is no longer dealing with a light structural assist and is instead forced to manage excess physical residue that slows clearance, holds water, traps nutrients, and increases pressure against the bowel wall. That shift happens more easily than people think because bulk is not a neutral passenger. It changes the mechanics of the meal from the moment fibrous plant matter begins swelling in fluid or preserving coarse fragments against breakdown. A thickened stomach contents delays emptying. A swollen intestinal mass slows mixing and diffusion, which means it slows the movement of enzymes toward food particles and the movement of liberated nutrients back toward the absorptive surface. Coarse residue keeps starch, protein, fat, and minerals partly enclosed inside plant structure longer than the nutrition label suggests. The meal now has more volume but less access. The bowel has more to push, and the body may have less to absorb. That is the point where bulk stops looking like digestive help and starts behaving like digestive drag.

Irritation begins when that drag turns into repeated mechanical and chemical stress at the mucosa, the living lining of the intestine. Coarse insoluble fragments can increase contact friction simply by moving as stubborn residue rather than as well-reduced digestible material. Soluble fibers can create a different kind of irritation by holding water, swelling into viscous gel, and prolonging the time that acids, fermentable carbohydrates, polyphenols, lectins, or other reactive plant compounds remain pressed into the same intestinal contents. The mucosa does not experience fiber in isolation. It experiences fiber carrying the rest of the meal with it. If the food is also releasing oxalate, phytate, tannins, poorly absorbed sugars, or enzyme inhibitors, then the swollen plant mass becomes a delivery system for prolonged contact with the same burden. The bowel wall has to keep moving that mixture, sensing its pressure, and tolerating its chemistry. At that point the problem is not that the gut failed to appreciate bulk. The problem is that the bulk turned the meal into a longer, rougher, less efficient exposure.

Slowed digestion follows naturally from the same mechanics. A stomach full of water-holding fiber empties differently than a stomach full of food that has been reduced cleanly into smaller particles. The pylorus, the muscular valve at the bottom of the stomach, meters out contents based partly on particle size and consistency. A bulky fibrous mass can remain longer, especially if soluble fractions have thickened the contents and insoluble fractions have kept large particles structurally intact. Farther down, the small intestine must work through a slower, denser mixture in which enzymes, bile salts, and nutrients are all moving less freely. Bile salts are the detergent-like molecules in bile that help emulsify fat and carry fat-soluble compounds through intestinal fluid. If the meal becomes too thick, too coarse, or too structurally resistant, digestive chemistry loses efficiency. The person experiences fullness that lasts too long, heaviness after meals, reflux from delayed gastric emptying, or the sense that food is sitting rather than moving. This is often described casually as poor digestion, but the physical sequence is specific. The bowel has been given too much structure to dismantle and too much swollen residue to clear smoothly.

Nutrient trapping is one of the most important hidden losses inside this process. When bulk increases because plant cell walls remain partly intact or because fibrous networks hold food particles inside a larger matrix, the nutrient is still in the bowel but no longer easily reachable. Minerals remain caught near oxalate or phytate. Proteins remain partly enclosed in plant particles that digestive enzymes have not penetrated well. Carotenoids and other fat-soluble compounds remain trapped in plant tissue and fail to enter micelles, the tiny bile-based transport particles that move fats and fat-soluble compounds through the watery contents of the small intestine. The food can look dense on paper and still deliver thinly because the intestine was asked to move bulk instead of extract value. The stool may increase. The nutritional return may not.

Symptom generation is what happens when these physical losses become sensory and mechanical problems the person can no longer ignore. Bulk holds water, volume rises, fermentation follows, gas accumulates, and the lumen, the hollow interior of the bowel, expands. Distension stretches the bowel wall. Stretch changes motility. Some people get urgency and loose stool because osmotic particles and water speed transit. Others get constipation because swollen residue, slowed movement, methane production, or poor muscular coordination leads to stalling and incomplete evacuation. Many get both at different times because the bowel alternates between holding and forcing. Bloating, cramping, visible distension, trapped gas, nausea, post-meal fatigue, reflux, and food aversion all grow out of this same sequence. Bulk becomes a symptom generator when the intestine is carrying more residue than it can process into a low-friction outcome. The claim that a food helps because it adds bulk ignores the more important question. What did that bulk force the gut to do, and what did the body actually get back for the effort.

Why Bowel Movement Rhetoric Often Ignores Digestion Quality

Most bowel movement rhetoric starts at the end of the process and mistakes output for success. A person eats a food, stool volume rises, transit changes, and the conclusion is drawn that the gut is working better. That skips the central question. What did digestion actually accomplish before that material reached the colon. A larger or more frequent bowel movement can reflect many different realities. It can reflect better hydration and smoother motility in one context. It can also reflect poor breakdown of plant structure, incomplete absorption of the meal, excess water being held in the lumen, the hollow interior of the bowel, and more undigested residue being pushed outward simply because the intestine could not extract much from it. The colon is receiving the leftovers. When rhetoric treats the size, softness, or frequency of stool as proof that the meal was beneficial, it often confuses disposal with nourishment. The bowel may be moving more material precisely because the body got less from it.

This confusion becomes worse with fiber because fiber is praised for what it does to stool without enough attention to what it may have done to the meal upstream. A bulky bowel movement may mean plant cell walls stayed partly intact, soluble fractions held water, insoluble fractions preserved coarse residue, and the small intestine moved a larger mass downstream while recovering less mineral, less amino acid, less fat-soluble material, or less usable energy than the label implied. A meal can look excellent by bathroom rhetoric and poor by digestive accounting. The stool is bigger. The mineral stayed bound to oxalate or phytate. The protein was only partly cleaved because protease inhibitors or structural resistance reduced enzyme access. The carbohydrate load fermented because too much escaped small-intestinal absorption. The colon then inherits a volume problem and bacteria finish the work the upper gut did not. The person may feel active, regular, even lighter afterward. That does not prove the digestive sequence was efficient. It may prove the opposite.

Good digestion is not defined by how much matter leaves the body. It is defined by how much useful material entered the body with minimal friction and how little residue, gas, pressure, and chemical burden the intestine had to manage on the way out. A well-moving bowel can be part of that. It is not the whole standard. Once bowel movement rhetoric is separated from digestive quality, the evaluation becomes stricter and more honest. Did the meal break down cleanly. Did nutrients remain available. Did the absorptive surface gain access to them. Did the gut avoid excess water retention, fermentation, cramping, reflux, or distension. Did the colon receive a modest remainder or a large undigested workload. The bathroom can tell you something. It cannot tell you everything. A bigger output may reflect smooth clearance. It may also reflect a meal the body never handled well in the first place.

Chapter 6

FODMAPs and the Fermentation Burden

FODMAP is a compression term for a group of small carbohydrates that share one important trait. They are either poorly absorbed in the small intestine, rapidly fermentable once they reach the colon, or both. The acronym stands for fermentable oligosaccharides, disaccharides, monosaccharides, and polyols. Fermentable means gut microbes can break them down and turn them into gas and short-chain fatty acids. Oligosaccharides are short chains of sugars, especially fructans and galacto-oligosaccharides, which are found in foods such as onions, garlic, wheat, and many legumes. Human digestive enzymes do not split these chains efficiently, so they pass through the small intestine largely intact. Disaccharides are two-sugar units, with lactose being the main example in this category when lactase activity is low. Lactase is the enzyme at the brush border, the enzyme-rich surface of the small intestine, that splits lactose into glucose and galactose for absorption. Monosaccharides are single sugars, but in the FODMAP framework the issue is mainly excess fructose, meaning fructose present in greater amount than the accompanying glucose and therefore more likely to exceed absorptive capacity. Polyols are sugar alcohols such as sorbitol and mannitol, which are absorbed slowly and incompletely. The important point is that these compounds are small, osmotically active, and poorly handled by many intestines even though they often arrive inside foods with a clean nutritional reputation.

What makes FODMAPs distinctive is not simply that they are carbohydrates. It is that they can escape the normal upstream digestive sequence. Starch, when well cooked and well handled, is usually reduced by amylase into smaller sugars that can be absorbed in the small intestine. FODMAP carbohydrates often avoid that clean sequence. Fructans and galacto-oligosaccharides resist human enzyme breakdown. Lactose remains intact when lactase is insufficient. Excess fructose may overwhelm transport capacity at the intestinal surface. Polyols move slowly across the intestinal wall and often remain in the lumen, the hollow interior of the intestine where digestion and absorption are taking place. Once these particles remain in the lumen, they begin behaving less like nutrition and more like fluid-retaining residue. Water moves toward them by osmosis, meaning water shifts toward the area with more dissolved particles. The intestinal contents become wetter, bulkier, and more distending before the colon has even entered the story. That is why FODMAP symptoms can begin before fermentation. The bowel is already carrying too much dissolved material that it could not clear cleanly.

The fermentation burden begins when that unfinished carbohydrate load reaches the colon. Bacteria now inherit what the small intestine failed to absorb. Microbes rapidly ferment these sugars and produce gases such as hydrogen, methane, and carbon dioxide along with short-chain fatty acids. The result is not abstract gut imbalance. It is volume, pressure, and stretch inside a tube. Gas expands the bowel wall. Water remains in the stool. Motility changes as the intestine tries to manage distension. In one person that means loose stool and urgency. In another it means slowed transit and constipation, especially when methane production is high enough to slow bowel movement. In many people it means some unstable combination of both. The same apple, onion, bean, or polyol-rich fruit that looked simple on the plate has now become osmotic load in the small intestine and bacterial substrate in the colon. The food may still contain vitamins, minerals, and plant compounds that nutrition language likes to praise. The gut is living inside a different reality. It is carrying retained water first and retained gas second.

This is why the FODMAP category matters so much in a book about plant burden. It shows that a food does not need a classical toxin to destabilize digestion. It only needs to leave enough poorly absorbed carbohydrate behind that the bowel is forced into fluid retention, fermentation, distension, and altered transit. The problem is mechanical and chemical at the same time. Small sugars and sugar alcohols hold water. Bacteria turn residue into gas. The mucosa, the living intestinal lining, and the muscular wall of the bowel then have to tolerate the pressure. That is not random sensitivity. It is a predictable consequence of where those carbohydrates are digested, or fail to be digested, and who ends up processing the remainder. In a resilient intestine, modest amounts may be tolerated. In a bowel already prone to bloating, pain, visceral hypersensitivity, or irregular transit, the same compounds stop behaving like harmless carbohydrate and start behaving like a daily fermentation problem.

Why Some Carbohydrates Remain Poorly Absorbed

Poor absorption is not an abstract food sensitivity. It usually begins with mismatch between the carbohydrate's structure and the machinery available to handle it. Some carbohydrates arrive as chains the human small intestine does not have the enzymes to split. Fructans in onions, garlic, wheat, and many other plants are one example. Galacto-oligosaccharides in legumes are another. These are short sugar chains, but human digestive enzymes still do not dismantle them efficiently. They pass through the upper intestine with much of their structure intact because the body lacks the specific tools to cleave them into absorbable units. That means the failure is built into the chemistry from the start. The bowel is not underperforming. It is encountering a carbohydrate it was never well equipped to finish.

Other carbohydrates are poorly absorbed not because the body lacks all the machinery, but because the machinery is limited, saturable, or easily overwhelmed. Fructose is the clearest example. Fructose uses a transporter called GLUT5, a membrane protein on the intestinal surface that moves fructose from the gut into the intestinal cell. That system has limits. When fructose arrives in modest amount and alongside glucose, absorption usually improves because glucose can help recruit additional transport through GLUT2, another sugar transporter that can appear at the intestinal surface under the right conditions. When fructose arrives in excess, especially without enough accompanying glucose, the transporter system can fall behind. The fructose then remains in the lumen, the hollow interior of the small intestine where digestion and absorption are taking place, instead of crossing cleanly into the body. The sugar is still there. The intestine simply cannot clear it fast enough.

Lactose makes the point through a different failure. Lactose is a disaccharide, a two-sugar unit made of glucose and galactose. It cannot be absorbed intact. It first has to be split by lactase, the enzyme anchored at the brush border, the enzyme-rich surface of the small intestine. When lactase activity is low, lactose remains whole. A whole disaccharide is too large and chemically wrong for direct uptake, so it stays in the intestinal contents, holds water there by osmotic force, and moves forward as unfinished carbohydrate. Polyols such as sorbitol and mannitol are different again. They do not require cleavage the way lactose does, but they cross the intestinal wall slowly and incompletely because their transport is inefficient and much of their movement depends on slow passive diffusion. Passive diffusion means molecules drift across a membrane without an active transport system pulling them through. That is a weak route for clearing a meal. When the dose rises, the intestine is quickly left with more polyol than it can move.

Dose, speed, and intestinal condition matter just as much as the molecule itself. A small amount of a poorly absorbed carbohydrate may remain tolerable because the bowel can dilute it, move it, and clear enough of it before pressure builds. A larger dose changes the whole mechanical problem. More dissolved particles remain in the lumen. More water follows. More material reaches the colon. Rapid eating, liquid delivery, juicing, blending, or a meal that empties quickly from the stomach can make that worse because the small intestine receives a larger carbohydrate load in less time. A damaged or inflamed intestinal surface can lower absorption further because the brush border enzymes and transport systems are part of the lining itself. If that lining is compromised, the bowel loses some of the very machinery it needs to finish digestion. The carbohydrate did not become toxic in a mystical sense. It arrived in more quantity, faster, or in a bowel with less reserve.

That is why some carbohydrates remain poorly absorbed. They are either built in a form human digestion does not split well, dependent on enzymes or transporters that may be weak or limited, or delivered in a dose that exceeds what the intestinal surface can clear before fluid and fermentation begin. Once that happens, the small intestine stops being a place of efficient transfer and becomes a holding space for dissolved residue. Water moves in. Volume rises. The colon inherits what the upper gut left behind. The symptom is felt later, but the first failure was simple. The carbohydrate stayed in the tube because the intestine could not convert it, transport it, or clear it fast enough.

Osmotic Pull, Bacterial Fermentation, Gas, Distension, and Altered Transit

Once a poorly absorbed carbohydrate remains in the lumen, the hollow interior of the intestine where digestion and absorption are still supposed to be clearing the meal, the chemistry shifts from nourishment to load. The first shift is osmotic. Small dissolved carbohydrates that have not crossed the intestinal wall keep water with them. Osmosis means water moves toward the area with more dissolved particles. In practical terms, the bowel starts retaining fluid around sugars and sugar alcohols it failed to absorb. The intestinal contents become wetter, heavier, and larger in volume. That larger volume stretches the intestinal wall sooner, increases the amount of material the gut has to move, and can speed transit before the body has had a fair chance to recover much value from the meal. The food may still be carrying vitamins, minerals, or plant compounds that looked favorable on paper. The intestine is already dealing with excess dissolved residue and excess water. The first symptom can begin here, before bacteria have even done much with the leftovers, because the tube is now under fluid pressure it was not meant to carry.

Bacterial fermentation begins when that unfinished carbohydrate escapes the small intestine and enters the colon. Now the problem changes hands. The human digestive system did not clear the substrate, so the microbiota take over. Colonic bacteria rapidly metabolize these residual sugars and produce gases such as hydrogen, methane, and carbon dioxide, along with short-chain fatty acids, which are small fats generated during bacterial carbohydrate metabolism. That process is often described in flattering terms because short-chain fatty acids can play useful roles in the colon. The bowel experiences the sequence less politely. Gas accumulates inside a limited space. The wall stretches. The lumen expands. Pressure rises segment by segment. If fermentation is brisk and the bowel is already carrying retained water from the upstream osmotic problem, the person now has a colon full of wet residue and newly generated gas at the same time. That is not a minor digestive quirk. It is a mechanical burden imposed by carbohydrate that failed to leave the intestinal tube when it should have.

Gas and distension matter because the bowel wall is not indifferent to stretch. It is supplied with sensory nerves that register tension, pressure, and movement. Distension is simply the expansion of the bowel by retained fluid, residue, or gas, but the body experiences it as fullness, tightness, bloating, cramping, visible abdominal enlargement, and sometimes pain that seems out of proportion to the meal itself. In people with visceral hypersensitivity, meaning a gut nervous system that reacts strongly to ordinary or modest stretch, the same amount of gas can produce far more discomfort than it would in a calmer bowel. That is why one person can tolerate onions, apples, beans, or polyol-rich fruit with little complaint while another gets marked bloating from a modest serving. The chemistry may be the same. The sensory response to distension is not. But the mechanism is still physical. Retained carbohydrate became retained water, then bacterial substrate, then gas, then stretch. The symptom follows the sequence.

Transit changes because the gut has only a few ways to respond to this kind of pressure. Sometimes it pushes faster. More water stays in the bowel, the contents move quickly, stool loosens, and urgency appears because the intestine is trying to clear an unstable load before more pressure builds. Sometimes it slows. Methane production is one reason this can happen, because methane-producing microbial patterns are associated with slower bowel movement and longer transit time. The colon holds the material longer, more gas accumulates behind partial stalling, and the person feels constipated, full, and blocked rather than urgent. Many people alternate between the two because different meals, different microbial activity, and different segments of bowel movement produce different pressures on different days. This is why altered transit is not random. The bowel is adapting to osmotic residue and fermentation pressure with the only tools it has, speed up, hold, squeeze harder, or segment the load. None of those responses means the meal was handled well. They mean the gut was forced to compensate for carbohydrate it could not absorb cleanly in the first place.

Common High-Burden Examples

The foods that create the clearest FODMAP burden are not obscure. They are ordinary staples that keep a clean public reputation while repeatedly overwhelming small-intestinal handling. Onions and garlic are among the strongest examples because they are rich in fructans, short chains of fructose molecules that human digestive enzymes do not split efficiently. The problem begins early. These carbohydrates are released from the plant tissue during chewing and digestion, but they are not cleared well at the brush border, the enzyme-rich surface of the small intestine where final carbohydrate breakdown and absorption are supposed to occur. They remain in the lumen, the hollow interior of the intestine, where they hold water by osmotic force and then pass into the colon for rapid bacterial fermentation. This is why even small amounts of onion and garlic can create disproportionate symptoms in sensitive people. The burden does not depend on a huge serving. It depends on how aggressively the bowel reacts to retained carbohydrate and the gas produced from it. A meal can taste richer because of onion and garlic while the gut is left carrying more fluid and pressure than the flavor was worth.

Apples and pears create a different but equally common problem because they often combine excess fructose with sorbitol, a sugar alcohol that crosses the intestinal wall slowly and incompletely. Fructose absorption depends on limited transport capacity, and sorbitol adds its own osmotic load while also worsening the traffic problem by remaining in the bowel longer. That makes these fruits especially effective at turning a simple snack into retained fluid, fermentation substrate, and abdominal distension. Watermelon and mango often look safer because they are juicy, sweet, and culturally protected as light wholesome foods, but sweetness does not guarantee clean absorption. Watermelon can deliver a significant fructose burden relative to what the intestine can clear comfortably in susceptible people, especially when eaten in large amounts. Mango can do the same. These fruits are often consumed quickly, in larger portions, and with little mechanical resistance, which means the small intestine may receive a rapid sugar load without the pace-control that denser foods sometimes impose. The pleasant texture makes the exposure easier to welcome. The intestine still has to absorb it.

Stone fruits such as peaches, plums, cherries, apricots, and nectarines are common high-burden foods for the same reason many people find them strangely unreliable. They can combine fructose with sorbitol or related polyols, which means they bring both poor absorption and strong fermentation potential in the same tissue. The problem is not that these fruits are poisonous in the acute sense. The problem is that they leave too much unfinished carbohydrate in the bowel. Water follows those dissolved particles into the intestinal contents. Bacteria later inherit the residue and turn it into gas. The person experiences bloating, cramping, visible distension, loose stool, or a swing toward constipation if the fermentation pattern slows transit. The fruit keeps its reputation because its sugars are natural and its color is attractive. The bowel is dealing with osmotic residue, gas expansion, and altered motility.

Legumes are one of the most important examples because they add a second kind of burden on top of fermentation. Beans, lentils, and many related legumes contain galacto-oligosaccharides, usually shortened to GOS, short sugar chains that human digestion does not break apart efficiently. Those carbohydrates move into the colon and ferment rapidly, which explains the familiar gas and bloating pattern. But legumes are rarely just a FODMAP issue. They also bring phytate, which can bind minerals, and they often bring protease inhibitors, which can interfere with protein digestion. That means the same food can create pressure in the bowel while also reducing the nutritional return from the meal. A bean can look high in protein, iron, magnesium, and fiber on paper while the intestine is simultaneously fermenting its carbohydrate residue, struggling with its protein yield, and absorbing less mineral than the chart suggested. The symptom pattern makes people think only about gas. The deeper problem is that the legume can burden both digestion and absorption at the same time.

These foods matter because they show how a common produce item or staple plant can become a daily fermentation problem without ever being labeled dangerous. Onions and garlic load the bowel with fructans. Apples, pears, watermelon, mango, and stone fruits can overload fructose handling, often with polyols riding beside it. Legumes push fermentable oligosaccharides into the colon while attaching mineral and protein penalties to the same meal. The food does not need a classical toxin to create real burden. It only needs to leave enough unfinished carbohydrate behind that the intestine becomes a site of retained water, bacterial gas, stretch, and unstable transit.

Why a Food Can Be Natural and Still Mechanically Destabilizing in the Bowel

Natural only tells you where the food came from. It tells you nothing about what the bowel has to do with it once it arrives. The intestine does not judge a food by whether it grew on a tree, came out of the ground, or kept a wholesome reputation on the plate. It judges by load, pressure, water movement, fermentability, particle structure, and how much of the meal can be cleared before the lumen, the hollow interior of the bowel, starts holding more residue than the gut can manage comfortably. A natural fruit can still deliver more fructose than the small intestine can absorb cleanly. A natural vegetable can still release fructans the human digestive tract does not split. A natural legume can still send galacto-oligosaccharides into the colon, hold water in the bowel first, and then become gas. The word natural does not alter transport capacity, reduce osmotic pull, or stop bacterial fermentation. It is a cultural reassurance placed on top of a mechanical problem.

Mechanical destabilization begins when the meal leaves behind material that changes the physical state of the intestinal contents. Poorly absorbed carbohydrates keep water in the bowel by osmosis, which means dissolved particles pull water toward themselves and prevent the lumen from clearing cleanly. Soluble plant fractions swell and thicken the meal. Insoluble fragments preserve bulk and structure. Fermentable residues reach the colon and become substrate for microbes, which convert them into gas and short-chain fatty acids. Gas expands the bowel wall. Water increases volume. Pressure changes motility. Some segments squeeze harder. Some stall. Some empty too fast. The person experiences bloating, visible distension, cramping, urgency, constipation, or the unstable alternation between them. None of that requires an artificial food, a contaminant, or a synthetic additive. It requires only a bowel receiving more fermentable, water-holding, pressure-generating material than it can turn into a low-friction result.

This is why the natural argument so often fails in practice. It confuses origin with handling. An apple is natural. If its fructose and sorbitol load exceed what the small intestine can transport, the colon still inherits the remainder. Onion and garlic are natural. Their fructans still pass through the upper gut largely undigested and become rapid fermentation fuel later. Beans are natural. Their galacto-oligosaccharides still produce gas, their fiber still contributes bulk, and their structure still makes the intestine work through a denser residue than the label implies. The bowel wall does not relax because the exposure came from a garden instead of a factory. It stretches when volume rises. It spasms when pressure and irritation rise. It changes transit when water and gas alter the load. Natural does not prevent a food from becoming physically disruptive inside a tube.

The deeper mistake is that people hear natural and assume biologically cooperative. But cooperation depends on whether the food clears the upper gut cleanly, whether it stays low enough in osmotic residue that water does not flood the lumen, whether it reaches the colon as a modest remainder rather than a large fermentable burden, and whether the bowel wall can tolerate the pressure that follows. A food can be natural and still ask the gut to carry too much water, too much gas, too much swollen residue, or too much retained carbohydrate. When that happens, the bowel loses mechanical stability. The food keeps the innocence. The intestine still has to survive the physics.

Sensitive Gut Versus Resilient Gut as Different Physiological Contexts

The same food is not the same digestive problem in every body because the bowel receiving it is part of the event. A resilient gut can clear a moderate carbohydrate load, mix secretions well, move contents at a steady pace, absorb enough before pressure builds, and tolerate the gas and fluid that do remain without turning the meal into a symptom pattern. A sensitive gut has less margin. The threshold for pressure, stretch, chemical contact, and altered motility is lower, so the same onion, apple, bean, pear, or mango that remains tolerable in one person can become retained water, fermentation, distension, and pain in another. This is not because the food changed moral category between bodies. It is because the bowel wall, the nerve signaling, the absorptive capacity, and the movement pattern changed the consequences of the exposure.

A resilient gut usually has several advantages working at once. Gastric emptying is paced well enough that the small intestine does not get flooded with poorly absorbed carbohydrate faster than it can handle. Brush border enzymes and transporters at the intestinal surface are functioning with enough reserve that sugars clear more effectively before they accumulate in the lumen, the hollow interior of the bowel. Motility is coordinated enough that contents move forward without stalling in one segment and rushing through another. The bowel wall also tolerates stretch better. Gas and fluid can build to a modest degree without the nervous system turning that stretch into bloating, cramping, or pain. In practical terms, resilience means the intestine can absorb more, dilute more, move more, and feel less from the same meal.

A sensitive gut loses ground in one or more of those same places. The issue may begin with weaker carbohydrate handling, where fructose, polyols, or oligosaccharides remain in the bowel longer because transport and clearance fall behind. It may begin with visceral hypersensitivity, meaning the bowel nerves register ordinary distension as discomfort or pain. It may begin with unstable motility, where the intestine alternates between holding contents too long and pushing them too quickly. It may begin with a mucosa, the living intestinal lining, that is already irritated and therefore less tolerant of repeated chemical and mechanical contact. Once that lower reserve is in place, the same FODMAP load becomes a different physiological sequence. More water stays in the lumen. More residue reaches the colon. More gas expands the bowel wall. The person feels the mechanics sooner and more intensely because the bowel cannot buffer the load quietly.

Microbial pattern matters too, but it matters through pressure and transit rather than through vague language about imbalance. If the colon ferments residue rapidly, gas production rises early and pressure builds faster. If methane-producing microbes are prominent, transit may slow, which can turn fermentation into stalling, fullness, and constipation rather than urgency. A resilient gut may still ferment the same food, but the combination of motility, absorption, and sensory tolerance prevents that fermentation from becoming a major symptom event. A sensitive gut can take the same residue and turn it into visible distension, griping pain, reflux, irregular stool, and food fear. The microbiota are part of the context, but they are acting inside a host bowel that either manages pressure well or does not.

This distinction matters because it changes how foods should be judged. A resilient gut can make a burden look small by compensating well. A sensitive gut exposes the burden faster because it has less room to absorb the mistake. That does not mean every symptomatic person is fragile in some abstract sense. It means the meal exceeded the handling capacity of that intestine. The clean question is not whether the food is healthy in theory. The question is what that specific bowel had to do when it received that specific plant load. If the answer is retained water, retained gas, altered transit, and repeated distress, then the food is no longer functioning as harmless carbohydrate in that host. It has become a daily fermentation problem wearing a wholesome reputation.

Chapter 7

Lectins and the Problem of Chemical Contact

Lectins are carbohydrate-binding proteins. That means they are proteins built to recognize and attach to specific sugar structures on the surface of cells, mucus, microbes, or other biological material. In plant tissue, that binding ability is not a decorative feature. It is part of defense. A plant cannot flee an insect, vomit out a predator, or close a wound with circulating immune cells the way an animal can. It has to manage contact where the contact happens. Lectins help do that by making the act of eating more complicated for the organism doing the eating. Some lectins bind to the gut lining of insects and animals. Some interfere with digestion indirectly by resisting breakdown long enough to remain chemically active in the intestine. Some help protect seeds and storage tissues from being turned quickly into someone else's nutrition. The important point is that lectins are not nutrients the plant accidentally stored in a useful food. They are part of the plant's contact chemistry. They are there because being eaten is a problem the plant has to solve.

The tissue that carries lectins tells you a great deal about why the plant uses them. Seeds, beans, and legumes are the major examples because these are storage organs with concentrated value packed into a compact biological structure. Protein, starch, minerals, and phosphorus are all sitting in one place waiting for the next growth cycle. The plant has every reason to defend that package. A lectin in a seed does not need to kill a predator outright. It only needs to make digestion less favorable, less efficient, or more irritating. That is often enough. The same logic applies to other defense compounds concentrated in seeds, such as protease inhibitors and phytate. The plant is protecting stored value by attaching costs to the act of extraction. Human nutrition language often strips that logic away and talks about beans as fiber and plant protein. The seed's chemistry is telling a different story. It is a guarded storage structure trying not to be digested easily.

Lectins matter because they operate through contact. Once the plant tissue is chewed, soaked, or partly digested, the lectin does not have to be absorbed into the bloodstream to create trouble. It can act at the gut surface if enough of its structure survives preparation and digestion. The gut lining is coated in glycoproteins, which are proteins with carbohydrate groups attached to them. Mucus is full of them. The brush border, the enzyme-rich surface of the small intestine that finishes digestion and mediates absorption, is full of them. Lectins are built to recognize carbohydrate structures, so this is precisely the kind of biological terrain where they become relevant. The plant uses that binding chemistry because the eater's intestine is not an empty tube. It is a sugar-decorated living surface. Once lectins reach that surface in an active enough state, the meal stops being only a question of nutrient content and becomes a question of how much chemical contact the intestine has to tolerate.

That is why lectins belong in a category different from simple antinutrients. An antinutrient such as phytate mainly reduces nutrient availability by binding minerals in the lumen, the hollow interior of the gut where digestion is taking place. A lectin can do more than reduce access. It can alter the quality of the contact between food and mucosa. That does not mean every lectin exposure becomes a dramatic poisoning event. Most do not. But it does mean the plant is using a protein whose job is to recognize and attach, and that kind of chemistry becomes more biologically serious the moment it reaches a living epithelial surface. Epithelium means the layer of cells lining the intestine. The plant is not just protecting itself with bitterness or hardness. It is using a molecule that can participate directly in the act of contact.

This is the deeper reason plants use lectins. They are a defense against being turned easily into animal tissue. They make the gut work harder, tolerate more, and in some cases react more violently. The seed keeps its stored nutrition under chemical guard. The eater has to overcome that guard with soaking, heating, fermentation, pressure, time, and digestive capacity. If that reduction is incomplete, the plant's defense strategy enters the bowel with the meal. The person may call it a healthy food. The intestine is dealing with a binding protein that was put there because the plant did not want its stored tissue surrendered cheaply.

Binding to Gut Surfaces and Why That Matters

The danger in a lectin is not simply that it exists in the food. The danger is that it is built to attach. Once a lectin survives preparation and enough of digestion to remain structurally active, it enters an intestine lined with carbohydrate-bearing surfaces. The mucus layer contains glycoproteins, which are proteins coated with sugar groups. The brush border, the dense enzyme-rich surface on the small intestine's absorptive cells, contains glycoproteins as well. The outer membrane of the enterocyte, the absorptive intestinal cell, is not smooth inert plastic. It is a chemically decorated living surface. Lectins recognize sugar patterns on that surface and bind to them. That matters because digestion depends on smooth contact between food particles, digestive enzymes, mucus, and the absorptive membrane. Once a binding protein begins attaching itself to that interface, the food is no longer simply moving past the intestinal wall. It is making directed chemical contact with it.

That contact matters first because the brush border is where much of the intestine's last-stage work is done. Enzymes anchored there finish carbohydrate and peptide digestion. Transporters embedded there move glucose, amino acids, minerals, and other small compounds into the cell. The surface area there is enormous because the intestine increases its absorptive reach through villi, which are finger-like projections, and microvilli, which are tiny projections on the absorptive cells themselves. Lectin binding introduces friction at precisely the surface where digestion is being completed and transport is supposed to be efficient. A nutrient already has to survive liberation from plant structure, avoid binding to inhibitors in the lumen, stay soluble, and reach the membrane. If the membrane itself is now being engaged by a plant defense protein, the intestine has inherited another layer of difficulty.

The problem is no longer just what was inside the meal. The problem is what the meal is doing to the surface that has to absorb it.

Binding also matters because the intestine is not only an absorptive organ. It is a barrier organ. Its lining has to decide what crosses, what stays out, what gets sampled by immune tissue, and what gets pushed onward. That requires intact mucus, coordinated cell turnover, controlled permeability, and stable local signaling. Permeability means how easily substances can cross the intestinal barrier. A lectin that attaches to epithelial surfaces, meaning the sheet of cells lining the intestine, can increase local stress even without being absorbed into blood in large amounts. The bowel may answer with altered secretion, changed motility, more mucus release, or local immune activity. The person may experience that as nausea, pressure, cramping, urgency, or the vague sense that a food feels aggressive rather than nourishing. The symptom often gets dismissed as sensitivity. The more precise description is that a binding protein made the intestinal surface part of the meal.

This is why lectins differ from a compound such as phytate. Phytate mainly acts in the intestinal contents by holding minerals in complexes that stay poorly available for absorption. Its damage is largely subtractive. Lectins can be subtractive too, but they also make the mucosa itself part of the chemical event. The contact is the mechanism. A bean or seed can therefore carry protein, starch, minerals, and calories while also delivering a molecule designed to interact directly with the surface that must process those nutrients. If preparation is thorough enough, much of that risk is reduced because heat can denature lectins, meaning it alters their three-dimensional structure enough that they lose much of their binding function. If preparation is weak, the intestine is left to finish a negotiation the kitchen should have handled first.

That is why binding to gut surfaces matters so much in a book about plant burden. It shows that the loss is not always happening only in the bowl of intestinal contents where minerals are being tied up or carbohydrates are being fermented. Sometimes the food reaches farther and engages the tissue itself. The intestine is built to extract value from a meal while preserving the boundary of the body. A lectin turns that boundary into a target. Once that happens, the cost of the food is no longer measured only by what failed to be absorbed. It is measured by how much chemical contact the absorptive surface had to endure while trying to do its job.

Kidney Beans as the Main Acute Case

Red kidney beans are the clearest ordinary-food example of lectin toxicity because they move the problem out of the slow chronic burden category and into an acute gastrointestinal poisoning pattern. The lectin is phytohaemagglutinin, usually shortened to PHA, a sugar-binding protein present at especially high levels in red kidney beans. FDA identifies raw or undercooked beans as the risk state and notes that properly cooked or canned kidney beans contain low enough levels that the toxin is not expected to affect the eater. The distinction matters because this is not a vague claim that beans are hard to digest. This is a specific protein toxin problem centered on one preparation failure.

Kidney beans make the main acute case because the dose needed to trigger illness is surprisingly small and the onset is fast. FDA's Bad Bug Book states that as few as four or five raw beans can trigger symptoms. The syndrome usually begins within one to three hours, most often with extreme nausea and vomiting, followed by diarrhea, and sometimes abdominal pain. FDA notes that vomiting may become severe. This is the opposite of the slow subtractive pattern seen with compounds such as phytate or moderate oxalate exposure. The body is not quietly losing mineral access over time. It is reacting violently to a plant defense protein that remained active when it should have been destroyed in preparation.

The mechanism is more aggressive than ordinary antinutrient language suggests. FDA describes lectins as proteins that bind carbohydrates and notes that some lectins, including PHA, can agglutinate mammalian red blood cells, alter cell-membrane transport systems, alter permeability to proteins, and interfere with cellular metabolism. The exact human toxicity pathway after eating undercooked kidney beans is not fully defined, and FDA says the mechanism is not known in complete detail, but oral lectin exposure is known to reduce intestinal absorption and produce diarrhea in animal species. That uncertainty is worth keeping because it sharpens the chapter rather than weakening it. The evidence is strong that the bean can cause abrupt illness. The precise sequence from intestinal contact to full symptom expression is not completely mapped in humans.

The practical lesson is simple and severe. Red kidney beans are not a food to undercook. FDA says soaking for at least five hours and then boiling in fresh water for at least thirty minutes removes and destroys the toxin. That instruction belongs in the biology of the food, not in a kitchen footnote, because it tells you what the seed is. It is concentrated storage tissue protected by a protein defense that has to be denatured before the meal becomes safe. Until that happens, the bean is not merely incomplete food. It is an active lectin exposure with a well-documented capacity to turn a common meal into acute upper and lower

Why Raw or Undercooked Beans Can Trigger Severe Gastrointestinal Symptoms

Raw or undercooked beans can trigger severe gastrointestinal symptoms because the bean's lectin remains active instead of being denatured by sufficient moist heat. In red kidney beans, the main lectin is phytohaemagglutinin, abbreviated PHA. Lectins are carbohydrate-binding proteins, and FDA identifies PHA in raw or undercooked beans as a natural toxin that can cause nausea, severe vomiting, and diarrhea when present at high levels. Proper soaking and then boiling in fresh water for at least 30 minutes reduces that risk by removing and destroying the toxin.

The reason the symptoms are so abrupt is that this is not mainly a fermentation problem or a slow antinutrient problem. It is a direct contact problem at the intestinal surface. PHA is built to bind carbohydrate-rich biological surfaces, and experimental work shows that phytohaemagglutinin can bind to brush border membranes and gut epithelium, disrupt mucosal organization, and impair gut function. That means the bean is not merely hard to digest when undercooked. It is carrying a protein that can make aggressive contact with the lining that is supposed to finish digestion and absorb nutrients. Animal and mechanistic studies support this mucosal-binding model, while FDA's food safety guidance establishes the human illness pattern clearly.

Once that lectin-rich bean enters the gut in an active form, the intestine reacts quickly. FDA's Bad Bug Book and related food safety guidance note that as few as four or five raw beans can trigger illness, with symptoms usually beginning within one to three hours. The early pattern is typically extreme nausea and vomiting, followed by diarrhea and sometimes abdominal pain. That timing matters because it shows the problem is happening before any long digestive sequence could explain it. The bean is hitting the gut as a toxin exposure, not simply as a heavy meal.

Undercooking is dangerous precisely because it leaves the bean in the worst middle state. The seed has softened enough to look edible, but the lectin has not been reliably destroyed. That is why slow or insufficient heating is a bad strategy for dried kidney beans. The person assumes the bean has become food. The chemistry is still defense chemistry. The stomach and small intestine then inherit a protein that was supposed to be neutralized in the pot, not at the mucosal surface.

The Difference Between Acute Lectin Poisoning and Lower-Grade Chronic Exposure

Acute lectin poisoning is a concentrated, short-window toxin event. The classic case is red kidney beans carrying active phytohaemagglutinin, abbreviated PHA, because the beans were eaten raw or undercooked. In that state the lectin remains active enough to produce a fast gastrointestinal illness pattern. EFSA identifies undercooked beans as a health concern when lectins remain in active form, and food safety authorities report that symptoms can begin within one to three hours, often with severe nausea and vomiting followed by diarrhea and abdominal pain. This is not a vague digestive complaint. It is an abrupt poisoning pattern driven by a high enough dose of active lectin making forceful contact with the small intestine.

Lower-grade chronic exposure is a different physiological situation. Here the food is not producing an obvious emergency. The person is not usually vomiting a few hours after a meal. The issue is repeated lower-level lectin contact that does not overwhelm the gut all at once but may keep adding friction at the intestinal surface. Mechanistic and animal literature show why that concern exists. Plant lectins can survive oral intake long enough to reach the small intestinal lumen, bind to the mucosal surface, and induce epithelial changes. Reviews of this work describe degeneration of the intestinal epithelium, altered glycoprotein turnover, villus injury, endogenous nitrogen loss, and impaired digestive enzyme activity in experimental models. That is a slower subtractive pattern, not an acute poisoning pattern.

The clean distinction is therefore one of dose, intensity, and visibility. Acute poisoning means enough active lectin survived preparation to trigger a sharp upper and lower gastrointestinal response in hours. Lower-grade chronic exposure means the lectin burden is lower, the contact is less explosive, and the cost is more likely to appear as repeated gut irritation, poorer digestive tolerance, incomplete extraction, or reduced absorptive efficiency rather than a dramatic toxic episode. The small intestine still matters in both cases. EFSA identifies the small intestine as the critical target organ in lectin risk assessment. The difference is that in acute poisoning the bowel reacts violently and immediately, while in lower-grade exposure the same surface may be asked to tolerate smaller repeated insults that are easier to overlook.

The most important caution is that the evidence is not equally strong in both categories. Acute kidney bean lectin poisoning in humans is well documented. The lower-grade chronic model is biologically plausible and supported by animal and mechanistic work, but it is less cleanly documented as a distinct long-term human syndrome from ordinary bean eating, especially when beans are properly processed. That is why the chapter should not overstate the case. Proper soaking and boiling move beans out of the acute poisoning category. The chronic question is narrower and more conditional. It concerns residual lectin activity, repeated exposure, host sensitivity, and whether the intestine is being asked to tolerate more chemical contact than it handles well.

What Soaking and Cooking Reduce, and What They Do Not Fully Solve

Soaking and cooking do real work because they begin dismantling the seed's defenses before the intestine has to face them. Water enters the dry seed, hydrates the tissue, softens the cell structure, shortens cooking time, and improves heat penetration. Then heat changes protein shape.

That matters most for lectins and protease inhibitors because these are heat-labile proteins, meaning their biological activity falls when enough heat unfolds them. EFSA states that proper soaking and boiling can render lectins biologically inactive, which means they lose the carbohydrate-binding activity that makes undercooked beans dangerous, and specifically recommends soaking beans for 6 to 12 hours, changing the water, and boiling for at least 30 minutes at 100°C. Food safety guidance makes the point even more sharply for kidney beans. Moist heat destroys the acute lectin hazard. Low-temperature cooking does not.

Cooking also lowers other parts of the seed's defensive package, especially trypsin inhibitors, the proteins that interfere with trypsin and related pancreatic enzymes that are supposed to cut dietary protein into absorbable fragments. One legume processing study found that cooking significantly reduced trypsin inhibitors in all legumes tested, while a broader review of enzyme inhibitors in pulses reported that cooking presoaked seeds produced very large reductions in inhibitor activity. That is an important improvement because once inhibitor pressure falls, protein digestion becomes less obstructed and the seed begins acting more like food and less like protected storage tissue. Soaking helps here too, but mostly by preparing the seed for effective heat treatment rather than by solving the problem on its own.

Soaking can also lower part of the fermentation burden, but this is where the limits become obvious. Raffinose-family oligosaccharides, the short sugar chains in legumes that human enzymes do not digest well, can leach into soaking water and fall with processing. That is one reason soaked beans are often better tolerated than unsoaked beans. But the reduction is often partial with soaking alone. A recent study reported only modest oligosaccharide reductions from soaking by itself, while older work showed that much larger reductions required a combination of soaking, dehulling, cooking, and fermentation. In other words, soaking can lower the load. It does not automatically clear the field. A bean can still arrive in the colon carrying enough fermentable residue to produce gas, distension, and altered transit, especially when the dose is large or the intestine is already sensitive.

The bigger limit is that soaking and ordinary cooking do not erase the seed logic. Phytate, the phosphorus storage compound that binds minerals such as zinc, iron, calcium, and magnesium, is often more persistent than lectins and trypsin inhibitors. Some studies show meaningful reduction with combined processing, but the reductions vary by legume, method, and duration, and fermentation or germination are often more effective than simple soaking and boiling. The same older legume study found that fermentation reduced phytic acid by roughly 30% rather than eliminating it, and a more recent study reported that soaking and roasting did not reduce phytic acid at all in the samples tested. Tannins show the same point from another angle. In that older study, dehulling eliminated tannins, which means removing the outer seed layers did work, but cooking alone was not described as a full solution. The lesson is clear. Heat can solve the acute lectin problem. It can markedly reduce enzyme inhibitors. It can improve tolerance. It does not automatically turn a defended seed into a low-burden food.

That is the distinction this chapter needs to keep. Soaking and cooking are not fake. They matter. They can make beans safe from the acute lectin hazard and materially improve digestibility. But they do not fully solve mineral binding, they do not always erase fermentable carbohydrate burden, and they do not remove every structurally protected or chemically persistent feature of the seed. Proper preparation moves the bean from dangerous toward more edible. It does not always move it all the way to nutritionally effortless.

Chapter 8

Protease Inhibitors and Poor Protein Yield

Protease inhibitors are proteins made by plants that block proteases, the enzymes that cut larger dietary proteins into smaller peptides and amino acids the intestine can absorb. In practical food terms, the most important targets are trypsin and chymotrypsin, two pancreatic proteases released into the small intestine to continue protein digestion after the stomach has done its first denaturing work. These inhibitors are concentrated especially in legumes and soybeans, where they function as part of the seed's defense system. The plant is storing nitrogen-rich tissue for its own future growth, and one way it protects that stored value is by attaching a protein that interferes with the eater's attempt to digest it. Reviews of legumes and pulse processing consistently identify trypsin inhibitors as major antinutritional factors because they reduce digestion and absorption of dietary protein.

That function makes sense once the seed is kept in view. A legume seed is not loose plant protein waiting to become human tissue. It is a compact storage organ holding amino acids, phosphorus, minerals, and energy for the next growth cycle. Protease inhibitors help defend that package by making protein extraction less efficient for insects, pathogens, and animals that eat the seed. Literature on legume protease inhibitors describes them explicitly as defense molecules and biopesticides, which is another way of saying they are part of the plant's anti-predation chemistry, not a nutritional gift to the eater. The same molecule that slows a pest's digestive proteases can also reduce human protein yield when enough inhibitor activity survives into the meal.

The nutritional cost is straightforward. If trypsin and chymotrypsin are being blocked, larger food proteins remain less completely cleaved in the lumen, the hollow interior of the small intestine where digestion and absorption are taking place. That means fewer amino acids and small peptides reach the brush border, the enzyme-rich surface of the intestine where final digestion and uptake occur. Reviews on plant protein digestibility and legume antinutrients describe this as reduced protein digestibility, reduced amino acid absorption, and in animal work, reduced nitrogen retention and compensatory pancreatic stimulation. The meal may still carry an impressive protein number on paper. The intestine is getting a lower return because the plant attached a brake to the digestive machinery required to unlock that number.

This is why protease inhibitors belong in a chapter about poor protein yield rather than overt poisoning. They usually do not announce themselves with the fast violent pattern seen in acute lectin poisoning. Their damage is more subtractive. They lower how efficiently the seed's protein becomes absorbable human nutrition. Processing matters because these inhibitors are generally heat-labile, meaning sufficient heat can unfold them and reduce their activity, which is why cooking, extrusion, and related treatments can improve protein digestibility in pulses and soy. But until that reduction happens, the seed is still behaving like defended storage tissue. The protein is present. The plant has simply made access more expensive.

Trypsin and Chymotrypsin as Digestive Enzymes That Must Break Protein Down

Protein does not enter the body as intact bean protein, soy protein, pea protein, egg protein, or meat protein. It has to be cut down first. The stomach begins that work by unfolding protein with acid and cleaving some of it with pepsin, but that first stage is incomplete by design. The larger burden falls on the small intestine, where pancreatic proteases take over. Trypsin and chymotrypsin are two of the main enzymes in that sequence. They are released by the pancreas as inactive precursors, trypsinogen and chymotrypsinogen, so the pancreas does not digest itself before the enzymes even reach the gut. In the duodenum, enteropeptidase, also called enterokinase, activates trypsinogen into trypsin, and trypsin then activates chymotrypsinogen and other pancreatic proteases. This is the handoff that turns partially digested protein from the stomach into a substrate the small intestine can finish reducing.

What these enzymes actually do is cut internal peptide bonds, the chemical links joining amino acids inside a protein chain. That matters because a large folded protein cannot cross the intestinal wall as food. It first has to be reduced into smaller peptides and free amino acids. Trypsin cuts at specific sites, especially after lysine and arginine. Chymotrypsin cuts at different sites, especially near aromatic or hydrophobic amino acids such as phenylalanine, tyrosine, and tryptophan. The two enzymes work as a coordinated dismantling system, not as duplicates. Their different cutting preferences break protein into a wider range of smaller fragments than either could produce alone. Those fragments are then handled further by brush border enzymes on the surface of the small intestine and by peptidases inside the enterocyte, the absorptive intestinal cell, until the meal has been reduced to units the body can actually transport into blood.

This is why protease inhibitors matter so much in legume and seed foods. If trypsin and chymotrypsin are being blocked, protein is still present in the meal but the digestive sequence cannot finish its work cleanly. Larger protein fragments remain in the lumen, the hollow interior of the intestine where digestion is taking place. Fewer amino acids and small peptides reach the absorptive surface in the form the body prefers. The food can still test high in protein on paper while producing a lower amino acid return in the intestine. The label keeps the number. The enzyme system loses access.

The deeper point is that trypsin and chymotrypsin are not side enzymes. They are central to the conversion of food protein into human nourishment. Once their activity falls, whether from pancreatic insufficiency, poor enzyme mixing, or plant protease inhibitors, the meal becomes structurally harder to finish. Protein digestion slows, absorptive yield falls, and more of the protein remains as unfinished residue rather than entering the body as usable amino acids. The seed keeps more of its stored nitrogen. The eater gets less of it.

How Plant Inhibitors Reduce Protein Digestion

Plant inhibitors reduce protein digestion by interfering with the enzymatic sequence that is supposed to turn food protein into absorbable amino acids and small peptides. In legumes and soy, the main inhibitors target trypsin and chymotrypsin, the pancreatic proteases that do much of the heavy protein-cutting work in the small intestine. Reviews of legume antinutrients describe trypsin inhibitors as major antinutritional factors specifically because they reduce digestion and absorption of dietary proteins, and recent soybean digestibility work continues to identify protease inhibitors as one of the main reasons plant protein yield can stay lower than the label suggests.

The loss begins in the lumen, the hollow interior of the small intestine where pancreatic enzymes are trying to attack protein fragments arriving from the stomach. A protease inhibitor binds the enzyme and blocks its active function, which means the enzyme can no longer cleave peptide bonds efficiently. The food protein is still present, but it remains in larger fragments for longer. That slows the conversion of intact or partly digested seed protein into the smaller peptides and free amino acids that can actually reach the brush border, the enzyme-rich absorptive surface of the intestine. The plant has not removed protein from the seed. It has attached a brake to the digestive machinery required to unlock it.

Once that brake is in place, the whole protein economy of the meal shifts downward. Less cleavage means less amino acid liberation. Less amino acid liberation means less transport across the intestinal surface. More of the meal remains as unfinished protein residue rather than usable human nutrition. This is why a bean, soy product, or seed can carry a respectable protein number and still underperform biologically. Gross content remains high. Digestive access falls. Some animal and feed studies make the cost visible at the whole-body level, showing reduced nitrogen digestibility, poorer amino acid utilization, and reduced growth or feed efficiency as trypsin inhibitor exposure rises. The mechanism is the same even when the endpoint differs. Protein stayed in the bowel longer because the enzyme system was held back.

The body also reacts to that inhibition rather than accepting it passively. Chronic exposure to trypsin inhibitors can stimulate increased pancreatic secretion as the body tries to overcome the blockade by pushing out more digestive enzyme. That compensatory move may partly recover some digestion, but it also confirms the central point. The food is not cooperating. The gut and pancreas are being forced to work harder just to approach the protein yield the label implied from the start. A defended seed is not merely giving you plant protein. It is making the intestine earn it.

That is the key distinction this chapter needs to keep in view. Plant inhibitors do not usually reduce protein digestion by poisoning the person in one dramatic step. They reduce protein digestion by slowing cleavage, prolonging the presence of larger protein fragments in the bowel, lowering amino acid release, and pushing the digestive system into compensation. The protein is still there. The body simply gets less of it.

Why Seeds and Legumes Often Carry These Inhibitors

Seeds and legumes often carry protease inhibitors because they are concentrated storage tissues, and concentrated storage tissue attracts predation. A seed is holding nitrogen, carbon, phosphorus, minerals, and the embryonic plant in one compact package. If that package is eaten and digested easily, the plant loses everything at once. So the seed defends the stored protein by attaching proteins that make protein extraction harder for the organism doing the eating. Reviews of legume protease inhibitors describe them as defense molecules concentrated in seeds and storage organs, especially the Kunitz and Bowman-Birk inhibitor families in legumes and soy. These inhibitors target digestive proteases in insects, pathogens, and animals, which means the same chemistry that protects the seed from predation also lowers protein digestibility in the human gut when enough activity survives into the meal.

The logic is structural before it is nutritional. Leaves are exposed tissues and often rely heavily on bitterness, phenolics, oxalate, or glucosinolate chemistry. Seeds have a different problem. They are dense storage bodies built to remain intact through time, dryness, microbial exposure, and attempted consumption. That is why they so often accumulate phytate, lectins, tannins, and protease inhibitors together. The plant is not only storing nutrients. It is storing them under guard. Experimental and review literature on plant protease inhibitors repeatedly frames them as anti-herbivore and anti-pathogen defenses because they inhibit gut proteases in insects and reduce nutrient availability to would-be predators. In plain terms, the seed is defending its protein by making the eater's protein digestion less efficient.

There is also a storage-side reason these inhibitors are found so often in seeds. Some plant protease inhibitors appear to have roles in seed development and protein preservation, not only in defense against predators. The seed has to hold its own proteins in a stable state until germination, then later mobilize those proteins in a controlled way as the new plant begins to grow. That makes the seed a natural place to concentrate protease-regulating proteins. The exact balance between storage function and defense function varies across species and inhibitor families, but the practical result for the eater is the same. The tissue carrying the plant's future nutrient reserve is also carrying proteins that make that reserve harder to digest.

This is why legumes and seeds can look protein-rich on paper and still yield that protein less generously in the bowel. The plant did not leave its stored amino acids exposed. It packed them into a defensive storage structure and attached inhibitors that interfere with the proteases required to unlock them. The seed keeps more control over its own protein than the nutrition label suggests. The intestine has to take that control away with soaking, sufficient heat, fermentation, grinding, and digestive capacity. Until then, the food is not simply carrying protein. It is carrying resistance to protein extraction.

Protein on the Label Versus Amino Acid Delivery in the Body

A protein number on a label is a crude inventory. It tells you how much nitrogen-containing material the food contains after laboratory analysis. It does not tell you how much of that protein will be broken down into absorbable amino acids, how much will actually reach the end of the small intestine in usable form, or which indispensable amino acid becomes the limiting step once digestion is finished. That distinction is important enough that the Food and Agriculture Organization moved away from treating crude protein digestibility as an adequate measure of protein quality and recommended focusing instead on digestible indispensable amino acids at the terminal ileum, the end of the small intestine, because fecal protein digestibility can overstate what the body actually absorbed and used. In other words, protein on paper and amino acid delivery in tissue are not the same biological fact.

The loss begins when the food reaches the small intestine. Trypsin and chymotrypsin have to cut larger protein chains into smaller peptides and amino acids before absorption can happen. If protease inhibitors from soy, beans, or other grain legumes are present in meaningful amounts, that cleavage slows down. The protein is still in the meal, but more of it remains in larger fragments for longer, which lowers amino acid release and lowers the amount that can cross the intestinal surface. Reviews on antinutritional factors report that dietary trypsin inhibitors from soybeans, kidney beans, and other legumes can cause substantial reductions in protein digestibility and amino acid availability. The seed keeps the protein number. The intestine gets less of the amino acid return.

This is why two foods with similar grams of protein can perform very differently in the body. The better question is not how much crude protein the food contains. The better question is how much digestible indispensable amino acid reaches the absorptive surface and enters the body after the full digestive sequence is over. FAO's DIAAS framework, the Digestible Indispensable Amino Acid Score, was built around this exact problem. It evaluates protein quality on the basis of digestible individual indispensable amino acids rather than assuming that total protein digestibility tells the whole story. That shift matters especially for plant proteins because the gap between crude protein content and true amino acid availability can widen when protease inhibitors, structural resistance, and other antinutritional factors remain part of the food.

So when this chapter talks about poor protein yield, it is not arguing that seeds and legumes contain no protein. It is arguing that the body does not live on listed grams of protein. It lives on amino acids actually liberated, actually absorbed, and actually retained after the intestine has fought through the plant's defensive structure and chemistry. A label can count protein that the gut never fully unlocked. The body only counts what crossed.

Processing Methods That Reduce the Burden

The methods that reduce protease-inhibitor burden are the ones that either denature the inhibitor protein directly or activate changes inside the seed that begin dismantling its storage defenses before the intestine has to do the work. Heat is the main method because most trypsin inhibitors in legumes and soy are heat-labile, which means their three-dimensional structure can be disrupted enough by sufficient moist or high-temperature processing that they lose much of their ability to block trypsin and chymotrypsin. Reviews of legume processing consistently identify boiling, autoclaving, and extrusion as the strongest routine tools for lowering trypsin inhibitor activity, with extrusion and adequately applied moist heat often producing especially large reductions.

Soaking helps, but it helps mostly by changing the seed so heat can work better. Water hydrates the tissue, shortens cooking time, improves heat penetration, and can leach out some soluble antinutritional material. On its own, soaking is usually not the decisive step for protease inhibitors the way proper cooking is. The important distinction is that a soaked seed is not the same thing as a neutralized seed. Soaking prepares the structure. Heat has to finish the job.

Germination, also called sprouting, reduces burden through a different route. Once the seed begins germinating, its own enzymes switch on to mobilize stored protein and starch for early plant growth. In that state, proteinaceous antinutritional factors such as trypsin inhibitors begin to fall because the seed is no longer trying to keep its storage package sealed as tightly. Reviews and older legume work both describe significant reductions in trypsin inhibitor activity during germination. Fermentation can help for a similar reason. Microbial and enzymatic activity begin dismantling storage structure and can lower multiple antinutrients at once, including some protease inhibitor burden, though the magnitude varies with the food, organism, and method used.

Dehulling and milling can reduce part of the burden too, but they work more by removing physical barriers and outer-layer antinutrients than by fully solving internal protease inhibition. Dehulling can improve digestibility by stripping away seed coat material and lowering some tannin and fiber load, which makes the protein more accessible to later processing. But if inhibitor proteins remain in the cotyledon, the main storage body of the seed, then dehulling alone does not fully rescue amino acid delivery. It changes access. It does not reliably eliminate the seed's internal protein-defense system.

The clean way to say it is this. Boiling, pressure cooking, autoclaving, and extrusion are the strongest routine methods for reducing protease inhibitor activity. Soaking helps the process but does not finish it. Germination and fermentation can lower the burden further by turning the seed from a protected storage organ into a metabolically changing tissue. None of these methods makes the original seed logic disappear. They make the seed less defended, more digestible, and less obstructive to protein extraction. That is a real improvement. It is not the same thing as the food having been low-burden from the start.

Chapter 9

Tannins, Polyphenols, and the Cost of Astringency

A plant makes astringent compounds because being eaten is a chemical problem long before it becomes a structural one. A leaf can be chewed once and lost. A seed can be crushed once and stripped of everything it stored for the next generation. The plant has to interfere with that extraction fast, often at the very first point of contact. Tannins are one of the ways it does that. They are polyphenolic compounds, meaning molecules built around multiple phenol groups that readily bind proteins and other biological surfaces. That binding property is the whole point. Astringency is not a flavor in the ordinary sense. It is the mouth physically registering protein binding. Salivary proteins lose their normal lubricating function when tannins attach to them, and the mouth begins to feel dry, rough, tight, and slightly scraped. The tissue has not stabbed the eater. It has changed the chemistry of contact. The plant is making the act of eating less smooth, less pleasant, and less efficient from the first bite.

That strategy makes sense in the tissues where tannins are commonly concentrated. Skins, seed coats, bark, hulls, unripe fruits, pods, and protective outer layers often carry more of this chemistry because those are the tissues most exposed to predators, insects, fungi, and repeated environmental damage. A ripe sweet fruit may lower astringency in the flesh to encourage consumption at the right time, while the peel, seed, or unripe stage still carries a harder chemical profile. The distribution is not random. The plant is controlling access. Unripe fruit often uses tannins to discourage early eating before the seed is ready. Seeds and hulls use them to make stored protein and starch less accessible. Outer tissues use them to resist microbial digestion, insect feeding, and physical degradation. The same compound that makes an unripe persimmon feel like it is turning the mouth inside out is serving a defensive purpose. The plant is not trying to nourish the eater yet. It is trying to preserve tissue value until the conditions of surrender favor the plant.

The important feature of tannins is that they do not merely taste unpleasant. They bind. They bind proteins in saliva. They can bind proteins in food. They can interfere with digestive enzymes by attaching to protein surfaces the gut needs to keep active. They can also interact with minerals in ways that reduce their availability. That means the mouth sensation is a preview of the deeper mechanism. The first dryness is the visible sign of a molecule whose whole strategy is to seize biological material and make it less usable. Once that tissue enters the stomach and small intestine, the same binding chemistry can continue shaping the meal. Protein digestibility can fall because digestive enzymes and dietary proteins are less free to interact normally. Mineral availability can narrow because the intestinal contents have become a less cooperative chemical environment. The astringent sensation feels sensory. Its real significance is mechanical and nutritional. The mouth is already showing you what the molecule does to proteins.

This is why plants keep returning to tannins and related polyphenols as defensive tools. They are versatile. They can reduce palatability, slow microbial attack, harden the economics of predation, and lower the digestive reward of a meal without requiring a dramatic toxin every time. A plant does not need to poison every animal that bites it. Often it only needs to make the bite less profitable. If the eater gets less protein, less mineral, less smooth digestion, and more chemical friction, the plant has defended itself cheaply and effectively. That is the real logic of astringency. It is not a culinary personality trait of certain foods. It is a defense signal carried by a binding chemistry built to make extraction harder.

Binding to Proteins and Minerals in the Gut

Tannins matter in the gut because they are built to bind. That is the center of their biology and the center of their nutritional cost. The same property that creates a dry, rough, puckering feeling in the mouth comes from tannins attaching to salivary proteins and stripping the mouth of its normal lubrication. In the intestine the setting changes, but the chemistry does not. Now the proteins in reach include dietary proteins, digestive enzymes, mucus glycoproteins, and protein-rich surfaces at the intestinal lining. Reviews of food tannins describe this protein affinity as one of their defining antinutritional properties, and experimental work on salivary proteins shows just how readily tannins attach to protein targets. The point is not simply that tannins taste harsh. The point is that they enter the gut carrying a strong tendency to seize proteins and make them less available for smooth digestion.

Once that binding chemistry enters the intestinal lumen, the hollow interior of the gut where digestion is unfolding, it can reduce protein value in two ways at once. First, tannins can bind directly to food proteins and make them harder for proteases to reach. Proteases are the enzymes that cut larger dietary proteins into smaller peptides and amino acids the body can absorb. Second, tannins can bind to the enzymes themselves and reduce their activity. That means the meal is losing access on both sides. The substrate becomes harder to digest, and the machinery meant to digest it works less efficiently. Review literature on tannins describes exactly this pattern: strong protein affinity, inhibition of digestive enzymes, and reduced protein digestibility. Astringency is therefore not a cosmetic trait riding along beside the meal. It is the sensory face of a molecule that is already showing you what it does to proteins.

Minerals are hit through a parallel route. Non-heme iron is the clearest case because tannins and related polyphenols can bind iron in the gut and lower the amount that remains soluble and available for absorption. Soluble matters here because a mineral has to stay dissolved in intestinal fluid if it is going to move toward the absorptive surface. Once tannin binds it into a poorly soluble complex, the iron is still physically present in the bowel but nutritionally farther away. Reviews on tannins and iron bioavailability describe this as the formation of insoluble or poorly available tannin-mineral complexes that reduce absorption before blood ever sees the meal. Recent work on plant polyphenols reaches the same conclusion more broadly: polyphenols can chelate, meaning bind and hold, iron strongly enough to alter its intestinal handling.

This is why tannin-rich foods can look respectable on paper and still underperform in the body. The gut is not absorbing the food's reputation, color, or antioxidant language. It is dealing with a binding compound that can grab proteins, slow enzymes, and hold minerals in the intestinal contents long enough that the body gets less amino acid and less iron than the label implied. The loss happens before the bloodstream has a chance to count anything as nourishment. Tannins do not have to poison acutely to matter. They only have to make extraction less profitable.

Reduced Digestibility and Reduced Iron Availability

Tannins reduce digestibility by changing the chemistry of the meal before absorption begins. Their main move is binding. They bind proteins in food, they bind digestive enzymes, and they bind to other organic material in the intestinal contents strongly enough that normal breakdown becomes less efficient. A protein that should have been exposed to trypsin and chymotrypsin, the pancreatic enzymes that cut larger food proteins into smaller absorbable fragments, is now partly shielded inside a tannin-protein complex. The enzyme can no longer reach the same cutting sites as easily, and the protein no longer behaves like open substrate waiting to be digested. The food still contains protein. The intestine is simply getting less access to it. That is the central deception of tannin-rich foods. The number stays high. The usable yield falls.

This same binding logic reaches the enzymes themselves. Tannins do not only wrap around the meal. They can also interfere with the protein surfaces of digestive enzymes and reduce their activity. That matters because digestion depends on repeated chemical contact between enzyme and substrate. Once tannins enter the lumen, the hollow interior of the small intestine where digestion is still taking place, they make that contact less clean. Larger peptides remain larger. More protein residue continues downstream only partly reduced. Less amino acid arrives at the brush border, the enzyme-rich absorptive surface of the small intestine, in the form the body actually wants. The loss is usually not dramatic enough to look like poisoning. It is quieter than that. The meal becomes less efficient. The gut works harder for smaller return.

Iron is lost through a related but distinct mechanism. Most iron in plant foods is non-heme iron, which means it is not packaged inside the heme structure found in animal tissue and is generally more vulnerable to interference from other compounds in the gut. For non-heme iron to be absorbed well, it has to remain chemically available in the intestinal contents and then reach the absorptive surface in the right form. Tannins disrupt that sequence by binding iron and creating complexes that stay poorly soluble. Soluble matters because a mineral has to stay dissolved in intestinal fluid if it is going to move toward the membrane and cross into the body. Once tannin has tied the iron up, the mineral is still physically present in the meal but nutritionally stalled. It remains in the bowel rather than entering blood. A plant food can therefore test rich in iron while delivering far less iron than the chart implies once tannin chemistry is counted.

This is why astringent foods can create two losses at once. They lower protein yield by interfering with digestion, and they lower iron yield by interfering with mineral availability. The body is not only breaking down a meal. It is fighting through a compound designed to make extraction harder. That is the real cost of astringency in nutritional terms. The mouth feels dryness first because salivary proteins are being bound. The intestine pays later because the same binding chemistry keeps protein from being reduced cleanly and keeps iron from remaining available long enough to be absorbed. A food like that may still carry nutrients on paper. The gut is already watching them slip out of reach.

The Difference Between Selective Pharmacologic Use and Staple Dietary Exposure

A tannin or polyphenol can make more sense as a selective pharmacologic exposure than as a staple dietary foundation because the biological goal changes when the dose changes and when the frequency changes. Pharmacologic use means a compound is being used for a specific effect, in a specific context, often for a limited period, with the understanding that the compound is active enough to change tissue behavior. That is very different from eating the same class of compounds every day in large amounts and calling the exposure nourishment. A selective exposure can tolerate tradeoffs because it is aimed at a purpose. A staple exposure has to nourish while it is asking the gut, liver, kidney, and mineral economy to keep absorbing the cost. That is where the distinction becomes important. A compound that can tighten tissue, slow microbial growth, reduce secretion, or alter signaling in a targeted context may still be a poor daily burden if it keeps binding proteins, lowering iron availability, and increasing friction in the digestive sequence meal after meal.

The gut feels that difference first. A limited astringent exposure may create only brief protein binding in the mouth and intestinal contents, with little lasting consequence if the meal is otherwise low burden and the person's nutritional reserves are strong. A staple exposure changes the whole terrain of digestion because the same binding event keeps recurring in the same lumen, the hollow interior of the intestine where food is being broken down and prepared for absorption. Tannins and related polyphenols keep meeting dietary proteins, digestive enzymes, and non-heme iron in the same chemical space. Protein digestibility falls a little here, iron availability narrows there, and the intestine keeps processing a meal that is chemically active in a way the nutrition label rarely admits. A single exposure and a staple exposure are not the same physiological event. The first may produce little more than a passing astringent effect. The second can become part of the intestine's regular workload.

This is why the public praise of polyphenol-rich foods often slips into confusion. It borrows the language of pharmacology and then applies it to everyday diet without keeping the tradeoffs visible. If a compound is biologically active enough to alter microbial behavior, protein interaction, enzyme function, or mineral handling, then that activity cannot be counted only when it sounds favorable. The same binding chemistry that gets praised in one context still exists when the food is eaten as a staple. The same capacity to precipitate proteins, meaning to pull them out of free solution into less available complexes, still matters when the meal is supposed to deliver amino acids and minerals efficiently. A limited medicinal use can justify some interference because the interference is part of the intended effect. A staple food has a different job. It is supposed to deliver nourishment with modest friction. Once the food keeps demanding compensation from the gut in order to express its supposed benefits, the category has already shifted away from simple nourishment.

The mineral story makes the difference even clearer. A selective plant extract or a short-term medicinal preparation may be tolerated because the person is not relying on that exposure as a primary source of iron, zinc, calcium, or protein at the same time. A staple dietary pattern built around tannin-rich foods is different because now the same person is asking the meal to nourish while the meal is still reducing mineral access. Iron is the cleanest example. Non-heme iron from plant foods is already more fragile in the gut than heme iron from animal tissue. Add repeated tannin exposure and the intestine keeps facing the same chemical handicap over and over. The food keeps its wholesome identity. The body keeps losing the mineral contest. A targeted exposure can be biologically acceptable because it is temporary, conditional, and not pretending to carry the whole nutritional load. A staple exposure has to survive a stricter standard. It has to keep feeding the body while being repeated often enough that any interference becomes cumulative.

That is the real difference. Selective pharmacologic use asks whether a compound can do something useful under controlled conditions. Staple dietary exposure asks whether repeated contact leaves the body with more nourishment than burden after digestion, absorption, and clearance are finished. Those are not the same question, and they should not receive the same answer. A plant compound can be interesting as a targeted tool and still be a poor foundation food if its daily presence keeps lowering digestibility, narrowing iron availability, and making the intestine fight through chemistry that was never designed to feed it generously in the first place.

Why "Antioxidant" Language Often Obscures Tradeoffs

The word antioxidant isolates one possible behavior of a plant compound and lets that behavior stand in for the whole food. That is the first distortion. A polyphenol can neutralize or modulate oxidative reactions under certain conditions and still bind proteins, chelate minerals, inhibit digestive enzymes, alter iron handling, or change microbial behavior in the gut. The antioxidant label highlights one laboratory or pharmacologic property and then lets the public imagination treat the molecule as if its other behaviors have stopped mattering. Review literature on polyphenols and tannins repeatedly describes this split. These compounds can show antioxidant activity, but tannins and related polyphenols are also recognized for antinutritional effects such as binding proteins and reducing mineral absorption, especially non-heme iron.

That matters because digestion does not encounter "antioxidants" in the abstract. It encounters chemically active compounds inside a meal. In the gut, tannins and polyphenols do not merely float past oxidative stress looking for radicals to neutralize. They meet food proteins, digestive enzymes, mucus glycoproteins, minerals, acids, and the absorptive surface. The same protein-binding chemistry that creates astringency in the mouth can continue in the intestine by reducing protein digestibility and interfering with digestive enzyme function. Reviews on tannins describe exactly this problem: strong affinity for proteins and the capacity to inhibit digestive enzymes, which lowers the efficiency of digestion even while the same compounds are praised for bioactive or antioxidant features.

Iron makes the tradeoff especially visible because the chemistry is hard to hide. Non-heme iron from plant foods is already more vulnerable to interference than heme iron from animal tissue. Polyphenols and tannins can bind that iron in the intestinal lumen, the hollow interior of the gut where digestion and absorption are still taking place, and reduce how much remains soluble and available for uptake. Reviews and mechanistic studies consistently report that tannins and polyphenols inhibit non-heme iron absorption, sometimes substantially, by forming poorly available complexes or by altering later steps in intestinal iron handling. That means a food can be praised for antioxidant content while still quietly lowering mineral return from the same meal.

The antioxidant frame also obscures dose and frequency. A selective exposure to a polyphenol-rich compound is not the same as building a daily diet around high repeated intake and then assuming the chemistry stays on the benefit side of the ledger. Public language often borrows from pharmacology, where a compound is interesting because it does something measurable, and then smuggles that language into everyday eating as if biological activity were automatically nutritional value. But a compound that is active enough to alter oxidation, microbes, enzymes, or metal handling is active enough to create tradeoffs when exposure becomes frequent. Even reviews that discuss potential benefits of polyphenols in health outcomes also note that the evidence base is mixed, context-dependent, and often drawn from models that do not settle what the net digestive and nutritional effect will be in ordinary food use.

So the problem with antioxidant language is not that the word is always false. It is that the word is too narrow for the biology it is trying to summarize. It spotlights one favorable property and lets the rest of the mechanism fall into shadow. A food does not become nutritionally cooperative because one class of molecules inside it can act as antioxidants in some settings. The gut still has to decide whether those same molecules bind protein, reduce iron access, slow digestion, or add friction to the meal. The antioxidant claim may be real. It is still only one piece of the chemical bill.

Tea, Legumes, Some Fruits, and Seeds as Examples of This Chemistry

Tea is one of the clearest examples because the chemistry is easy to feel before the digestion story even begins. The dryness, roughness, and tightening sensation in the mouth are not metaphors. They are the first visible sign that tannins and related polyphenols are binding proteins at the surface. The saliva loses part of its lubricating quality, the mouth feels less coated, and the tissue starts to feel slightly stripped. That same binding logic does not stop at the tongue. Once tea enters the stomach and small intestine, those compounds are still chemically active. If iron from the meal is present in the intestinal contents, especially non-heme iron from plant foods, tea polyphenols can lower how much stays soluble and available for absorption. This is why tea can look refined, light, even medicinal in reputation while still functioning as a mineral-limiting exposure when paired repeatedly with meals. The cup is not only delivering aroma and fluid. It is carrying a protein-binding and iron-binding chemistry into the same digestive space where the body is trying to recover nutrients.

Legumes show the same chemistry inside a denser and more complicated tissue. Beans, lentils, and many related seeds do not carry only starch and protein. They often arrive with tannins in the seed coat, phytate in the storage tissue, lectins, protease inhibitors, and fermentable carbohydrates all in the same package. That means the tannin problem in legumes is not isolated. It joins a broader defensive system. The outer tissues can bind proteins and reduce digestibility. The inner storage chemistry can reduce mineral availability. Fermentable carbohydrate can continue downstream and become gas. This is one reason legumes often look better on paper than they behave in the gut. Their protein number, iron number, and fiber number are all counted cleanly in nutrition language. Digestion has to work through a seed that is still acting like protected storage tissue. Tannins are part of that resistance. They make the act of extraction less favorable by lowering the freedom of proteins and minerals in the intestinal contents.

Some fruits carry this chemistry most clearly when they are unripe, concentrated, or especially skin-heavy. An unripe persimmon is the classic lesson because its astringency is so forceful that the mouth tells the truth immediately. The fruit may be sweet later, but in its more defended state it is chemically announcing that the tissue is not yet ready to be surrendered easily. Pomegranate, cranberries, some grapes, and other fruits with notable skin or seed polyphenol load show the same principle in milder form. The flesh may be edible and attractive while the peel, seed, or unripe phase still carries compounds that bind proteins and alter the mineral environment of the meal. Fruit often escapes scrutiny because sweetness softens the public reading of the food. But sweetness and astringency can exist in the same structure at different intensities, and a fruit can still be chemically active in the gut even when it no longer tastes aggressively resistant in the mouth.

Seeds and seed-derived foods may be the most important example because they combine concentrated nutrition with concentrated defense. A seed has no reason to surrender its stored protein, phosphorus, and mineral content cheaply. Tannins in the seed coat or outer layers help harden that barrier. They bind proteins, lower palatability, interfere with digestive access, and work alongside phytate and enzyme inhibitors to reduce the profitability of the meal for the eater. Nuts, legumes, cacao, some grains, and many seed-rich plant foods all express some version of this logic. The important point is not that every tannin-rich seed is equally problematic in every person. The point is that the chemistry is not accidental. The plant is defending concentrated value with molecules that make extraction harder. Tea shows that chemistry in a fluid. Fruit shows it in a ripening tissue. Legumes and seeds show it in stored food meant for the plant's future, not the eater's convenience.

Chapter 10

Saponins and Detergent-Like Plant Chemistry

Saponins are amphiphilic glycosides, which means they are built from two chemically different parts joined into one molecule. One part is the sapogenin, the non-sugar core that is fat-compatible and relatively nonpolar. The other part is one or more sugar chains, which are water-compatible and polar. That split structure is the whole reason saponins behave the way they do. They are not just bitter plant compounds floating through tissue. They are molecules built with one end that interacts well with lipids and another that interacts well with water, which is why reviews repeatedly describe them as plant surfactants, meaning surface-active compounds that behave in a detergent-like way at interfaces.

The main structural classes are triterpenoid saponins and steroidal saponins. In triterpenoid saponins, the sapogenin core is a triterpene skeleton, typically built on a 30-carbon framework. In steroidal saponins, the core is steroid-like, more compact, and classically based on a 27-carbon framework. In both cases the sugar portion is attached by glycosidic bond, and the number, identity, and attachment position of those sugars change the molecule's solubility, membrane activity, bitterness, and biological behavior. Some saponins carry a single sugar chain. Others carry more than one, which changes how strongly they interact with membranes and aqueous environments.

That architecture is why the detergent comparison is not metaphor. A detergent works because it contains a water-loving region and a fat-loving region in the same molecule. Saponins are built the same way. Their polar sugar chains let them remain active in water, while their nonpolar sapogenin core lets them insert into lipid-rich structures such as cell membranes. Reviews on saponin chemistry and surfactant behavior describe this amphiphilic design as the basis for their foam-forming properties, their ability to lower surface tension, and their membrane-disrupting potential. This is also why many saponins are hemolytic, meaning they can disrupt red blood cell membranes under the right conditions.

In plant tissue, that structure makes biological sense. A molecule that can engage both water and membranes is useful at the plant-environment boundary. It can deter insects, interfere with fungi, make tissue less palatable, and change what happens when another organism tries to digest or penetrate the plant. In food terms, the same structure means a saponin-rich tissue is not just carrying nutrients. It is carrying a compound class built to interact with membranes in a physically aggressive way. The sugar portion helps the molecule travel in watery digestive contents. The sapogenin portion helps it engage lipid surfaces. The chemistry is already telling you why the gut may experience it as irritation rather than as simple nourishment.

Soap-like Interaction with Membranes

The detergent comparison is not metaphor. It comes directly from the molecule's architecture. Saponins are amphiphilic, with a water-friendly sugar portion and a fat-friendly sapogenin core, so they behave like surfactants at the boundary between water and lipid. That allows them to lower surface tension, organize into micelle-like structures, and insert themselves into biological membranes instead of remaining passive in the intestinal contents. Reviews of saponin chemistry describe this membrane activity as one of their defining physical traits, and experimental work shows that many saponins interact strongly with membrane cholesterol and phospholipids rather than merely passing by them in solution.

That interaction matters because the intestinal lining is a lipid membrane system, not a neutral wall. The outer membrane of the enterocyte, the absorptive intestinal cell, is built from phospholipids, cholesterol, membrane proteins, and a surface glycocalyx, the carbohydrate-rich outer coating that helps regulate contact with the intestinal contents. A saponin can embed its hydrophobic core into that lipid layer while its sugar chains remain oriented toward the watery environment of the lumen, the hollow interior of the gut. Once that happens, membrane organization can change. Fluidity can shift. Permeability can rise. In stronger cases, pores can form or membrane integrity can break down far enough to allow leakage of cell contents. Multiple membrane studies report that saponins perturb membrane structure, alter conductance and boundary properties, and in cholesterol-rich systems can become frankly membranolytic, meaning membrane-breaking.

This is why the classic laboratory sign of saponin activity is hemolysis, the rupture of red blood cells. Red cell membranes are rich in cholesterol, and many saponins bind cholesterol strongly enough to destabilize the membrane and cause leakage or lysis. That red-cell model matters for food chemistry because it reveals the underlying principle cleanly. A molecule that can disrupt cholesterol-containing membranes in one setting is not nutritionally neutral when it reaches the gut. It may not destroy intestinal tissue the way it destroys isolated red cells in vitro, but it is still bringing a membrane-active chemistry to the mucosal surface. The intestine then has to absorb nutrients across a surface that is simultaneously being asked to tolerate a plant compound built to behave like soap.

That is the real burden of saponins. They do not only taste bitter or ride along as abstract phytochemicals. They change the quality of contact between plant tissue and the gut surface by engaging the lipid layer itself. A food carrying meaningful saponin load is not just delivering carbohydrate, minerals, or protein. It is delivering a compound class whose structure is suited to mixing water with lipid boundaries and, under the wrong conditions, making those boundaries less stable than the intestine would like.

Why Some People Tolerate Them and Others React Poorly

Saponin tolerance is not a simple yes-or-no trait because the burden depends on how much of the molecule reaches the gut surface, how long it stays there, what form it is in, and what kind of intestinal lining receives it. Saponins are poorly absorbed overall and tend to remain in the gastrointestinal tract for a relatively long time, which means their main biological action is often local rather than systemic. That alone creates variability. A person with a calm bowel, intact barrier function, and modest exposure may experience little more than bitterness or no obvious symptom at all. A person receiving a larger dose, repeated exposure, or a more membrane-active saponin profile may experience much more contact at the mucosal surface before the molecule is cleared or transformed by gut microbes.

The chemistry of the membrane matters because saponins do not act like neutral food particles. They interact with membrane cholesterol and can increase membrane permeability, and that effect depends on the specific saponin structure and the composition of the membrane it meets. Reviews describe cholesterol interaction, pore formation, and increased permeability as central features of saponin behavior. That means one bowel may tolerate a given exposure better because the dose is lower, the food matrix slows contact, or the mucosal surface remains more resilient. Another bowel may react poorly because the same compound makes stronger contact with the epithelial membrane and the intestine has less margin for that disruption.

Food form and processing also change tolerance. Quinoa is the cleanest example because its surface saponins contribute much of the bitterness, and processing methods such as washing and milling are used specifically to lower that burden. Even there, the reduction is variable. Review literature notes that washing alone is not always highly efficient at removing quinoa saponins, which means two people can both say they ate quinoa while receiving very different actual saponin exposure depending on how the grain was processed. The same principle applies more broadly to legumes and other saponin-containing plant foods. The category name does not tell you the delivered dose.

Gut context matters just as much as food chemistry. Experimental work has shown that some saponins can increase intestinal permeability and inhibit active nutrient transport, and animal work with soy saponins has linked them to increased gut permeability and intestinal injury under the wrong conditions. Those are not direct proof that every human gut will react the same way to every saponin-containing food, but they do show why host context changes the outcome. A bowel that is already irritated, permeable, inflamed, or dealing with other dietary burdens has less reserve when a membrane-active compound arrives. A more resilient bowel may absorb the hit with little obvious symptom.

Microbial handling adds another layer. Reviews on gastrointestinal behavior report that saponins are poorly absorbed and can be transformed by gut microbes into sapogenins, which may have different bioactivity from the parent compounds. That means people are not all exposed to exactly the same chemistry after ingestion. One person may leave more of the original saponin in the lumen. Another may generate more sapogenin downstream. Because microbial composition, transit speed, and colonic fermentation patterns differ from person to person, the same food can produce different local exposures and different symptoms even before questions of systemic benefit or harm enter the picture.

So the short answer is that some people tolerate saponins better because the delivered dose is lower, the food was processed more thoroughly, the intestinal barrier is more resilient, membrane contact is handled with less disruption, and microbial transformation or transit reduces the burden before symptoms build. Others react poorly because the same compound stays in the gut longer, makes harsher contact with the epithelial surface, and lands in a bowel that is already easier to destabilize. The food can be the same. The intestinal context is not.

Legumes and Certain Pseudo-Grains as Recurring Examples

Legumes recur in this chemistry because they are storage seeds, and storage seeds rarely arrive carrying only protein and starch. Reviews of plant antinutritional factors identify saponins as common in cultivated legumes such as soybean, peanuts, chickpeas, broad beans, and lentils. That matters because these foods are already dense with other seed defenses, including phytate, lectins, protease inhibitors, and fermentable carbohydrates. Saponins therefore do not arrive alone. They arrive as part of a stacked defense package inside a tissue the plant was trying to keep from being digested cheaply. A bean can look like a straightforward protein-and-fiber food on the label while still carrying membrane-active compounds that add another layer of contact burden to the gut.

Soy is one of the clearest recurring legume examples because it is both widely used and chemically defended. Reviews of legume-based protein sources identify soybean as rich in multiple bioactive and antinutritional compounds, including saponins, and broader reviews of food saponins continue to list soy and other legumes as major dietary sources. That makes soy useful as a model food in this chapter. It shows how a staple protein crop can still carry detergent-like plant chemistry even after processing has made it socially legible as a health food, ingredient isolate, or meat substitute base. The protein keeps the reputation. The seed chemistry stays attached unless processing removes enough of it.

Certain pseudo-grains belong beside legumes because they are often marketed as clean alternatives while still carrying the same kind of surface-active burden. Quinoa is the main case. Reviews of quinoa chemistry describe saponins as major seed-surface compounds that contribute bitterness and are often removed before human consumption precisely because they are an obstacle to palatability and use. Quinoa is therefore a very useful example for this chapter. It makes the chemistry visible. The seed coat is carrying membrane-active compounds strongly enough that industry and home preparation both treat removal as normal practice rather than as an eccentric precaution. Some broader pseudo-cereal reviews also describe saponins in quinoa and related pseudo-cereal categories, though quinoa remains the clearest and most established example.

That is why legumes and certain pseudo-grains keep returning in a discussion of saponins. They are concentrated storage tissues that often combine nutritional density with chemical resistance. In legumes the burden sits inside a broader seed-defense system. In quinoa the burden is obvious enough that washing, abrasion, or other removal methods are built into normal preparation. The lesson is the same in both cases. A food can be high in protein, minerals, or fiber and still arrive carrying detergent-like plant compounds that make the gut earn the meal more than the label admits.

Gut Irritation, Bitterness, and Reduced Comfort as Practical Outcomes

Saponins often announce themselves before digestion has gone very far. They taste bitter because the mouth is already detecting a chemically active plant defense, not a neutral nutrient. That bitterness is useful to the plant. It discourages feeding before the intestine has even had a chance to meet the molecule. In quinoa this is easy to notice when the seed coat has not been washed well enough. In legumes it is often less dramatic because the food matrix is denser and other flavors are covering part of the signal, but the chemistry is still there. The point is not that bitterness always proves danger. The point is that the taste is part of the defense logic. The plant is telling the eater that the tissue is carrying compounds meant to make contact less favorable.

Once saponins reach the gut, the problem shifts from taste to surface behavior. These molecules carry a fat-compatible core and water-compatible sugar chains, so they interact with membranes instead of remaining passive in the intestinal contents. The mucosa, the living lining of the intestine, is a membrane surface covered in mucus, transport proteins, and lipid-rich cell boundaries. A membrane-active compound does not have to poison acutely to create discomfort there. It only has to increase friction at the surface, alter permeability, or make the bowel work around a more irritating contact than it was built to prefer. The result may be nausea, vague abdominal unease, post-meal heaviness, burning, or the sense that a food feels rough rather than nourishing. That is one reason people often describe certain legumes or poorly prepared pseudo-grains as foods that sit badly even when they cannot name a dramatic symptom.

Reduced comfort also comes from the fact that saponins rarely arrive alone. In legumes they are usually part of a larger seed-defense package that includes phytate, protease inhibitors, lectin activity, fermentable carbohydrate, and coarse structural residue. That means the bowel is not only dealing with membrane-active chemistry. It is also dealing with reduced protein digestion, altered mineral availability, water retention in the lumen, which is the hollow interior of the intestine, and later fermentation in the colon if enough carbohydrate escapes absorption. The meal can therefore become uncomfortable through several routes at once. The intestinal lining gets more chemical contact. The digestive sequence gets less efficient. The bowel carries more residue, more gas, or more fluid than it wanted. A person does not need to experience a dramatic toxic event to know the food was costly. Reduced comfort is often the first honest report the gut gives.

This is why gut irritation and reduced comfort should be treated as real biological outcomes rather than as vague sensitivity language. A bitter saponin-containing food may be tolerated in one person, in one dose, after good preparation, and still become a poor staple when the exposure is larger or more frequent. The question is not whether the food can be eaten at all. The question is what kind of contact it creates at the intestinal surface and how much digestive effort it demands relative to what it returns. When a food keeps leaving the bowel with more friction than nourishment, discomfort is not random. It is the intestine describing the chemistry in plain terms.

Why the Plant's Defense Function Matters More Than the Marketing Language Around It

Marketing language begins outside the body and usually ends there too. It calls a food clean, antioxidant-rich, plant-based, heart-healthy, nutrient-dense, ancestral, colorful, or full of beneficial phytochemicals. None of those phrases tells you what the plant tissue is doing once digestion starts breaking it apart. The seed does not stop being a defended storage organ because the package says protein. The leaf does not stop carrying oxalate, nitrates, glucosinolates, or tannin-rich outer tissue because the label says greens. The pseudo-grain does not stop carrying surface saponins because it has been reintroduced as a modern superfood. Marketing speaks in reputation. The intestine is dealing with structure, release, binding, inhibition, fermentation, membrane contact, and clearance burden. That is why the plant's defense function matters more. It follows the food into the gut. The slogan does not.

Defense function also predicts the real friction points better than praise language ever can. If a food is a seed, you should expect protected storage chemistry. If it is a leaf, you should expect exposed-surface chemistry, mineral management chemistry, or compounds built to make chewing and digestion less favorable. If it is a peel or hull, you should expect boundary chemistry concentrated where the plant meets insects, fungi, and abrasion. That gives you a map before the first symptom ever appears. Lectins point toward contact problems. Protease inhibitors point toward poorer protein reduction. Phytate points toward mineral trapping. Tannins point toward protein binding and lower iron availability. Saponins point toward membrane-active friction and bitterness. FODMAP-rich carbohydrates point toward osmotic pull and fermentation. The plant's defense logic tells you what kind of burden is likely to appear. Marketing language usually erases that logic and replaces it with a category claim that hides the mechanism.

This matters because the body does not care why the eater wanted the food. It does not care that the bean was sold as plant protein, the tea as antioxidant-rich, the quinoa as ancient grain, or the berry as a polyphenol source. The gut still has to break the tissue down, move liberated compounds through the lumen, the hollow interior of the intestine, keep nutrients soluble, protect the mucosa, which is the living intestinal lining, and clear whatever the body cannot use. If the plant's defense chemistry keeps binding proteins, trapping iron, slowing enzyme access, irritating membranes, or feeding fermentation, then the food is behaving according to its biology, not according to its branding. The label can keep the virtue. The bowel still has to absorb around the obstacle.

That is why this book keeps returning to plant defense instead of public reputation. Defense function explains why a food can be edible and still low-yield. It explains why a food can test dense and still undernourish. It explains why symptoms keep showing up in the gut, the thyroid, the kidney, or the mineral economy while the food itself continues to enjoy a protected image. The plant is built to preserve its own tissues first. That is the truer starting point. Once that is kept in view, the rest of the digestive sequence becomes easier to read. The marketing language tells you what the seller wants the food to mean. The defense chemistry tells you what the body is actually meeting.

Part III

Mineral Theft and Nutritional Loss

Chapter 11

Oxalates: Mineral Traps and Urinary Burden

Oxalates are small organic acids or their salts built around the oxalate ion, a two-carbon dicarboxylate structure that binds readily to positively charged minerals. In food and physiology, the word usually covers both oxalic acid itself and oxalate salts. That distinction matters because oxalate is not floating in isolation once it enters a plant or a meal. It is already looking for a mineral partner. Sodium, potassium, and ammonium oxalates are more soluble in water. Calcium and magnesium oxalates are far less soluble. That one chemical preference explains much of the burden that follows. The same molecule that can remain dissolved in the intestinal contents under one set of conditions can become a poorly soluble mineral complex under another.

In plants, oxalate is often part of tissue architecture rather than a stray contaminant. Reviews of plant oxalate biology describe calcium oxalate crystals as common plant structures involved in calcium regulation, protection, tissue support, and defense. That means a high-oxalate leaf is not simply carrying a free pool of calcium and a separate free pool of oxalate waiting to be judged kindly by a nutrient chart. Much of the chemistry is already prearranged inside the tissue. The plant has used oxalate to manage calcium on its own terms, often in crystalline form, and those crystals or dissolved oxalate fractions then become part of what digestion has to handle.

The soluble versus insoluble distinction is where the physiology becomes real. Insoluble oxalate, especially calcium oxalate, tends to stay less available for absorption and more likely to pass outward in stool. Soluble oxalate is more mobile. It can stay dissolved in gut fluid, interact with minerals present in the meal, and under the wrong conditions remain available for absorption. Reviews on oxalate homeostasis and food oxalate chemistry note that oxalate absorption depends strongly on whether it is in soluble form, and that calcium can block absorption by shifting oxalate into insoluble complexes. That is the first reason oxalate is not just a plant chemistry issue. It becomes a digestive chemistry issue the moment the meal enters the lumen, the hollow interior of the intestine where nutrients and binding compounds are being mixed together in fluid.

Once absorbed, oxalate stops being only a gut problem and becomes a urinary solute, meaning a dissolved compound the kidney has to filter and excrete. NIDDK notes that calcium oxalate stones are a major kidney stone type and specifically advises stone-formers to reduce high-oxalate foods such as spinach and rhubarb because oxalate in food can raise the amount of oxalate in urine. That is why oxalate belongs in a chapter about both mineral trapping and urinary burden. In the gut it can reduce the value of the meal by binding calcium. In the body it becomes something the kidney must keep dissolved well enough to prevent crystal formation. The same molecule changes organs as it moves.

Why Plants Accumulate Them

Plants accumulate oxalate because oxalate solves several plant-side problems at once. The first is calcium control. Calcium is essential to plant life, but it is also dangerous when left too freely available inside cells because it changes membrane behavior, cell wall structure, and intracellular signaling. Reviews of plant calcium oxalate biology describe crystal formation as one of the major ways plants regulate excess calcium, store it in a less reactive form, and keep ionic balance inside tissues. In plain terms, the plant uses oxalate to lock calcium down on its own terms. What becomes a nutritional problem in the eater begins as a regulatory solution in the leaf.

The second reason is defense. Calcium oxalate crystals can make plant tissue less pleasant and less profitable to chew. Needle-like raphides and other crystal forms are not inert decorations. They harden tissue, add abrasive contact, and in some plants work as part of a broader anti-herbivore system. Experimental work in Medicago truncatula and review literature both support a defensive role for calcium oxalate crystals against herbivory, while broader reviews continue to list plant defense as one of the major proposed functions of oxalate accumulation. The plant does not need every crystal to poison the attacker. It only needs feeding to become more irritating, more damaging, or less rewarding.

Oxalate also helps plants manage difficult mineral environments. Plant crystal studies describe calcium oxalate formation as a route for removing excess calcium and, in some cases, participating in detoxification of metals such as aluminum and other heavy elements. That matters especially in tissues exposed to variable soil conditions or high mineral loads. A plant rooted in place cannot walk away from a calcium-rich or metal-rich environment. It has to immobilize part of that burden inside its own tissues. Oxalate is one of the ways it does that.

In some plants, oxalate may do even more than storage and defense. Research on calcium oxalate crystal turnover in leaves suggests that these crystals can also act as an internal carbon reserve, breaking down under drought or stomatal closure to release carbon dioxide for continued photosynthetic metabolism. That role is not the main point of this chapter, and it is not established as the universal explanation for oxalate accumulation across all plants, but it shows how integrated the chemistry can be on the plant side. Oxalate is not there by accident. It is part of the plant's operating system.

That is why high-oxalate foods have to be judged from the plant outward rather than from the nutrient chart inward. The spinach leaf, beet green, or rhubarb stalk did not accumulate oxalate to nourish the eater. It accumulated oxalate to regulate calcium, defend tissue, and manage its own mineral economy. Once digestion breaks that tissue apart, the plant's solution becomes the eater's problem. In the gut, oxalate can bind calcium and lower mineral availability. If enough soluble oxalate remains free and is absorbed, the same compound becomes a urinary burden the kidney has to clear. The plant solved one set of problems. The body inherits another.

Soluble Versus Insoluble Oxalate

The distinction between soluble and insoluble oxalate is the distinction between oxalate that stays chemically mobile in gut fluid and oxalate that is already locked into a mineral complex that moves very differently. Oxalate forms soluble salts when it is paired with sodium, potassium, or ammonium, and it forms far less soluble salts when it is paired with calcium or magnesium, especially calcium oxalate. Reviews of food oxalate chemistry and oxalate homeostasis both make this point clearly. Soluble oxalate is the fraction more likely to remain dissolved in the intestinal contents. Insoluble oxalate is the fraction more likely to remain as poorly dissolved mineral-bound material.

That chemical difference matters first in the gut. Soluble oxalate can move through the lumen, the hollow interior of the intestine where digestion is taking place, and it can bind calcium released from the meal before that calcium reaches the absorptive surface. Insoluble oxalate, especially calcium oxalate, is less available for absorption and more likely to pass outward in stool. Human oxalate reviews state that intestinal oxalate absorption depends heavily on how much oxalate is present in soluble form, and that calcium in the gut lowers oxalate absorption by shifting it into insoluble oxalate-calcium complexes.

This is why a high-oxalate food can behave in two different ways at once. If the food carries a substantial soluble fraction, that fraction is more able to alter the mineral chemistry of the meal and, if it remains unbound, more able to cross into the body. If the oxalate is already present largely as insoluble calcium oxalate, it is less absorbable, but it is also not delivering that calcium generously to the eater because calcium oxalate remains poorly soluble. A review on calcium absorption from food matrices notes that even the low pH of the stomach, which helps solubilize many calcium salts, does not fully rescue calcium oxalate because calcium oxalate complexes remain insoluble.

The urinary consequence follows the same chemistry. Soluble dietary oxalate is the fraction more likely to be absorbed, enter circulation, and then appear in urine, where it can contribute to calcium oxalate supersaturation and stone risk. Insoluble calcium oxalate formed in the gut is more likely to stay in the intestinal stream and leave in stool instead. Clinical nephrology sources describe this sequence directly. Usually dietary oxalate binds dietary calcium and leaves as insoluble calcium oxalate, but when oxalate remains unbound and soluble, more of it can be absorbed and later excreted in urine. That is why soluble versus insoluble oxalate is the hinge point for the whole chapter. The first form is more reactive in the gut and more dangerous to the kidney later. The second is less absorbable, but it also represents calcium already trapped in a form the body does not use well.

Binding of Calcium and Other Minerals in the Gut

Oxalate becomes a gut problem the moment plant tissue breaks open and releases it into the same intestinal fluid where minerals are trying to stay dissolved long enough to be absorbed. Oxalate is a negatively charged ion with a strong attraction to positively charged minerals, especially calcium. In the lumen, the hollow interior of the intestine where digestion is taking place, that attraction changes the chemistry of the meal. Calcium that might have remained free and transportable is pulled into calcium oxalate complexes instead. If enough calcium is present, more oxalate is shifted into an insoluble form and leaves in stool. If less calcium is present, more soluble oxalate stays available for absorption. Either way, the food's mineral story has already changed before blood ever sees the meal.

This is why a high-oxalate food can carry calcium on paper and still deliver little usable calcium in the body. Spinach is the model case. Human calcium-absorption work found that calcium from spinach was absorbed far less efficiently than calcium from milk, which is exactly what you would expect from a food carrying a heavy oxalate burden. The calcium is present inside the leaf, but much of it is chemically trapped in a form the intestine cannot use well. The plant kept the mineral. The label kept the number. The gut lost the value.

Calcium is the main clinical story, but it is not the only mineral affected. Oxalate can also bind magnesium, and human data show that magnesium absorption falls when a meal is served with spinach compared with a low-oxalate vegetable such as kale. More broadly, oxalate chemistry can interact with other cations such as iron and zinc, though the most consistent dietary and stone-related evidence centers on calcium and magnesium. The important point is that oxalate does not simply add a burden of its own. It changes the whole mineral environment of the meal by seizing minerals the intestine was supposed to recover.

The downstream effect is why calcium intake and oxalate intake cannot be judged separately. Calcium in the gut is protective against oxalate absorption because it binds oxalate before oxalate can cross into the body. That is why low-calcium diets can backfire in calcium oxalate stone disease. Less calcium in the intestinal contents means less oxalate is trapped there, more oxalate is absorbed, and more oxalate later reaches the kidney in urine. So the same binding event has two meanings at once. In the gut it lowers mineral availability from the meal. At the same time, when enough dietary calcium is present, it also protects against a larger urinary oxalate burden later. The chemistry is the same. The consequence depends on where the oxalate ends up.

Why Spinach Can Test High in Calcium and Still Deliver Little Usable Calcium

Spinach tests high in calcium because chemical analysis can measure how much calcium is present inside the leaf after the tissue has been fully broken apart. The intestine does not receive spinach in that state. It receives a leaf carrying calcium and oxalate in the same structure. Once digestion ruptures the cells and releases those compounds into the intestinal lumen, the hollow interior of the gut where digestion is taking place, the calcium number on paper stops meaning what most people think it means. Oxalate has a strong affinity for calcium. It binds it and shifts it toward calcium oxalate complexes that are poorly soluble and poorly available for absorption. The calcium is still physically in the meal. It is no longer behaving like freely available calcium the intestine can move into the body. Clinical and review sources describe this directly, and the National Academy's bone-health table uses spinach as the textbook example of oxalate preventing absorption of the calcium present in the same food.

This is not a theoretical concern. Human absorption data made the point decades ago and it remains one of the strongest examples in nutrition. In the classic crossover study by Heaney and colleagues, calcium absorption from spinach was dramatically lower than calcium absorption from milk, despite spinach containing calcium. The problem was not the absence of the mineral. The problem was the chemical form in which the gut encountered it. The oxalate-rich leaf released calcium into an environment where that same leaf was also releasing the molecule that traps it. The plant kept the mineral in its tissue. The body did not recover much of it.

The soluble versus insoluble distinction sharpens the mechanism further. Some oxalate in spinach is present in soluble forms that remain chemically mobile in gut fluid. That soluble fraction can bind calcium from the spinach itself and calcium from the rest of the meal. Brogren and Savage describe this directly in work on spinach oxalate bioavailability: soluble oxalates from spinach can bind calcium in the spinach and calcium eaten with it, reducing calcium availability and changing what remains free for absorption. This is why a food can look calcium-rich in a database and still act as a poor calcium source in the bowel. The nutrient chart records content. The gut experiences competition, binding, and loss of solubility.

So the contradiction is only apparent. Spinach is high in calcium as composition. It is low in usable calcium as delivery. The leaf is built around oxalate chemistry that serves the plant's own calcium management and defense needs. When that chemistry enters the intestine, it changes the whole mineral environment of the meal before blood ever sees it. The calcium number survives on paper. The body gets much less of the calcium than the number suggests.

Oxalate Absorption and Urinary Oxalate Load

Oxalate becomes a urinary problem only after it escapes the gut first. That escape depends mainly on how much oxalate remains in soluble form inside the intestinal contents. Soluble oxalate stays dissolved and mobile enough to cross the intestinal lining. Insoluble calcium oxalate is less available for absorption and is more likely to leave in stool. This is why calcium in the gut matters so much. Calcium does not simply add another mineral to the meal. It changes oxalate handling by shifting more oxalate into insoluble complexes before it can cross into the body. NIDDK reflects this same logic in practical form when it notes that enough dietary calcium can block stone-forming substances in the digestive tract, and controlled human work has shown that restricting dietary calcium can increase oxalate absorption and urinary oxalate excretion rather than protect against stones.

Once oxalate is absorbed, the body has no meaningful nutritional use for it. It enters circulation and becomes part of the kidney's filtration workload. The kidney then has to excrete it into urine while keeping it dissolved well enough that it does not combine with calcium and fall out as crystals. That is why urinary oxalate matters so much in stone disease. About 75% of kidney stones are predominantly calcium oxalate, and urinary oxalate is considered a crucial risk factor for their formation. The gut may have started the problem, but the kidney is where the chemical cost becomes visible. A leaf that looked mineral-rich on the plate can end as a urinary solute burden the kidney has to manage under concentration pressure.

The size of that urinary oxalate load is not determined by diet alone. Urinary oxalate comes from two major sources: dietary oxalate that was absorbed from the intestine and endogenous oxalate synthesis, meaning oxalate the body makes internally through metabolism. Older estimates suggested diet contributed only a minor fraction of urinary oxalate, but more recent reviews note that dietary contribution can rise substantially, in some contexts approaching half of urinary oxalate excretion. That matters because it means the food burden is neither trivial nor absolute. The kidney is handling a combined load from what the intestine allowed across and what the body generated on its own.

This sequence becomes much more dangerous in enteric hyperoxaluria, a condition in which the intestine absorbs abnormally high amounts of oxalate, often because fat malabsorption changes the mineral chemistry of the gut. Unabsorbed fat binds calcium, leaving less calcium available to trap oxalate inside the bowel, so more oxalate remains free for absorption. The 2024 review on enteric hyperoxaluria describes the result plainly: oxalate is excessively absorbed in the gut and then excreted in urine, where it forms calcium oxalate crystals and can drive stones and crystalline kidney injury. This is the full oxalate sequence in one line. In the gut, oxalate lowers mineral value or escapes binding. In blood, it becomes a transported waste compound. In urine, it becomes a crystallization risk.

Calcium Oxalate Crystal Formation

A calcium oxalate crystal begins as a solubility failure. Urine is carrying calcium and oxalate in dissolved form, moving them through a fluid system that is supposed to keep them separated, diluted, and in motion until they leave the body. That arrangement holds only while the concentration stays below the point where the fluid can keep those ions comfortably dissolved. Once that threshold is crossed, the chemistry changes. The urine becomes supersaturated, meaning it is now holding more crystal-forming material than it can keep stable in solution. At that point calcium and oxalate are no longer just being excreted. They are becoming candidates for solid formation.

That first shift is invisible to the person, but it is the decisive step. A dissolved burden becomes a crystal burden when ions begin organizing into a stable nucleus. Nucleation is the moment the first microscopic crystal seed appears. Once that seed exists, the rest of the sequence becomes easier. More calcium and oxalate can deposit onto the same structure. The crystal grows. Other crystals form nearby. Small crystals begin aggregating, which means they cluster together into larger masses that are harder to wash away. The kidney is no longer handling only dissolved waste. It is now handling particulate matter forming inside its own fluid system.

Whether that crystal becomes a stone depends on retention as much as formation. Crystals can form and still leave in the urine stream if flow, dilution, and urinary inhibitors of crystallization are strong enough to keep them moving. Stone disease begins when the crystals stop leaving. They lodge against renal tissue, remain trapped in tubular fluid, or anchor to papillary surfaces long enough to keep enlarging. That is the transition from chemistry to structure. A transient crystal can pass unnoticed. A retained crystal becomes a growth site.

This is why urinary oxalate matters disproportionately. Oxalate is not merely one more dissolved waste compound among many. Small rises in urinary oxalate can shift calcium oxalate supersaturation sharply because calcium oxalate is poorly soluble to begin with. Once oxalate has escaped the gut, entered blood, and reached urine, it becomes part of a system where concentration and retention decide whether the kidney clears waste or starts building crystal. The same molecule that trapped calcium in the intestine can now meet calcium again in the urinary tract under far more dangerous conditions.

So the stone is not a random hard object that appeared one day in the kidney. It is the end of a sequence. Oxalate survived the gut. The kidney filtered it. The urine concentrated it. Solubility failed. A nucleus formed. Crystals enlarged. Clearance failed. Retention turned chemistry into structure.

High-Oxalate Foods: Spinach, Swiss Chard, Beet Greens, Beets, Rhubarb, Almonds, and Sweet Potatoes

These foods matter because they are not just carrying oxalate as a minor side compound. They are among the ordinary foods most likely to deliver a meaningful oxalate load in real diets, especially when they are eaten often, blended into smoothies, juiced, concentrated into powders, or treated as staple health foods rather than occasional ingredients. National Kidney Foundation guidance specifically identifies spinach, Swiss chard, almonds, rhubarb, and beets as very high oxalate foods, and its calcium oxalate meal-planning guide also lists beet tops and greens, sweet potatoes, and Swiss chard in the avoid or very-high category for calcium oxalate stone prevention.

The leafy greens in this group are the strongest trap foods because they combine a nutrient-dense reputation with a heavy oxalate burden in the same tissue. Spinach, Swiss chard, and beet greens are all sold as mineral-rich greens, but once the cells rupture in the gut, the oxalate changes the mineral chemistry of the whole meal. Calcium that looked present on paper is no longer simply available for absorption. The green keeps the calcium number. The lumen becomes a binding field. This is why these leaves are worse as daily smoothie ingredients than as occasional foods cooked and eaten in smaller amounts. The leaf is not merely carrying nutrients. It is carrying a strong mineral trap inside the same structure.

Beets, rhubarb, and sweet potatoes show a different version of the same burden. These foods are not leafy, but they still deliver enough oxalate to matter, especially when they are eaten repeatedly or in large servings. Rhubarb is one of the classic high-oxalate foods. Beets are listed with their tops, roots, and greens in the Kidney Foundation guide, which is useful because it shows the burden is not confined to one decorative part of the plant. Sweet potatoes matter for the same reason. They often keep a clean public image as a safer starch, but for people with calcium oxalate stone vulnerability or high urinary oxalate, they are not a neutral substitute. They can still push the oxalate load upward while carrying a healthy reputation that hides the tradeoff.

Almonds belong in this group because nuts are often treated as concentrated health foods while their concentrated chemistry gets ignored. Almonds are energy-dense, mineral-dense, and easy to overeat. They also show up in almond flour, almond butter, snack bars, dairy substitutes, and low-carbohydrate baking, which means the real exposure can become much larger than a small handful of nuts. When a food like that is high in oxalate, concentration matters. A few almonds are one event. Almond flour used daily as a staple ingredient is another. The same problem appears with green powders and superfood blends made from high-oxalate ingredients. The chemistry gets concentrated while the marketing language gets cleaner.

The practical point is not that everyone must permanently avoid every food on this list. The practical point is that these are the foods most likely to distort the meal's mineral economy in the gut and, in the wrong host, add meaningfully to urinary oxalate burden later. For someone with calcium oxalate stone risk, the National Kidney Foundation advises limiting very high oxalate foods rather than trying to eliminate all oxalate from plant foods, and it stresses that enough calcium with meals helps reduce oxalate absorption. That is the right physiological frame. The food list matters, but the bigger question is exposure pattern: which foods are repeatedly delivering the highest soluble oxalate burden, in what form, and into what kind of body.

Why the Oxalate Problem Is Both Nutritional and Renal

Oxalate matters twice because it creates loss in two different organs and at two different stages of the food's passage through the body. The first loss is nutritional. The second is renal. In the gut, oxalate reduces what the meal can yield. In the kidney, absorbed oxalate becomes a waste solute that has to be filtered, concentrated, and excreted without being allowed to crystallize. The same molecule changes jobs as it moves. It begins as a mineral trap in the intestinal contents and ends as a crystal-forming burden in urine. That is why oxalate cannot be judged only as a kidney stone topic or only as an antinutrient topic. It is both at once.

The nutritional problem begins before blood ever sees the meal. Once a high-oxalate leaf, root, nut, or tuber is broken down in the gut, oxalate enters the same luminal fluid where calcium and other minerals are trying to stay soluble long enough to be absorbed. If calcium meets oxalate there, calcium oxalate complexes form and the available calcium pool shrinks. The food may still test high in calcium on paper, but the intestine is now working inside a mineral environment that has already been altered against absorption. This is why oxalate-rich foods can look nutrient-dense and still feed poorly. The chart records the mineral inside the plant. The lumen records how much of that mineral remained reachable after the plant chemistry was released.

The renal problem begins with whatever oxalate escapes that first intestinal checkpoint. Soluble oxalate that is not trapped in the gut can cross into the body, enter circulation, and then reach the kidney, which has no nutritional use for it and must remove it in urine. At that point the question is no longer whether the meal delivered calcium well. The question is whether the urine can carry oxalate safely in dissolved form. Reviews of dietary oxalate and hyperoxaluria show the same sequence clearly. Absorbed oxalate is excreted in urine, and once urinary oxalate rises, calcium oxalate supersaturation rises with it. That is the chemical condition that pushes the urinary system toward crystal formation.

This is what makes oxalate different from many other antinutrients. A compound such as phytate mainly lowers mineral return in the gut. Oxalate does that, then keeps going. If intestinal calcium is low, or fat malabsorption leaves more oxalate free for absorption, the problem shifts downstream and becomes enteric hyperoxaluria, meaning excessive oxalate absorption from the intestine followed by excessive urinary oxalate excretion. The 2024 review on enteric hyperoxaluria states the consequence plainly: oxalate is excessively absorbed in the gut and then excreted in urine where it forms calcium oxalate crystals, driving stones and crystalline kidney injury. The same molecule therefore creates a failed meal first and a filtration burden later.

So the oxalate problem is both nutritional and renal because the body pays for the same chemistry twice. It pays in the intestine when calcium and other minerals become less available. It pays again in the kidney when absorbed oxalate must be cleared under concentration pressure. A food like spinach can therefore disappoint on the way in and injure on the way out. That is the full oxalate story. The plant keeps control of its mineral chemistry. The body inherits the cost in digestion first and urine second.

Chapter 12

Phytates: Mineral Locking in Seeds, Nuts, Legumes, and Grains

Phytic acid is the seed's phosphorus vault. Chemically, it is myo-inositol hexakisphosphate, also written as InsP6, a six-phosphate molecule built on an inositol ring. In mature seeds and grains it serves as the main storage form of phosphorus, and it is commonly deposited as mixed mineral salts rather than as a free floating acid. When phytic acid is bound to minerals such as potassium, magnesium, calcium, iron, zinc, or manganese, that salt form is called phytate.

That chemistry is why phytate matters so much in food. The molecule carries multiple phosphate groups, which give it a high negative charge and a strong tendency to bind positively charged minerals. A seed uses that property to pack phosphorus and associated minerals into a stable storage form for germination later. The plant is solving a storage problem. The eater inherits a binding problem, because the same molecule that preserves mineral value for the seed can hold those minerals tightly enough in the gut that human absorption falls.

This is also why phytate shows up most heavily in the tissues that matter most to the next generation of the plant. It is concentrated in seeds, grains, legumes, nuts, and other reproductive or storage structures, not mainly in watery fruit flesh or most leafy tissues. A 2024 review notes that phytic acid is the principal phosphorus reservoir in mature seeds and is minimal in vegetables, fruit, and starchy roots, which is exactly what you would expect from a molecule designed for stored growth potential rather than immediate metabolic turnover.

Inside human digestion, phytic acid is not a vitamin, not a fuel, and not a meaningful nutrient source unless the molecule is broken down first. Humans do not produce enough endogenous phytase, the enzyme that cleaves phosphate groups off phytate, to rely on raw seed phytate as an efficient phosphorus delivery system. So the molecule often passes through the gut still doing what it was built to do: holding onto minerals. That is why phytate is such a central antinutrient in seed foods. It does not need to poison the eater. It only needs to keep zinc, iron, calcium, and magnesium from becoming freely available in the intestinal contents.

So the cleanest way to think about phytic acid is this: it is not random plant chemistry and it is not a side issue in seeds. It is the seed's mineral-and-phosphorus storage architecture. The food keeps the nutrient count because the minerals are present. The intestine gets a lower return because the seed stored them in a form designed to stay put until the plant, not the person, needed them.

Why Seeds Store Phosphorus This Way

A seed has to store phosphorus in a form that is dense, stable, and hard to lose. Free phosphate would be too chemically exposed for that job. It would move too easily, interact too freely with other cell components, and fail as a long-term storage solution for a dry tissue that may sit for months before germination begins. Phytic acid solves that storage problem by packing six phosphate groups onto an inositol ring, creating a molecule that can hold a large phosphorus load in a compact form and bind mineral cations into stable salts at the same time. That is why seed physiology literature describes phytic acid as the main storage form of phosphorus in seeds and grains, often accounting for most of the seed's total phosphorus.

The seed is not storing phosphorus only for its own chemistry in the dry state. It is storing it for the first burst of life after water arrives. During germination, the seedling needs phosphorus for membrane phospholipids, nucleic acids, phosphorylation reactions, and energy transfer through adenosine triphosphate, or ATP, the cell's main immediate energy currency. It also needs mineral cofactors and inositol-derived compounds for rapid early growth. Phytate is useful because it stores all of that potential in one place until phytase and related enzymes begin breaking it down during germination. Seed biology sources describe phytate precisely this way, as a phosphorus reserve that serves the biosynthetic needs of the growing seedling.

This storage form also helps the seed survive as a seed. A mature grain, legume, or nut is a dry storage organ, not an actively growing leaf. It needs chemical stability more than immediate metabolic flexibility. Depositing phosphorus as mixed phytate salts with potassium, magnesium, calcium, iron, zinc, and manganese lets the plant lock phosphorus and minerals into a relatively inert reserve that can sit through dryness and time without being spent prematurely. The same reviews that describe phytic acid as the principal phosphorus reserve also note that it is commonly deposited as mineral phytate salts in seed tissues.

That is why phytate is concentrated in seeds, nuts, legumes, and grains rather than in most fleshy fruits or watery leaves. The tissues that need long-term storage and future growth potential are the tissues that accumulate it most heavily. A fruit flesh is built to attract dispersal. A leaf is built for immediate metabolic work. A seed is built to hold concentrated future life in suspended form. Phytic acid belongs to that architecture.

The plant's solution becomes the eater's problem because the molecule keeps doing in the gut what it was built to do in the seed. It keeps holding onto phosphorus and minerals. Humans do not break phytate down efficiently enough to treat that stored reserve as freely available nutrition, so the seed's storage chemistry enters the intestine still acting like storage chemistry. The food keeps the phosphorus and mineral numbers on paper. The body gets a lower return because the seed stored them for germination, not for generous human absorption.

Chelation of Zinc, Iron, Calcium, and Magnesium

Phytate locks minerals by charge. Its six phosphate groups carry enough negative charge that the molecule behaves like a mineral trap in the intestinal contents, especially once seed tissue has been broken apart and the stored phytate is free to meet positively charged ions. Zinc, iron, calcium, and magnesium are the main nutritional casualties. They may all be present in the same meal, but once phytate binds them, they are less likely to remain soluble and less likely to reach the absorptive surface in a form the body can use. Reviews of phytate chemistry describe exactly this high-affinity chelation behavior and identify phytate as a potent inhibitor of mineral absorption in seed-heavy diets.

Zinc is one of the minerals most consistently impaired by this chemistry. Zinc absorption falls when phytate rises because zinc-phytate complexes remain poorly available in the gut. In some settings, calcium can worsen that problem further by helping form calcium-zinc-phytate complexes that are even less soluble than zinc-phytate binding alone. That is why seed- and legume-heavy diets can look respectable in zinc content while still delivering weak zinc status over time. The mineral is present. The intestinal chemistry is hostile to its uptake.

Iron is trapped through the same basic mechanism, but the cost can be especially severe because plant foods are already relying mainly on non-heme iron, which is more vulnerable to interference than heme iron from animal tissue. Once phytate binds non-heme iron, the intestine loses access to a mineral that was already harder to absorb. This is why phytate is repeatedly identified in the literature as a major inhibitor of iron absorption, especially in diets built heavily from grains, legumes, nuts, and seeds. The food keeps the iron number. The body gets less iron across the membrane.

Calcium and magnesium are caught in the same net. Phytate can bind both and lower their bioavailability, though the most consistent human concern in the literature is still strongest for zinc and iron. Calcium is complicated because it can both become less available itself and, in some contexts, participate in larger phytate-mineral complexes that worsen the absorption problem for other minerals. Magnesium is also vulnerable because it is another divalent cation the highly charged phytate molecule can hold tightly in the intestinal lumen. The important point is not that every mineral is blocked equally in every meal. The important point is that phytate changes the mineral economy of seed foods before blood ever sees them.

This is why phytate belongs in a chapter on mineral locking rather than simple nutrient content. Seeds, nuts, legumes, and grains can test dense in zinc, iron, calcium, and magnesium precisely because they stored those minerals in a chemically guarded form. Digestion breaks the tissue open, but the storage logic does not disappear. The plant built a phosphorus reserve that also holds minerals tightly. The eater inherits the same binding chemistry in the gut.

Why Mineral Density and Mineral Availability Are Not the Same Thing

Mineral density tells you how much of a mineral is present inside a food sample when the laboratory has fully broken the tissue apart and counted what is there. Mineral availability asks a different question. After chewing, acid exposure, enzyme contact, dilution into intestinal fluid, binding with other compounds, and transport across the intestinal surface, how much of that mineral is still reachable by the body. Those are different measurements because the first describes composition and the second describes outcome. Reviews on mineral bioavailability from whole foods make this distinction directly. The amount present in the food does not by itself predict how much will be absorbed, because the food matrix and the interactions inside that matrix change what the intestine can actually recover.

The gap opens as soon as the tissue is broken down in the gut. A mineral has to be released from the plant structure, remain soluble in the lumen, the hollow interior of the intestine where digestion is taking place, and avoid being trapped by compounds that keep it from reaching the absorptive surface. If the mineral remains enclosed in plant architecture, or if it is liberated only to be tied up immediately by oxalate or phytate, then the food can stay mineral-dense on paper while behaving as a poor mineral source in the bowel. Phytate-rich diets based on cereals and legumes are repeatedly identified in the literature as a classic case of high mineral content paired with poor mineral bioavailability, especially for zinc and iron.

Spinach makes the distinction brutally clear because the leaf carries calcium and oxalate in the same tissue. The calcium number survives chemical analysis, but once digestion opens the leaf, oxalate changes the fate of that calcium in the gut. Human absorption work found that calcium absorbability from spinach was far lower than from milk, about 5.1% from spinach versus 27.6% from milk in the classic study, because the calcium in spinach was effectively tied up by oxalate. The food kept the calcium content. The body received very little of the calcium as usable mineral.

The same logic applies to seed foods built around phytic acid. A grain, nut, legume, or seed can test rich in zinc, iron, calcium, and magnesium precisely because those minerals are present in stored form inside the tissue. But phytic acid, stored as phytate salts, was built to hold phosphorus and associated minerals tightly for the seed's future growth. In the intestine that same storage chemistry becomes a liability. The minerals are still there, but they are not freely surrendered. This is why food scientists and nutrition researchers keep separating nutrient content from bioaccessibility and bioavailability. Presence is a chemical fact. Access is a physiological contest.

So mineral density is the gross number. Mineral availability is the number that survives digestion. A food can look rich because the mineral is physically inside the plant. It becomes nourishing only if the gut can liberate that mineral, keep it dissolved, move it to the brush border, the enzyme-rich absorptive surface of the small intestine, and transport it into the body before the plant's own chemistry locks it away. Until that sequence is completed, density is only a promise. Availability is the part the body actually gets.

The Special Burden on Diets Heavily Built From Plant Staples

Phytate becomes a much larger problem when seeds, grains, legumes, and nuts stop being part of the diet and become the diet's structural base. An occasional seed-heavy meal can lower mineral availability in that one digestive window. A staple diet built around cereals, legumes, and other seed foods keeps returning the same binding chemistry to the same intestine day after day. That matters because phytic acid is not a minor side compound in these tissues. It is their main phosphorus storage architecture, concentrated precisely in the foods most plant-staple diets rely on most heavily. Reviews of phytate in plant foods describe cereals, legumes, nuts, and oilseeds as the main dietary sources and identify phytate as a potent inhibitor of iron, zinc, and calcium absorption in plant-based staple foods.

The burden is amplified because these diets often stack the same mineral problem on both sides of the equation. They raise phytate exposure while also leaning more heavily on the minerals most vulnerable to phytate binding. Iron is more often present as non-heme iron, which is already harder to absorb than heme iron from animal tissue. Zinc may be present in reasonable gross amounts while staying chemically trapped in the intestinal contents. Calcium and magnesium can be drawn into the same complexes. The food therefore looks mineral-bearing on paper while the intestine keeps meeting those minerals inside a seed-storage chemistry that was built to hold them tightly until germination.

This is why the burden becomes cumulative rather than theoretical. In a mixed diet, a high-phytate exposure may be diluted by other meals carrying more available minerals or by a lower total phytate load across the day. In a diet dominated by unrefined cereals and legumes, the same binding event keeps recurring at breakfast, lunch, and dinner. The International Zinc Nutrition Consultative Group thresholds cited in the phytate literature make the consequence visible: diets with phytate:zinc molar ratios above 18, typical of unrefined cereal-based patterns, are associated with low zinc absorption, around 18%, while FAO materials describe high-phytate diets in several countries as providing only about 15% zinc absorption. That is not a subtle penalty. It means the diet can carry zinc and still deliver little of it.

The problem also deepens because staple use changes exposure from periodic to structural. A few lentils beside a mineral-rich mixed meal are one physiological event. A diet where grains and legumes provide most of the calories and much of the iron, zinc, calcium, and protein is another. Now the same foods that carry the minerals are also carrying the compound that reduces their availability. The body is being asked to build itself out of materials that remain partly locked during digestion. That is why phytate-heavy staple diets are discussed so often in the context of complementary foods and mineral vulnerability. The issue is not only what the food contains. The issue is whether the diet keeps forcing the intestine to pull essential minerals out of storage chemistry that was never designed to surrender them easily.

So the special burden is not simply that plant staples contain phytate. It is that reliance changes the scale of the problem. The same compound keeps returning in the same foods that are supposed to supply the bulk of the diet's phosphorus, iron, zinc, calcium, and magnesium. The person is not just eating a defended seed occasionally. They are asking defended seed tissue to serve as the foundation of mineral nourishment. That is where phytate stops being a footnote and becomes a governing feature of the diet's biological yield.

Soaking, Sprouting, Fermenting, and Phytase Activation

Phytate is not removed by willpower or by wholesome intention. It has to be enzymatically cut apart. The enzyme that does that is phytase, which hydrolyzes phytic acid by cleaving phosphate groups off the inositol ring. Once that cleavage begins, the seed's phosphorus reserve starts breaking down and some of the minerals held in phytate complexes become less tightly trapped. That is why the real question is not whether a grain or legume was traditionally prepared in a vague sense. The real question is whether the preparation created enough water, time, temperature, and acidity for phytase activity to rise meaningfully before the food was eaten.

Soaking is the mildest version of that process. Water enters the dry seed, softens the structure, and in some grains and legumes can activate endogenous phytase, meaning phytase the seed already contains. But soaking alone is inconsistent. Its effect depends on the species, the intactness of the grain or legume, temperature, and duration. In some cases it reduces phytic acid only modestly, and intact kernels soaked for a short period may show little change. Soaking is best understood as opening the door. It hydrates the tissue and begins the biochemical shift, but it often does not finish the mineral problem on its own.

Sprouting, or germination, is a more serious biological event because the seed has now entered early growth mode. At that point phytase activity rises for a reason. The plant is trying to mobilize its stored phosphorus and minerals for the seedling. The same process that helps the new plant feed itself also helps dismantle the phytate burden for the eater. This is why germination usually outperforms simple soaking. Recent and older studies both report increased phytase activity and meaningful phytate reduction during germination, though the magnitude still varies by seed type and germination time. The seed stops behaving like fully locked storage tissue and starts spending its reserves.

Fermentation often goes further because it does not rely only on the seed's own enzymes. It can bring microbial phytases into the system while also lowering pH into a range that favors phytate breakdown. That is why fermentation frequently produces the largest reductions. In the rice work by Liang and colleagues, fermentation was the most effective treatment, reducing phytic acid by roughly 56% to 96%, while germination and soaking were less effective overall. Review literature on fermentation and germination reaches the same general conclusion: fermentation can improve mineral bioavailability because both endogenous and microbial phytase activity are working on the same storage chemistry under better conditions for hydrolysis.

The limit is important. These methods reduce burden. They do not create a universal guarantee. Some grains are naturally low in phytase, some seeds hold onto phytate stubbornly, and some processing methods trade phytate reduction for losses of dry matter or even minerals leached into soaking water. Soaking, sprouting, and fermenting are best understood as tools that change the seed from a closed storage organ into a partially opened one. They can improve zinc, iron, calcium, and magnesium availability by breaking down the molecule that was holding them back. They do not turn every grain, nut, or legume into a low-burden mineral food automatically. The chemistry improves when phytase is activated. The seed still decides how much it gives up.

What Preparation Can Partially Improve and What It Cannot Fully Reverse

Preparation can improve the phytate problem only when it changes the seed from a closed storage organ into a tissue that has begun spending its own reserves. That is the real dividing line. Water alone softens the grain or legume and can begin activating endogenous phytase, the enzyme already present in some seeds that cleaves phosphate groups off phytic acid. But soaking by itself is inconsistent. Its effect depends on the species, the duration, the temperature, whether the grain is intact or milled, and how much native phytase the food carried to begin with.

Review work on grains and legumes shows that soaking can reduce phytate, but usually modestly compared with stronger methods, and some studies show little change when conditions are weak or the food itself is low in active phytase.

Sprouting and fermentation usually go further because they shift the food into a more active biochemical state. During sprouting, the seed begins early germination and starts mobilizing the phosphorus and minerals it stored for growth. Phytase activity tends to rise, phytate begins to fall, and mineral bioaccessibility can improve. Fermentation can push this farther still because it does not rely only on the seed's own enzymes. Microbes bring additional phytase activity, lower pH into a range that often favors phytate breakdown, and continue opening the storage chemistry the intestine would otherwise have to fight through on its own. Across reviews and comparative studies, fermentation and germination repeatedly outperform simple soaking, with fermentation often giving the largest reductions.

Cooking helps, but it helps differently. Heat can soften structure, improve starch digestibility, reduce lectins, and lower trypsin inhibitor activity, which is why a cooked bean is safer and easier to handle than a raw one. But phytic acid is not just another heat-labile defense protein. It is a phosphorus storage molecule, and ordinary cooking does not reliably dismantle it the way boiling dismantles lectin toxicity in kidney beans. Some processing studies show additional phytate reduction when heat is combined with soaking, germination, or fermentation, but thermal treatment alone is usually a partial measure rather than a full reversal. The kitchen can soften the seed and make it more edible without fully unlocking the minerals it was storing under phytate control.

That is the limit people miss when preparation gets romanticized. A soaked, sprouted, or fermented grain or legume is often improved, sometimes substantially improved, but improvement is not the same thing as complete surrender. The amount of phytate reduction varies widely across cereals and legumes, and even when phytate falls, mineral bioavailability does not always rise in a clean proportional way because minerals can also be lost into soaking water, dry matter can be lost during wet processing, and other antinutrients may still remain in the food. One comparative study found that fermentation could remove much more phytate than soaking, yet the best phytate reduction did not necessarily produce a dramatic increase in predicted mineral bioavailability. The seed can be opened and still remain a guarded source of minerals.

So the honest conclusion is narrower and stronger than the usual food-prep slogans. Soaking can help. Sprouting usually helps more. Fermentation is often the most effective routine method because it activates phytase more aggressively and breaks the storage chemistry down further. But none of these methods automatically turns a grain, nut, or legume into a low-burden mineral food. They can reduce the lock. They do not always hand the minerals over freely. The preparation changes the seed's resistance. It does not erase the fact that the seed stored its phosphorus and minerals this way precisely to keep them from being given up cheaply.

Chapter 13

When a Food Tests Dense but Nourishes Poorly

A nutrient database is a record of composition after the food has been chemically reduced to analyzable matter. Human physiology is not receiving the food in that condition. It is receiving a plant tissue or an animal tissue that still has to be torn apart, acidified, mixed with enzymes, exposed to bile, held in solution, and carried across a living intestinal surface without being trapped, precipitated, fermented, or excreted first. That is the first mismatch. The database tells you what is in the sample. The body is dealing with what digestion can actually liberate from structure and keep available long enough to absorb. Those are not the same question, and once they are confused, whole foods begin looking far more nourishing on paper than they behave in the gut.

The database also strips away opposition. It counts the calcium and does not feel the oxalate that will bind it in the lumen, the hollow interior of the intestine where digestion is taking place. It counts the iron and does not register the phytate or tannins that will hold part of that iron back before it reaches the absorptive surface. It counts the protein and ignores the protease inhibitors that can slow the enzymes meant to cut that protein into absorbable amino acids. It counts carotenoids and folate after laboratory destruction of the tissue, while the bowel is still trying to fracture cell walls, soften fibrous structure, and move fat-soluble compounds through a watery environment that requires bile and micelle formation before transport can even begin. The database is not lying. It is answering a narrower question than people think.

That narrowing becomes more misleading when a food carries both nutrients and the chemistry that lowers their yield. Spinach can look calcium-rich while behaving as a poor calcium food because the same leaf carries the oxalate burden that changes the mineral environment of the meal. Seeds and legumes can look impressive in zinc, iron, magnesium, phosphorus, and protein because those compounds are truly present in storage tissue, but the storage chemistry was built for the seed's future, not for generous human absorption. Phytic acid holds phosphorus and associated minerals in a compact reserve. Protease inhibitors slow access to stored protein. Tannins can bind proteins and reduce iron availability. The database reports the inventory. Physiology has to negotiate with the defense system attached to it.

Human physiology is also dynamic in a way the database can never be. Absorption changes with bile flow, gastric acidity, pancreatic output, transit time, mineral competition, intestinal surface health, and the state of the mucosa, the living lining of the intestine. A food can behave one way in a calm bowel with strong digestive output and another way in a person with fat malabsorption, low enzyme reserve, unstable transit, or repeated gut irritation. A nutrient database has no place to record that the same fructose load is trivial in one intestine and a fermentation problem in another. It has no column for osmotic pull, retained gas, slowed gastric emptying, or the kidney's later filtration burden when a compound crosses into blood and becomes urinary work. The chart ends at composition. Physiology keeps going until the organs are done paying for the meal.

This is why a food can test dense and still nourish poorly. The laboratory can prove presence. It cannot prove usable yield. The body has to do that. It has to break the tissue, separate nutrients from inhibitors, keep minerals soluble, reduce proteins into transportable fragments, carry fats and fat-soluble compounds through intestinal fluid, absorb what remains available, and clear what it cannot use without paying too much for the process. Until that full sequence is accounted for, the database is only an opening description. It is not yet a biological verdict.

The more a diet relies on charts, the easier it becomes to confuse stored compounds with delivered nourishment. Human physiology is harsher than that. It does not care what the spreadsheet admired. It cares what crossed the membrane, what stayed available, what was lost in the lumen, what irritated the mucosa, what entered portal blood on the way to the liver, and what the kidney later had to excrete. A food earns its value in tissue, not in the database.

Calcium in Spinach as the Model Example

Spinach is the cleanest demonstration of why a food can look mineral-rich and still nourish poorly. The leaf contains calcium. That part is true. But the same leaf also contains a heavy oxalate burden, and once digestion opens the tissue, the calcium is no longer entering an empty intestinal field. It is entering a fluid mixture where oxalate is being released at the same time and can bind that calcium before the intestine has a fair chance to absorb it. Reviews of calcium bioavailability identify spinach as the classic high-oxalate exception among calcium-containing vegetables for exactly this reason.

The important point is that the calcium number in spinach is a composition number, not a delivery number. The database can measure how much calcium is present after the leaf has been chemically dismantled. The gut does not receive spinach in that state. It receives a leaf carrying calcium and oxalate together. In the lumen, the hollow interior of the intestine where digestion is taking place, oxalate changes the mineral environment of the meal by pulling calcium into poorly soluble complexes. Once that happens, the calcium is still physically present in the food mass but is less available to move toward the absorptive surface.

The human absorption data made this point decisively. In the classic Heaney study, fractional calcium absorption from spinach averaged 5.1%, while absorption from milk in the same subjects averaged 27.6%. The investigators also measured calcium and oxalate in the spinach and concluded that the oxalate burden was high enough that essentially all of the spinach calcium was effectively bound. That is the whole problem in one result. The leaf keeps the calcium reputation. The body gets a fraction of the calcium the number seemed to promise.

The contrast with low-oxalate greens makes the mechanism even harder to ignore. Kale, a low-oxalate vegetable, showed excellent calcium absorbability in a later Heaney study, averaging about 40.9%, which was actually higher than milk in that trial. The plant category did not decide the result. The chemistry did. One green traps much of its calcium inside an oxalate-heavy matrix. Another green leaves far more of its calcium available for uptake. This is why "contains calcium" and "functions as a calcium food" are not the same statement.

So spinach works as the model example because the contradiction is easy to see and hard to explain away. The calcium is real. The poor calcium yield is also real. The difference lies in what digestion is actually handling. A nutrient chart sees calcium inside the leaf. Human physiology sees calcium entering the intestine with the very compound most likely to lock it down before absorption can happen.

Iron in Legumes and Greens Versus Inhibitory Context

Legumes and greens can both test as iron-containing foods and still deliver that iron poorly because the iron in these foods is mostly non-heme iron, the form most exposed to the chemistry of the meal around it. Non-heme iron is not carried inside the protected heme structure found in animal tissue, so its absorption rises or falls depending on what else enters the intestinal lumen with it. Reviews of iron absorption make this point repeatedly: phytate and polyphenols are among the strongest inhibitors of non-heme iron uptake from plant foods.

Legumes carry the heavier built-in penalty because they bring iron inside a seed-storage system that is already loaded with phytate. Phytate is the seed's phosphorus reserve, but in the gut it also binds minerals tightly enough to lower their availability. Hurrell's review notes that phytic acid is a strong inhibitor of iron absorption and reports that iron absorption may be as low as 2 to 3 percent from porridges based on whole-grain cereals and legumes, even in iron-deficient subjects. That is the whole problem in one number. The food contains iron. The seed chemistry keeps much of that iron from becoming human iron.

Greens look different on the plate but can fail for related reasons. They also provide non-heme iron, so their yield depends on the intestinal context rather than on the iron number alone. Spinach is the clearest caution here, but not in the simplistic way people usually repeat. A human stable-isotope study comparing kale and spinach meals found that oxalic acid itself did not explain the reduction in iron absorption. Spinach was higher in calcium and polyphenols than kale, and iron absorption from the spinach meal was lower, while added oxalic acid to kale did not reduce absorption. That is an important correction. The inhibitory context in greens is real, but oxalate does not appear to be the main iron-blocking mechanism in humans the way it clearly is for calcium. In leafy vegetables, polyphenols, calcium, the non-heme form itself, and the broader food matrix matter more than the raw iron number suggests.

This is why legumes and greens are often misread in exactly the same way. The database sees milligrams of iron. Human physiology sees non-heme iron entering a crowded intestinal field. In legumes, phytate dominates that field. In greens, polyphenols, calcium, and matrix effects often matter more, with oxalate playing a much less important role for iron than popular nutrition rhetoric implies. The outcome is the same in practical terms. A food can carry iron chemically while delivering much less iron physiologically.

So the useful question is not whether legumes and greens contain iron. They do. The useful question is what kind of iron they contain and what kind of meal that iron is forced to survive. Once the iron arrives as non-heme iron inside phytate-rich seeds or polyphenol-rich greens, the number on the label stops being the verdict. The intestine still has to get the mineral free, soluble, and across the membrane before the food earns the right to be called a meaningful iron source.

Zinc Loss in Phytate-Heavy Meals

Zinc is one of the cleanest examples of how a meal can carry a mineral and still fail to deliver it. The reason is chemical, not rhetorical. Phytate has a dense negative charge, and zinc is a positively charged divalent mineral, so once both are present in the intestinal lumen, the hollow interior of the small intestine where digestion and absorption are still unfolding, they are drawn into complexes that remain poorly available for uptake. Zinc does not disappear. It simply stops behaving like a freely absorbable mineral. Reviews of dietary zinc absorption identify phytate as one of the strongest dietary inhibitors of zinc uptake from composite meals, especially when the diet is built around cereals, legumes, and other seed foods.

This matters because zinc absorption is already a narrower physiological process than the label suggests. The intestine has to transport zinc across the apical surface of the enterocyte, the absorptive intestinal cell, and that transport depends on the mineral arriving at the membrane in an available form. If the meal is rich in phytate, the zinc is still present chemically but arrives tied up inside a storage-derived complex the gut handles poorly. That is why the literature keeps returning to the phytate:zinc molar ratio rather than to zinc content alone. It is not enough to know how many milligrams of zinc are present. The gut is asking how much phytate is arriving beside them. WHO and zinc-assessment guidance classify diets with phytate:zinc molar ratios below 5 as high bioavailability, ratios from 5 to 15 as moderate, and ratios above 15 as low bioavailability, with roughly 50%, 30%, and 15% zinc absorption, respectively.

That is where staple use becomes dangerous. In a mixed diet, one phytate-heavy meal may lower zinc absorption only in that digestive window. In a diet built heavily from whole grains, legumes, nuts, and seeds, the same binding event keeps repeating in meal after meal. The intestine keeps meeting zinc inside the same seed-storage chemistry that was designed to hold minerals tightly until germination. Gibson's review of phytate and mineral nutrition describes phytic acid as a potent inhibitor of zinc absorption in plant-based complementary and staple foods, and IZiNCG-based dietary modeling treats high-phytate diets as low-zinc-bioavailability diets for exactly that reason. The food keeps the zinc number. The bowel keeps losing access to it.

The loss is not only theoretical. Mathematical modeling of human zinc absorption shows that the quantities of zinc and phytate in the diet are the primary determinants of how much zinc is actually absorbed, and recent reviews continue to describe phytate as the major dietary antagonist of zinc bioavailability. This is why plant-heavy menus can look nutritionally responsible while still pushing the body toward marginal zinc delivery. The problem is not that zinc is absent. The problem is that the meal keeps presenting zinc in a chemically defended form.

So zinc loss in phytate-heavy meals is the same broader story you have been building through the chapter. The seed stores phosphorus in phytic acid. The stored phosphorus holds minerals with it. The meal reaches the intestine carrying zinc and the molecule that locks zinc down. The database records density. The gut records access. When that pattern becomes habitual, a respectable zinc intake on paper can still behave like a low-zinc diet in tissue.

The Idea of Gross Content Versus Retained Biological Value

Gross content is what the food contains when the laboratory tears it all the way down. Retained biological value is what the body still has after chewing, acid, enzymes, bile, binding chemistry, transport, and clearance have all finished taking their share. Those are not competing theories of nutrition. They are two different accounting systems. The first counts what was present inside the food. The second counts what survived the digestive sequence and actually became part of the body.

This is where nutrient language starts lying by omission. A food can carry calcium, iron, zinc, magnesium, carotenoids, folate, and protein in measurable quantity and still deliver far less of each than the chart suggests because the intestine does not absorb presence. It absorbs what remains accessible. A mineral has to be released from the food matrix, remain soluble in the lumen, the hollow interior of the intestine, avoid being trapped by oxalate, phytate, or polyphenols, reach the brush border, the enzyme-rich absorptive surface of the small intestine, and then cross into the body. A protein has to be unfolded, cleaved, and reduced into amino acids and small peptides before the intestine can use it. A fat-soluble compound has to be liberated, emulsified, and carried through intestinal fluid in micelles before transport can even begin. Gross content says the compound is somewhere inside the food. Retained biological value asks whether digestion ever got it out cleanly enough to matter.

Spinach is the cleanest demonstration because the contradiction is built into the same leaf. The calcium is real. The poor calcium yield is real too.

In the classic human absorption study, calcium absorption from spinach averaged about 5.1%, compared with 27.6% from milk, because the oxalate-rich leaf delivered calcium inside a chemistry that trapped much of it before absorption could happen. The database recorded density. The intestine recorded loss.

Seed foods show the same split through a different mechanism. A grain, legume, nut, or seed can test rich in zinc and iron and still behave like a low-zinc or low-iron food once phytate enters the same meal. Reviews of phytate-rich plant foods use phytate-to-zinc and phytate-to-iron molar ratios precisely because the gross mineral number is not enough to predict what the body will retain. The seed stored the mineral under chemical guard for germination. The eater inherits the guard in the gut.

Polyphenol-rich foods and drinks make the same point in plain sight. Tea can be praised for antioxidant content while still lowering non-heme iron absorption because the same polyphenol chemistry that sounds favorable in one frame becomes inhibitory in the intestinal one. That is why gross content is always the easier number and the less important one. A food earns retained biological value only after the gut has broken it down, kept the nutrient available, moved it across the membrane, and handed the tissues something they can actually keep. Until then, density is only stored potential. The body lives on what remained after the fight.

Why Nutrition Tables Hide the Cost of the Plant Matrix

A nutrition table begins after the food has already been defeated. The tissue has been dried, milled, dissolved, burned, extracted, or otherwise broken down until its components can be measured. That is useful for composition. It is useless as a picture of digestion. The body does not meet spinach, beans, almonds, grains, or seeds as liberated calcium, iron, zinc, magnesium, carotenoids, and protein entries on a chart. It meets a matrix, a physical domain in which nutrients are enclosed, attached, or interacting with cell walls, fibers, protein bodies, starch granules, oils, oxalate, phytate, and polyphenols. Reviews on food matrices and micronutrient bioavailability make this point directly: the matrix changes release, accessibility, and absorption, and plant foods often deliver minerals less efficiently because of entrapment in cellular structures and binding by antagonists such as phytate, oxalate, polyphenols, and fiber.

That is the first hidden cost. The table can count a mineral that digestion never actually gets free. A nutrient can be present in the sample and still remain physically enclosed inside plant structure or chemically trapped once the meal reaches the intestinal lumen, the hollow interior of the gut where digestion is taking place. Bioaccessibility research uses this exact distinction. A nutrient must first be released from the food matrix before it is even potentially available for absorption, and only after that can bioavailability become the question. The table collapses both steps into one flattering number. It shows presence and lets the reader assume delivery.

The second hidden cost is opposition inside the meal. Nutrition tables do not show the mineral-binding or protein-binding chemistry that arrives beside the nutrient. They do not show that phytate in seeds and legumes can chelate zinc and iron, that oxalate in certain leaves can trap calcium, or that phenolic compounds can reduce mineral bioaccessibility by binding metals in the same digestive fluid where absorption is supposed to occur. They also do not show when fibrous cell walls and food structure slow enzyme access or keep nutrients physically encapsulated long enough that the bowel pushes them onward before the body has extracted much value. Reviews focused on mineral bioaccessibility in plant foods describe exactly this discrepancy between measured mineral content and the smaller amount that can actually be released and absorbed during digestion.

A table also hides the cost of processing and preparation. Milling, cooking, fermenting, sprouting, soaking, or juicing can change the matrix, the particle size, the hydration state, the phytate burden, the accessibility of starch and protein, and the fraction of nutrients that become bioaccessible. That means the same food name can correspond to very different digestive realities depending on how the tissue was handled before it entered the mouth. Reviews of food matrices and plant-food bioavailability stress that processing alters release kinetics and nutrient accessibility, sometimes improving them and sometimes creating new tradeoffs. The label rarely tells that story clearly because the label is built to standardize content, not to follow what digestion has to do.

The deeper problem is that nutrition tables reward storage chemistry as if it were nourishment. A seed stores phosphorus as phytate and locks minerals into the same architecture. A leaf stores calcium in tissue that may also carry oxalate. The table counts those stored compounds as if the intestine were a laboratory furnace with no friction, no barriers, no binding chemistry, and no failed transport. Human physiology is harsher than that. It has to liberate, keep soluble, move across a membrane, and retain. If the food matrix keeps the nutrient enclosed or ties it up once released, the number on the chart survives while the biological value collapses. The table records what the plant possessed. The body only keeps what digestion could actually take.

Part IV

Direct Plant Toxins in Common Foods

Chapter 14

Glycoalkaloids in Potatoes and Nightshades

Glycoalkaloids are steroidal defense molecules built into the tissue of nightshades. Chemically, they are alkaloids attached to sugar chains, which means they combine a nitrogen-containing steroid-like core with one or more carbohydrate groups. In potatoes, the main glycoalkaloids are alpha-solanine and alpha-chaconine. Both are built on the same aglycone, the non-sugar core, called solanidine. The sugar chains differ, and that difference matters because the attached sugars are part of what shapes solubility, membrane behavior, and biological activity. These are not loose bitter residues sitting on top of the food. They are structured plant defense compounds built into the tuber itself.

That chemistry fits the tissue that carries it. A potato tuber is a storage organ. It is holding carbohydrate for the plant's own use, and that stored energy has to be protected from insects, fungi, and animals. The tuber may read to the eater as a bland starch food, but to the plant it is defended reserve material. Glycoalkaloids are part of that defense system. They are especially concentrated in the outer parts of the tuber and rise in tissues that are sprouting, damaged, or exposed to light. That is why peel, sprout, and greened tissue matter later in the chapter. The starch makes the potato look nutritionally simple. The glycoalkaloids show that it is still biologically guarded.

The structure of these molecules is what makes them physiologically serious. Glycoalkaloids are not only bitter. They are membrane-active. Toxicology reviews describe potato glycoalkaloids as capable of disrupting cell membranes, especially in the gastrointestinal tract, and also of inhibiting acetylcholinesterase, the enzyme that normally breaks down the neurotransmitter acetylcholine after a nerve signal has been sent. That means the same molecule can act locally at epithelial surfaces and, at high enough exposure, contribute to systemic effects as well. The important point is that these compounds are not just flavor warnings. They are active plant defense chemistry with mechanisms that matter in human tissue.

This is why glycoalkaloids sit in a different category from simple antinutrients. A compound such as phytate mainly lowers mineral availability in the intestinal contents. Glycoalkaloids can do more than reduce yield. They can turn the food itself into a toxic contact problem when levels rise high enough. EFSA's assessment and other toxicology sources treat alpha-solanine and alpha-chaconine as the dominant potato glycoalkaloids of concern and link elevated exposure to acute gastrointestinal symptoms such as nausea, vomiting, and diarrhea, with neurologic effects possible at higher intake. The molecule is part of the plant's strategy for making predation costly. The eater inherits that cost when the chemistry climbs.

So when this chapter uses the word glycoalkaloids, it is naming a specific class of steroidal nightshade defense molecules, not a vague natural-toxin category. In potatoes, the main forms are alpha-solanine and alpha-chaconine. They are built on a solanidine core, modified by sugar chains, concentrated in the parts of the tuber most exposed to stress and attack, and capable of disturbing membranes and normal physiology when exposure becomes high enough. The potato keeps its identity as a starch. The plant keeps its chemistry as a defense organ. The body ends up dealing with both at once.

Alpha-Solanine and Alpha-Chaconine in Potatoes

The potato does not carry one dominant glycoalkaloid. It carries two, and the pair matters more than either molecule alone. Alpha-solanine and alpha-chaconine are the principal steroidal glycoalkaloids in potato tubers, usually making up about 95 percent of total potato glycoalkaloids. They share the same aglycone, solanidine, which is the non-sugar steroidal core, but they differ in the carbohydrate side chains attached to that core. That difference sounds small until the biology is followed. The sugars help determine how the molecules interact with membranes, how bitter they taste, and how toxic the mixture becomes once the tissue is stressed or eaten.

These compounds are not distributed evenly through the tuber. They concentrate toward the outer tissues, especially the peel, and rise sharply in sprouts, eyes, and tissue exposed to light or damage. That is why a potato can look like a bland starch source in the center while its surface chemistry is telling a much harder story. Greening itself is chlorophyll, not glycoalkaloid, but the same light exposure that drives greening often drives glycoalkaloid accumulation as well, which is why greened potatoes are treated as warning signs rather than harmless cosmetic defects. The plant is reinforcing the exposed parts of the storage organ, not seasoning the tuber for the eater.

Alpha-chaconine is often the more membrane-disruptive of the two, while alpha-solanine contributes strongly to the overall toxic burden through related but not identical behavior. Together they damage more effectively than either alone. Older membrane studies showed synergistic destabilization when the two were combined, which is important because potatoes do not present these compounds separately in real life. The eater gets the pair. That pair can interact with membrane sterols, especially cholesterol-containing membranes, and undermine barrier integrity in a way that helps explain the gastrointestinal pattern of glycoalkaloid poisoning.

This is why the first symptoms of excess potato glycoalkaloid exposure are usually gastrointestinal. EFSA notes acute effects in humans such as nausea, vomiting, and diarrhea, and toxicology reviews continue to describe two main mechanisms: disruption of cell membranes and inhibition of acetylcholinesterase, the enzyme that normally clears the neurotransmitter acetylcholine after nerve signaling. The membrane side helps explain the local bowel injury. The acetylcholinesterase side helps explain why higher exposures can move beyond stomach upset into neurologic symptoms. The potato stops behaving like food and starts behaving like defended tissue once enough of this chemistry is present.

So alpha-solanine and alpha-chaconine should be read together as the potato's main chemical guard system. One tuber can look ordinary, calorically simple, and nutritionally familiar while still carrying a paired alkaloid defense concentrated where the plant most needs protection. That is the real reason peel, sprouts, and greened tissue matter. The potato is not only storing starch. It is storing starch under chemical guard, and the guard is built largely from alpha-solanine and alpha-chaconine.

Why Greening, Sprouting, and Plant Stress Raise Concern

A green potato is not dangerous because it is green. It is dangerous because the green color can be the visible sign that the tuber has shifted back toward active defense. The green pigment itself is chlorophyll, which is not the toxin. What matters is that light exposure, the same signal that drives chlorophyll production under the skin, also tends to increase steroidal glycoalkaloid production in potato tissues. EFSA's risk assessment identifies light as an important factor in glycoalkaloid accumulation, and USDA materials note that light exposure can raise glycoalkaloid content in harvested tubers.

That is why greening matters even though greening itself is not the toxic molecule. The potato tuber is a storage organ, but once it is exposed to light it begins expressing chemistry more typical of active plant tissue rather than quiet buried reserve. Recent mechanistic work describes light exposure of tubers as driving both greening and increased steroidal glycoalkaloid production. The visible color change is therefore useful as a practical warning, even if it is not a perfect chemical measurement by itself. USDA documents are careful on this point: greening does not always correlate precisely with glycoalkaloid concentration, but it often travels with the same stress conditions that push those compounds upward.

Sprouting raises concern for a harder reason. A sprout is active growth. The potato is no longer sitting in a dormant storage state. It is reallocating resources into a vulnerable new shoot that needs chemical protection. That is why glycoalkaloids concentrate especially in sprouts, eyes, and nearby outer tissue. USDA and related technical materials note higher glycoalkaloid levels in sprouts and in the skin and green parts of sprouted potatoes. The plant is defending the new growth and the exposed tissues around it. The eater is inheriting a higher concentration of the very compounds the tuber uses to make predation more costly.

Stress matters more broadly because glycoalkaloids are part of the potato's injury-and-exposure response, not just part of its normal background chemistry. Light is the most familiar trigger, but physical damage, age, and other environmental stressors also raise concern. USDA draft positions on potato quality note that elevated glycoalkaloid levels are associated not only with light exposure but also with physical damage and age. Once the tuber is bruised, cut, aging, or pushed back toward active defense, the chemistry can shift upward in exactly the tissues people are most likely to peel shallowly, trim casually, or overlook.

So the practical reading is straightforward. Greening means pay attention. Sprouting means the warning is stronger. Damaged, aged, and stressed potatoes deserve more caution because the tuber may be acting less like a simple starch reserve and more like a defended plant organ again. The starch remains. The chemistry around it has changed.

Membrane Disruption and Cholinesterase Interference

The first damage potato glycoalkaloids do is often local and physical. Alpha-solanine and alpha-chaconine are membrane-active molecules, and toxicology reviews identify cell membrane disruption as a major mechanism behind their gastrointestinal effects. That is why the earliest poisoning pattern is so often nausea, vomiting, abdominal pain, and diarrhea. The bowel is the first tissue forced into contact with the chemistry.

That membrane effect is not vague. Glycoalkaloids interact strongly with sterol-containing membranes, especially membranes rich in cholesterol. Experimental membrane studies show that potato glycoalkaloids can bind sterols and destabilize the membrane enough to increase permeability and promote leakage of cellular contents. This is the mechanism that makes the potato stop behaving like a starch food and start behaving like a defended storage organ. The chemistry is not just bitter. It is physically disruptive at the cell boundary.

The pair matters here. Potatoes do not usually expose the eater to alpha-solanine alone or alpha-chaconine alone. They expose the eater to both, and the mixture is more important than either molecule in isolation. Reviews of potato glycoalkaloid toxicity describe the major acute mechanisms as membrane disruption and acetylcholinesterase inhibition, and they also note that the relative contribution of the two major glycoalkaloids can differ. In practical terms, the tuber is carrying a combined defense chemistry, not a single isolated toxin.

The second mechanism is cholinesterase interference. Glycoalkaloids can inhibit acetylcholinesterase, the enzyme that normally breaks down acetylcholine after a nerve signal has been delivered. Once that enzyme is inhibited, acetylcholine is cleared less efficiently, and cholinergic signaling can begin to persist longer than it should. Reviews of steroidal glycoalkaloids identify inhibition of cholinesterase activity in neurons as the second major toxic mechanism, and human and experimental literature supports this as part of the explanation for the neurologic side of glycoalkaloid poisoning.

This is why the symptom pattern can widen when exposure rises. At lower or more common toxic exposures, the gut often shows the problem first because the intestinal lining is the first membrane field the glycoalkaloids hit. At higher exposures, the nervous-system side becomes easier to see because cholinesterase inhibition adds to the injury pattern. The same compounds that strip membrane stability in the bowel can also interfere with normal acetylcholine regulation. The food is no longer merely irritating. It is disrupting tissue on one side and signal clearance on the other.

Gastrointestinal and Neurologic Symptoms

Potato glycoalkaloid poisoning usually declares itself through the gut first and the nervous system second. That split is not accidental. The intestine is the first tissue forced into direct contact with alpha-solanine and alpha-chaconine, so the earliest pattern is usually gastrointestinal. EFSA identifies nausea, vomiting, and diarrhea as the characteristic acute human effects, and food-safety sources describe onset anywhere from about 30 minutes to 12 hours after ingestion, usually after eating greened, sprouted, damaged, or otherwise high-glycoalkaloid potatoes.

The bowel symptoms are usually blunt and physical. Nausea, stomach pain, abdominal cramps, vomiting, and diarrhea dominate because the glycoalkaloids are disturbing the epithelial surface and membrane integrity of the digestive tract before anything else has had time to unfold. This is why the first human stories of potato glycoalkaloid poisoning sound like foodborne gastroenteritis even though the chemistry is different. The person feels the meal as a toxic contact event in the gut, not as a subtle digestive intolerance.

Neurologic symptoms appear when the burden rises beyond local bowel distress and starts affecting cholinergic signaling more broadly. More severe cases are reported with drowsiness, apathy, restlessness, shaking, confusion, weakness, headache, and visual disturbance. MedlinePlus and poison-center sources also note delirium, hallucinations, slowed breathing, paralysis, and shock in serious poisoning. The nervous-system picture is less common than the gut picture, but it is what makes glycoalkaloids more than just irritating plant compounds. They can move from intestinal toxicity into systemic dysfunction.

Severity is partly a dose question and partly a tissue-exposure question. EFSA's assessment and related toxicology summaries identify gastrointestinal symptoms as the main acute pattern at lower toxic exposures, while neurologic findings become more visible in more severe poisoning. The older toxicology review by Mensinga and colleagues links this symptom split to the two major mechanisms already discussed: membrane disruption helps explain the gut injury, and acetylcholinesterase inhibition helps explain the neurologic spillover. The same defended tuber can therefore produce two layers of illness, first by damaging the bowel surface, then by interfering with normal signal clearance if exposure is high enough.

So the symptom pattern should be read as a sequence rather than a list. The potato hits the gut first. If the chemistry is concentrated enough, the nervous system starts showing the burden next. That is why greened and sprouting potatoes deserve more respect than they usually get. They are not just bad-tasting potatoes. They are potatoes whose defense chemistry has risen far enough that the meal can turn into vomiting, diarrhea, confusion, weakness, and in rare severe cases, collapse.

Why Peeling and Cooking Help but Do Not Make a Bad Potato Good

A potato becomes chemically worse before it becomes culinarily worse. The starch is still there. The tuber still looks like food. But once light, sprouting, bruising, age, or other stress has pushed glycoalkaloid production upward, the potato is no longer behaving like quiet storage tissue. It is behaving like threatened plant tissue again. Alpha-solanine and alpha-chaconine rise most heavily in the peel, just under the peel, in the eyes, and in the sprouts, which is why trimming and peeling help in the first place. You are physically cutting away the zones where the plant concentrated more of its chemical guard. Greening matters for the same reason. Chlorophyll itself is not the toxin, but the same light exposure that drives greening often raises glycoalkaloids with it, so the green color is useful as a warning that the tuber has shifted back toward defense chemistry. A normal potato can tolerate ordinary preparation. A stressed potato is already asking for damage control before the pan is even hot.

Peeling can lower the burden substantially because the burden is not distributed evenly. EFSA reports that peeling can reduce glycoalkaloid content by roughly 25 to 75 percent, which is a real reduction, not a cosmetic one. But that number is also the reason peeling does not solve the whole problem. A bad potato is not simply a good potato with a contaminated wrapper. Once glycoalkaloids have risen, especially in a greened or sprouting tuber, the chemistry is no longer confined neatly to a disposable skin. The outer tissues still carry the highest concentration, but the rest of the potato has already moved away from the chemistry of a calm starch reserve. Cooking has the same limit. Glycoalkaloids are more heat-stable than people assume. They are not like lectins in raw kidney beans, where proper boiling can collapse the acute hazard decisively. EFSA reports only partial reductions with boiling and frying. That means heat can lower exposure, but it cannot be trusted to erase a tuber that has already become chemically aggressive. The knife and the stove can reduce the load. They cannot restore a stressed potato to its original biological state.

That is why a bad potato stays bad in a deeper sense even after preparation improves it. The stomach will still receive whatever glycoalkaloids remain. The intestine will still be the first membrane field forced to tolerate them. The local cost is usually gastrointestinal first because these molecules disrupt membranes in the gut before the body has done anything useful with the starch around them. If the remaining burden is high enough, the chemistry can keep moving past irritation and into overt poisoning territory. So the practical rule has to stay harder than kitchen optimism wants it to be. A slightly compromised potato may be made more tolerable by aggressive peeling and proper cooking. A clearly green, bitter, heavily sprouted, or aged potato has already crossed into a different category. At that point you are not refining a food. You are cutting back a plant defense that has risen too far, and the part that remains still carries the same chemistry into the bowel.

Potatoes as Ordinary Examples of Defended Plant Tissue

The reason potatoes matter so much in this book is that they look ordinary while still carrying the full logic of plant defense. A potato does not present itself as a chemically aggressive food. It presents as starch, comfort, softness, and familiarity. That public reputation is exactly what makes it useful as an example. The tuber is a storage organ. It exists to hold reserve material for the plant's future growth, which means it is holding concentrated value in one place. Any plant structure doing that has a predation problem. The stored starch has to be protected from insects, fungi, animals, and decay. So the potato does what defended plant tissue does. It surrounds stored carbohydrate with chemistry that makes feeding riskier and less profitable. The eater sees a side dish. The plant sees buried reserve under guard.

That guard is not abstract. It sits in the tissue. Glycoalkaloids concentrate toward the peel, the eyes, the sprouts, and the stressed outer parts because those are the places where the tuber is most exposed and most vulnerable. Once the potato is cut, bruised, greened by light, or pushed into sprouting, the storage organ is no longer behaving like quiet reserve. It is behaving like active plant tissue again, and the chemistry rises with that shift. This is why the potato is such a useful corrective to shallow nutrition language. It forces the point that a food can be calorically simple and chemically defended at the same time. The starch does not cancel the alkaloid. The familiarity does not erase the plant's need to protect stored energy.

It also exposes a broader mistake in the way people judge foods. The public tends to separate plant toxins into exotic categories and everyday foods into safe categories, as if ordinary use proves biological innocence. Potatoes break that illusion cleanly. They are ordinary enough to disappear into the background of the diet, which means their defense chemistry is often treated as a minor technicality rather than as part of the food's real identity. But the intestine does not care that the potato was common, cheap, or socially invisible. Once glycoalkaloid levels rise, the bowel still receives a membrane-active compound from a stressed storage organ. The same tuber that looked like bland carbohydrate on the plate can become nausea, cramping, vomiting, or neurologic spillover if the chemistry climbs far enough. That is defended plant tissue in its simplest visible form. The food keeps the reputation. The plant keeps the chemistry.

Potatoes also make the structural principle easier to follow because the defense is attached to a food that people do not usually romanticize as medicinal. With tea, berries, greens, seeds, or legumes, the discussion often gets lost in praise language about antioxidants, fiber, phytonutrients, or plant diversity. Potatoes cut through that. The tuber is easier to read. It stores energy. It protects energy. It shifts its chemistry under stress. It punishes careless handling when the protective compounds rise too far. That is the same logic already seen in leaves that carry oxalate, seeds that carry phytate and protease inhibitors, and legumes that carry lectins. The plant stores something valuable. The plant attaches resistance. The person eats both together.

That is why potatoes deserve more attention than they usually get in discussions of plant defense. They are ordinary enough to teach the central lesson without distraction. A plant food does not need a dramatic image, a bitter medicinal taste, or a reputation for toxicity to be chemically defended. It only needs stored value inside tissue that the plant cannot afford to surrender easily. The potato shows that the most familiar foods can still follow the same biological law as every other plant organ in this book. Stored tissue invites predation. Plant chemistry pushes back.

Chapter 15

Cyanogenic Glycosides: Plants That Can Release Cyanide

A cyanogenic glycoside is a plant storage-and-defense molecule built to stay relatively quiet inside intact tissue and then become dangerous when that tissue is broken. Chemically, these compounds are glycosides of alpha-hydroxynitriles, which means they contain a sugar-linked cyanide-bearing structure held in a more stable form until the plant is crushed, chewed, grated, bruised, or otherwise damaged. They are widely distributed in the plant kingdom, with well-known food examples including linamarin and lotaustralin in cassava and amygdalin in apricot kernels and other stone-fruit seeds. FDA identifies cassava and apricot kernels among the familiar food cases, and toxicology reviews describe cyanogenic glycosides as amino-acid-derived plant defense metabolites present in thousands of plant species.

The key to the whole chemistry is separation. In intact plant tissue, the cyanogenic glycoside is often kept apart from the enzymes that can break it down. Once the tissue is damaged, that separation fails. Beta-glucosidase, the enzyme that cleaves the sugar from the molecule, now gains access to it. The glycoside is hydrolyzed, a sugar is released, and an unstable cyanohydrin intermediate forms. That cyanohydrin can then decompose further and release hydrogen cyanide, the small rapidly acting poison that makes this chemistry clinically serious. EFSA's review of cyanogenic glycosides describes this sequence directly, and recent reviews of plant cyanogenic chemistry describe the same two-step liberation process from damaged tissue to cyanide release. The plant is not storing free cyanide. It is storing a triggerable cyanide system that becomes active when the tissue is disrupted.

That is why cyanogenic glycosides belong in a different category from simple antinutrients. A compound such as phytate mainly lowers mineral return in the gut. A cyanogenic glycoside can cross from defended tissue chemistry into outright toxin chemistry once the release sequence runs far enough. The biological target is cellular respiration, the process by which cells use oxygen to make energy. Cyanide binds to cytochrome c oxidase, the terminal enzyme of the mitochondrial electron transport chain, and blocks that final oxygen-using step. When that happens, oxygen may still be present in blood, but the cell cannot use it normally to sustain energy production. Reviews of cyanide toxicology and plant food toxicants describe exactly this mechanism. So when this chapter uses the term cyanogenic glycosides, it is naming a class of plant defense compounds that store the potential for cyanide release inside ordinary tissues and seeds. The food may still look like starch, fruit, kernel, or flour. The chemistry inside it is a latent respiratory poison waiting for tissue damage, enzyme contact, and inadequate preparation to let it out.

Tissue Damage, Enzyme Action, and Cyanide Release

A cyanogenic plant is dangerous only when its internal separation fails. In intact tissue, the cyanogenic glycoside and the enzyme system that can break it down are often kept in different compartments. That spatial separation is the plant's way of storing a latent toxin without poisoning itself. The chemistry is loaded, but it is not yet firing. Once the tissue is cut, chewed, grated, bruised, crushed, or otherwise ruptured, those compartments break open and the glycoside comes into contact with plant beta-glucosidase, the enzyme that clips the sugar off the molecule and starts the release sequence.

That first break matters more than most people realize. A whole seed, an intact cassava root, or an unbroken kernel does not present the same toxic problem as a ground flour, grated pulp, or chewed tissue, because the act of fracturing the plant multiplies contact between substrate and enzyme. The plant is using damage itself as the trigger. When the tissue is left intact, the molecule can remain comparatively quiet. When the tissue is broken aggressively, the defense chemistry becomes active at exactly the moment another organism is trying to eat the plant.

Once beta-glucosidase reaches the cyanogenic glycoside, the sugar is cleaved away and the molecule is converted into a cyanohydrin, an unstable intermediate that still contains the cyanide-bearing structure. That intermediate is not the end of the process. It is the unstable bridge between stored defense chemistry and free cyanide release. In foods such as cassava, this is the crucial middle step. The plant is not storing free hydrogen cyanide in large open pools. It is storing a compound that can be converted into a cyanohydrin and then pushed the rest of the way toward cyanide once the tissue has been broken down.

The last step is decomposition of that cyanohydrin into hydrogen cyanide, the small rapidly acting toxin that interferes with cellular respiration, the oxygen-using process by which mitochondria make energy. That breakdown can occur spontaneously under the right conditions, and in some plants it can also be accelerated by hydroxynitrile lyase, an enzyme that speeds cyanohydrin cleavage. By that point the chemistry has moved out of the storage phase and into the poisoning phase. The plant's quiet reservoir has turned into a respiratory toxin because the tissue was opened and the enzyme sequence was allowed to run.

This is why preparation matters so much with cassava and similar foods. Grating, pounding, soaking, fermenting, drying, and thorough processing are not cultural decorations around the food. They are part of managing this release chemistry. Some steps increase rupture first, which can increase cyanide liberation, but then allow volatilization, leaching, or further removal before the food is eaten. Poor preparation does the opposite. It damages the tissue enough to activate the system without carrying the process far enough to clear the cyanide burden safely. FDA's food-safety guidance specifically flags cassava as a food in which cyanogenic glycosides can become dangerous if preparation is inadequate.

So the sequence is clean. Intact tissue stores the toxin potential in separated form. Tissue damage collapses that separation. Beta-glucosidase removes the sugar. Cyanohydrin forms. Cyanohydrin breaks down and releases hydrogen cyanide. The meal stops being only starch, kernel, or root and becomes a plant tissue whose internal defense chemistry has been switched on by fracture.

Cassava as the Central Staple Example

Cassava is the central staple example because it looks most clearly like food while still carrying one of the hardest plant-defense burdens in the book. The root is built as a carbohydrate reserve. It reads as starch, flour, porridge, bread, chips, paste, meal. It is not socially coded as a medicinal plant or an obviously toxic one. That is exactly why it matters. Cassava is ordinary enough to become a foundation food, and that changes the scale of the problem immediately. FDA identifies cassava as a plant food containing cyanogenic glycosides that can release cyanide if improperly prepared, and specifically notes that the levels in cassava can lead not only to death from uncooked use but also to chronic neurologic disease. Once a defended root becomes a staple, the chemistry stops being an exotic toxicology footnote and becomes part of daily human intake.

The root carries this burden mainly through linamarin and lotaustralin, the two principal cyanogenic glycosides in cassava, with linamarin making up the great majority of the total cyanogen load. In intact tissue those compounds remain comparatively quiet because the glycosides are separated from the enzymes that break them down. Once the root is peeled, grated, pounded, chewed, or otherwise damaged, the plant's own enzyme system gains access, cyanohydrins form, and hydrogen cyanide can be released. Food-safety authorities also distinguish between sweet cassava and bitter cassava, not because one is harmless and the other poisonous in some absolute sense, but because the cyanogenic load differs sharply. The Hong Kong Centre for Food Safety notes that sweet cassava generally contains less than 50 mg hydrogen cyanide per kilogram fresh weight, while bitter cassava may reach up to 400 mg/kg. The root is still the same species. The defensive burden is not the same.

This is why processing is not an optional culinary refinement with cassava. It is part of the biology of making the food edible. FDA, CDC, and FAO all describe the same logic from slightly different angles: proper preparation methods such as peeling, grating, soaking, fermenting, drying, scraping, and thorough cooking are used to reduce cyanogenic burden before consumption. That sequence is easy to misunderstand if cassava is treated as a simple starch. The damage step can increase cyanide liberation by collapsing the plant's internal separation, but the later steps are what allow cyanide and cyanogenic intermediates to leach out, volatilize, decompose, or otherwise fall to safer levels before the food is eaten. Poor preparation therefore produces the worst middle state. The tissue has been fractured enough to activate the defense chemistry, but not processed far enough to clear the burden.

Cassava belongs at the center of this chapter because it shows what happens when defended plant tissue becomes a staple rather than an occasional exposure. An occasional cyanogenic seed or kernel matters. A root that can anchor the diet matters more because the cost can be repeated meal after meal. CDC has documented fatal outbreaks from cassava flour that was not properly detoxified, and FDA's policy statement is explicit that cassava can produce not only acute cyanide poisoning but chronic neurologic disease when preparation is inadequate. The chemistry is simple and severe. The root stores carbohydrate for the plant. The plant protects that reserve with cyanogenic glycosides. The person eats the starch and the defense together unless processing has done enough to separate them again before the bowel receives the meal.

Why Traditional Processing Exists

Traditional cassava processing exists because the root is not born edible in the generous sense. It is born as defended storage tissue. The flesh looks like carbohydrate reserve, but that reserve is held inside a root carrying linamarin and lotaustralin, cyanogenic glycosides that can release cyanide once the tissue is broken and the internal chemistry is allowed to run. That is why cassava cultures did not need modern toxicology to discover that the root had to be handled in stages. The danger is built into the tissue itself. A whole root can sit comparatively quiet. A grated or chewed root is already moving toward cyanide release because tissue damage collapses the separation between substrate and enzyme. Traditional processing is the accumulated answer to that plant chemistry, not a layer of folklore draped over a harmless starch.

The first purpose of processing is to control what happens immediately after rupture. Peeling removes outer tissues that carry higher cyanogen concentrations. Grating, pounding, and crushing then do something that seems contradictory at first. They increase tissue damage, which increases contact between cyanogenic glycosides and the plant enzymes that break them down. But that step is necessary because an intact root keeps too much of its cyanogen system sealed inside itself. Once the tissue is opened thoroughly, the chemistry can finally be driven outward instead of staying trapped in the food. Codex background material states this directly: proper grating is used to rupture cassava tissue for rapid breakdown of cyanogenic glycosides, while peeling removes rind and peel tissue known to contain high cyanogenic concentrations. Traditional processors were not merely softening the root. They were opening the defense system so it could be discharged before eating.

That is why soaking, pressing, and fermenting keep appearing across cassava traditions. Once the root has been opened, the next problem is removal. Hydrogen cyanide can diffuse out. Water can leach cyanogenic material and breakdown products away from the mash or chips. Fermentation lowers pH, changes the chemical environment, and can help drive further cyanogen reduction, while pressing physically forces liquid out of the grated mass. FAO materials describe prolonged soaking and fermentation as ways dissolved cyanide can move into water and later evaporate during drying, and Codex notes that soaking for one to three days allows hydrogen cyanide to diffuse out and makes the product safer for consumption. These methods are not redundant. They are separate removal steps aimed at a chemistry that was already activated by fracture.

Fermentation matters especially because cassava is often a staple, not an occasional hazard. Once a root like this becomes daily food, the preparation cannot merely make it look edible. It has to drive the cyanogen burden down hard enough that repeated intake does not keep returning the same toxin problem to the same body. That is why longer, more aggressive traditional sequences developed where cassava was foundational. The literature describes cyanogen reductions above 90 percent with sufficiently extended soaking and fermentation sequences, and one Codex background summary cites a process of soaking followed by grating and fermenting that achieved about 98 percent cyanide removal. That kind of reduction is not culinary ornament. It is what it takes to turn a defended staple root into something the intestine and mitochondria can tolerate repeatedly.

Drying and cooking belong to the same logic, but they are not interchangeable with the earlier steps. Drying helps because liberated hydrogen cyanide is volatile, meaning it can escape into the air once the root has been properly opened and processed. Cooking can help too, but only after the chemistry has been managed correctly upstream. Codex warns that if cassava pieces are exposed to high heat too early, cyanogenic glycosides can remain in the product instead of being adequately broken down and removed first. That is a crucial detail. Heat is not a universal rescue. In cassava, timing and sequence matter. A root that has not been peeled, opened, soaked, pressed, fermented, or otherwise detoxified enough cannot be trusted merely because it was cooked.

So traditional cassava processing exists for the same reason any serious detoxification sequence exists. The food arrives with a problem built into its tissue. The preparation has to remove peel burden, collapse the plant's internal separation, allow enzyme breakdown to proceed, move cyanide and cyanogenic intermediates out into water or air, and only then finish the root into something resembling safe human food. The sequence persisted because it matched the chemistry. A plant that stores carbohydrate under cyanogenic guard cannot be made safe by taste, custom, or optimism alone. It has to be worked open until the defense has somewhere to go other than the body.

Improper Preparation as a Route to Acute and Chronic Toxicity

Cassava becomes dangerous when preparation stops halfway through the chemistry. The root is peeled, grated, pounded, or milled, which is enough to rupture the tissue and bring cyanogenic glycosides into contact with the enzymes that begin their breakdown, but the later steps needed to clear that burden are shortened, weakened, or skipped. That is the worst position to leave the food in. The plant's internal separation has already collapsed, so linamarin and related compounds are no longer sitting quietly in intact tissue, yet the mash or flour has not been soaked, fermented, pressed, dried, or otherwise detoxified long enough to let the released cyanide and its intermediates leave the food. CDC's Uganda outbreak report states this plainly: cassava can cause fatal cyanide poisoning if it is not properly detoxified by steps such as soaking, drying, and scraping before consumption.

That is the route to acute toxicity. The chemistry is concentrated enough, the release is fast enough, and the person eats the product before the burden has been driven down. Acute cassava poisoning then looks like a respiratory toxin hitting the body through a staple food. CDC documented an outbreak in western Uganda involving 98 cases and 2 deaths after inadequately processed cassava flour was eaten, and food safety sources describe acute cyanide intoxication from cassava with symptoms such as rapid breathing, vomiting, abdominal pain, dizziness, weakness, and in severe cases collapse or death. The root is still being treated as starch by the eater, but at the mitochondrial level, cyanide is blocking cytochrome c oxidase, the enzyme complex cells need to use oxygen for energy production. The bowel receives the food first. The respiratory poison declares itself next.

Chronic toxicity appears when the same preparation failure is smaller but repeated. The person may not receive a single overwhelming cyanide load, but day after day the diet keeps delivering enough residual cyanogen from poorly processed cassava to force continual detoxification and tissue stress. The strongest chronic association in the cassava literature is konzo, a sudden-onset, non-progressive spastic paralysis syndrome linked to high dietary cyanogen intake from insufficiently processed bitter cassava, especially in populations also burdened by low sulfur amino acid intake, which weakens cyanide detoxification capacity. FDA also notes that inadequately prepared cassava is linked not only to acute poisoning but to chronic neurologic disease. That is what makes cassava so important in this chapter. It is not merely a root that can poison if eaten raw. It is a staple that can keep returning a smaller cyanide burden to the same nervous system until the cost stops being episodic and becomes part of the body's daily metabolic workload.

Apricot Kernels, Apple Seeds, and Other Seed Tissues as Secondary Examples

The seed examples matter because they show the same cyanogenic logic in a smaller, more concentrated package. The edible flesh and the protected reproductive tissue are not the same biological object. Apricot kernels, bitter almonds, apple seeds, peach pits, and plum kernels all contain amygdalin, a cyanogenic glycoside that can be converted into cyanide during digestion. FDA states this plainly: the chemical is found in the seeds or pits, not in the fruit flesh itself, and while accidentally swallowing a seed or pit is not expected to harm you, consuming larger amounts can become dangerous because intestinal enzymes can turn amygdalin into cyanide. That is the key distinction. The sweetness or familiarity of the fruit does not extend to the chemistry of the seed. The plant made the flesh to invite handling. It kept a harder chemistry around the next generation.

Apricot kernels are the clearest secondary case because the concentration is high enough that the risk stops being theoretical quickly. EFSA concluded that eating more than three small raw apricot kernels, or less than half of one large kernel, in a single serving can exceed the safe acute exposure level for adults, and that even one small kernel can exceed that level for toddlers. FDA issued a 2024 warning on apricot seed products for the same reason, noting that the amygdalin burden in some products was high enough to create a risk of fatal cyanide toxicity. This is why apricot kernels belong in the chapter but remain secondary to cassava. Cassava matters because a defended root becomes a staple and can create both acute and chronic toxicity through daily use. Apricot kernels matter because they reveal the same chemistry in a smaller, more concentrated seed tissue that can become dangerous fast when people treat it as a health product or medicinal food instead of as protected plant reproductive tissue.

Apple seeds and similar fruit seeds belong in the section as quieter examples. They carry the same class of molecule, but ordinary incidental exposure is usually too small to matter because people do not normally chew and consume large numbers of seeds. FDA makes that distinction clear by noting that accidentally eating a seed or pit will not harm you, while larger amounts can become problematic. That is the right physiological frame for the subsection. These seeds are not daily staple burdens on the scale of cassava, and they are not all equal in cyanogenic load. They still belong in the architecture of the chapter because they show the same design principle. The fruit can be edible. The seed can still be chemically defended. Once the seed is crushed, ground, chewed, or concentrated into a product that defeats its natural packaging, the hidden chemistry stops being incidental and starts behaving like what it always was: a reproductive tissue the plant did not intend to surrender cheaply.

Why Edible Flesh and Reproductive Tissue Are Different Biological Structures

A fruit is not one biological object wearing one flavor profile. It is a layered structure built for different jobs at once. The soft outer flesh is one tissue. The seed, pit, or kernel inside it is another. The outer tissue can become sweet, fragrant, pigmented, watery, and physically yielding because one of its functions is to invite contact at the right stage of ripeness. The reproductive core has the opposite problem. It has to remain chemically and structurally intact long enough to protect the next generation. That is why the public reading of a fruit becomes so unreliable. The eater keeps judging the whole structure by the softness and sweetness of the outer tissue, while the plant has built the center under a very different logic.

The flesh is allowed to become metabolically expendable in a way the seed cannot. Cells in the pulp can swell with sugars, organic acids, water, pigments, and aroma compounds because that tissue is serving dispersal. It can afford to be eaten under the right conditions. Its architecture reflects that. The walls soften. Starch can be converted. Acidity can shift. Volatile compounds rise. The texture changes from resistance to surrender. None of that means the plant has abandoned defense. It means the defense has been redistributed. The invitation is concentrated in the tissue meant to be handled. The protection is concentrated in the tissue that cannot afford to be digested.

The seed, pit, or kernel is carrying a different economic problem for the plant. It is storing embryonic tissue, reserve material, and the structural possibility of another plant. So its chemistry stays harder. The outer covering is tougher. The storage compounds are denser. The defensive molecules are often sharper. Cyanogenic glycosides in apricot kernels and similar reproductive tissues fit that pattern cleanly. The fruit can ripen into sweetness while the kernel remains a latent cyanide system. There is no contradiction there. The flesh was built to be approached. The reproductive tissue was built to survive the approach. One tissue can welcome contact. The other has to make contact costly.

That difference only becomes dangerous to the eater once the plant's compartmentalization is defeated. A whole pit or seed moving intact through the gut is not the same physiological situation as a chewed kernel, a crushed seed, or a ground meal made from reproductive tissue. Intact structure limits enzyme access. Rupture changes everything. The moment the seed is cracked, chewed, milled, or otherwise broken open, the interior chemistry is no longer protected from moisture, plant enzymes, digestive enzymes, and mechanical mixing. The plant's internal separation collapses. What was stored as guarded reproductive chemistry begins behaving like active toxic or antinutritional chemistry in the eater. That is why people get into trouble when they stop eating the fruit and start eating the reproductive tissue as though the two belonged to the same food category.

So the useful distinction is not fruit versus seed in the abstract. It is expendable outer tissue versus defended reproductive tissue. The soft flesh can carry one message to the eater while the pit carries another. Sweetness in the pulp says nothing reliable about the kernel. The pleasant outer tissue does not clear the chemistry of the center. Once that is understood, the structure becomes easier to read across the whole plant world. The plant can make the outside edible without surrendering the inside. The body pays the price when people mistake the invitation of the flesh for permission to consume the guarded reproductive core.

Chapter 16

Cucurbitacins: When Bitter Squash Becomes Dangerous

Bitterness is the first clue, but bitterness is not the molecule. In squash, zucchini, cucumbers, gourds, and related cucurbits, the bitter warning comes largely from cucurbitacins, a family of highly oxygenated triterpenoids, meaning thirty-carbon plant compounds built from terpene chemistry and then heavily modified with oxygen-containing groups. Recent reviews describe them as common secondary metabolites in the Cucurbitaceae family, and toxicology summaries note that they are the principal natural toxins known in these plants. The fruit can still look watery, soft, and ordinary. The chemistry inside it can still be a defense system.

What makes cucurbitacins matter is not just that they are bitter. It is that the plant uses them to make feeding less profitable. These molecules are concentrated forms of resistance. Extension and crop-disease sources describe cucurbitacins as plant-produced bitter compounds selected down in cultivated edible lines because high levels make the fruit unpleasant and, at high enough concentrations, dangerous to humans and animals. In other words, the mild modern zucchini or squash people expect to eat is already the result of human selection against a stronger ancestral defense chemistry. The soft edible fruit did not begin as a neutral water-and-fiber package. It began as cucurbit tissue carrying a more aggressive deterrent system.

The structure of these molecules helps explain why the warning is so forceful. Cucurbitacins are not simple flavor compounds drifting through the flesh. They are highly modified, strongly bitter triterpenoid molecules whose biological activity sits close to their toxic range in many reviews. Some are present as glycosides, meaning sugar-linked forms, and different cucurbits can accumulate different members of the family, such as cucurbitacin B, C, or E and related compounds. The common thread is the same. The fruit carries a chemically active deterrent that can shift from unpleasant to overtly toxic when concentrations rise high enough. That is why "bitter squash" is not a culinary complaint first. It is a plant-defense signal that has become intense enough for the eater to notice.

This is also why cucurbitacins belong in a chapter about dangerous plant tissue rather than in a chapter about flavor. The molecule is telling you what kind of tissue you are eating. A cultivated squash with low cucurbitacin expression behaves like a mild fruiting body. A stressed, crossed, or aberrant squash with high cucurbitacin expression behaves like defended plant tissue again. The eater may still see zucchini, pumpkin, cucumber, or bottle gourd. The bowel receives a bitter triterpenoid defense chemistry that the plant never meant to surrender cheaply.

Why Unusual Bitterness Is a Warning Sign

The mouth often catches the problem before the stomach has to. A squash, zucchini, cucumber, or bottle gourd that tastes sharply and abnormally bitter is not simply off-flavor produce. It is usually showing you that cucurbitacin expression has risen beyond the mild range expected in cultivated edible varieties. Food-safety and horticulture sources treat this bitterness as a practical warning sign because cucurbitacins are the major bitter toxic compounds in cucurbits and their presence at unusually high levels correlates with poisoning risk.

That warning matters because bitterness in this case is not a culinary preference issue. It is the sensory face of a defense molecule. Cucurbitacins are highly oxygenated triterpenoids with extremely bitter taste, and they were bred down in normal food cultivars precisely because the stronger ancestral chemistry made the fruit less edible and, at high concentrations, unsafe. When that bitterness reappears strongly, the fruit is no longer behaving like the soft, selected, low-burden vegetable people think they are eating. It is behaving more like defended cucurbit tissue again.

The biology behind the warning is straightforward. Modern edible cucurbits were selected for low cucurbitacin content in the flesh, but that selection can be disrupted. Cross-pollination with ornamental gourds, reversion in saved seed, environmental stress, or other breeding irregularities can restore bitter chemistry in the fruit. Extension sources describe toxic squash poisoning exactly this way: an edible-looking squash or zucchini can develop abnormal cucurbitacin levels and taste intensely bitter even though it still looks ordinary from the outside. The appearance stays familiar. The chemistry changes first.

That is why the advice around bitter cucurbits is harsher than people expect. The correct response is not to cook it longer, season it harder, or eat around the bitterness. Heat does not reliably make the problem disappear because cucurbitacins are not just volatile aroma compounds that can be cooked off casually. Poison-center and clinical case literature describe severe gastrointestinal poisoning after ingestion of unusually bitter squash or bottle gourd, often with abrupt vomiting, diarrhea, abdominal pain, and in some cases bleeding or shock. When the bitterness is strong and abnormal, the plant has already done the useful diagnostic work for you.

So unusual bitterness matters because it is one of the few warning systems in plant food chemistry that is still readable without a laboratory. The fruit may still look soft, fresh, and edible. The mouth is telling you the tissue has shifted back toward defense. In this chapter that makes bitter squash a valuable example. It shows that a common vegetable can remain visually ordinary while the chemical profile has moved into a range where the safest interpretation is simple: the plant is no longer offering food first. It is showing you its deterrent chemistry.

Squash, Zucchini, and Gourds as Examples

The useful thing about squash, zucchini, and gourds is that they look so normal. They are watery fruiting bodies, soft-fleshed, kitchen-friendly, easy to slice, roast, sauté, juice, or blend. They do not read like chemically defended tissue in the way a bitter medicinal herb or a hard seed does. That is exactly what makes them strong examples. In the cucurbit family, the same tissue that can look mild and edible can still shift back toward a harder defensive chemistry if cucurbitacin production rises. Extension guidance for toxic squash treats zucchini and summer squash this way, not as exotic poisons but as ordinary garden foods that can become dangerous when bitter chemistry returns.

Zucchini is the clearest household example because people expect it to be bland. When a zucchini turns sharply bitter, the change is not culinary personality. It is chemical reversion. The fruit is no longer behaving like the selected low-cucurbitacin tissue people buy at the store. It is behaving more like defended cucurbit tissue again. Oregon State Extension warns that even a couple grams of extremely bitter squash can cause stomach cramps and diarrhea lasting up to three days, and the Pacific Northwest handbook warns not to eat unusually bitter zucchini or squash at all. The flesh may still look tender and harmless. The mouth is already telling you the chemistry has shifted.

Bottle gourd shows the same chemistry in a harsher form because it is often consumed as juice or in larger concentrated servings. That changes the exposure immediately. A bitter bottle gourd is not merely unpleasant produce. Clinical case reports and reviews describe rapid-onset nausea, vomiting, diarrhea, abdominal pain, gastrointestinal bleeding, and hypotension after ingestion of unusually bitter bottle gourd or its juice. Once the fruit has been juiced, the tissue is no longer buffered by much structure, and the bitter compounds have been delivered in a form the stomach receives quickly. The fruit kept its ordinary identity. The preparation increased the speed and density of chemical contact.

Squash and gourds also matter because the same family contains both the familiar edible forms and the more obviously hard-edged warning forms. That family relationship helps explain why the danger can reappear in the garden without changing the fruit's shape enough to warn the eater visually. Cross-pollination with ornamental gourds, volunteer growth, seed saving from unstable crosses, and plant stress are all cited by extension sources as routes by which cucurbitacin burden can rise again in home-grown fruits. The skin can still look marketable. The interior can still cook down like an ordinary vegetable. The defensive chemistry has already moved before appearance catches up, if appearance ever does.

That is why squash, zucchini, and gourds belong together in this chapter. They show the same rule inside different kitchen forms. A soft green zucchini, a yellow squash, or a pale bottle gourd can still be defended fruit tissue under the wrong conditions. The warning is not rarity. The warning is bitterness. Once the flesh tastes abnormally bitter, the plant has stopped offering a mild cultivated fruit and has started reasserting the chemistry it uses to make feeding costly. The bowel receives the fruit as ordinary only when the defense has been bred down and stays down. When that fails, the same soft flesh becomes a delivery system for deterrent chemistry instead of a low-burden vegetable.

Acute Nausea, Vomiting, Diarrhea, and Toxicity Reports

Cucurbitacin poisoning usually announces itself through the gut first, and it does so fast. The person eats a squash, zucchini, cucumber, or bottle gourd that tastes sharply and abnormally bitter, and within a short window the bowel begins reacting as though it has been hit with chemically aggressive plant tissue rather than ordinary produce. Nausea comes first in many reports, then repeated vomiting, abdominal pain, cramping, and diarrhea. The bitterness matters because it is the sensory face of the toxin burden. In the Indian review of bitter bottle gourd poisoning, the authors describe abrupt gastrointestinal toxicity with severe abdominal pain, vomiting, diarrhea, and in some cases hematemesis, meaning vomiting of blood, because the mucosa, the living gastrointestinal lining, is being injured hard enough that the problem is no longer just food intolerance. The German assessment of bitter zucchini reports the same direction of injury from a different cucurbit tissue, noting that ingestion of about 3 g of bitter zucchini was sufficient in one case to trigger nausea, collapse, severe stomach cramps lasting three days, and diarrhea. These are not subtle post-meal complaints. They are the body reacting to cucurbit tissue whose deterrent chemistry has risen back into the humanly dangerous range.

The toxicity reports become more serious once the bitter tissue is concentrated or the mucosal injury is stronger. Bottle gourd juice is the clearest example because juicing removes much of the plant structure that would otherwise slow intake and delivers the bitter chemistry quickly to the stomach. Case reports describe hypotension, hematemesis, shock, and severe gastrointestinal distress after ingestion of bitter bottle gourd juice, and poison reviews on toxic squash syndrome describe the same broader pattern for cucurbit poisoning in general: violent vomiting, diarrhea, cramping, and systemic deterioration when the toxin burden is high enough. The reason these reports matter in the chapter is that they show the fruit does not need to look exotic or medicinal to become dangerous. It can still look like ordinary kitchen produce. The bowel is the first membrane field forced to absorb the mistake. Once the cucurbitacin load is high enough, the fruit stops behaving like soft edible flesh and starts behaving like defended plant tissue that is stripping comfort, fluid balance, and epithelial stability from the gut.

Why Taste Can Function as a Defense Alarm the Eater Ignores at Their Own Risk

Taste is not only about preference. It is part of the body's first-contact screening system. Bitter taste receptors exist because plant tissues and other environmental materials can carry compounds that are chemically active enough to injure, disrupt, or poison if swallowed in the wrong amount. Reviews of bitter taste biology describe bitterness as a signal strongly tied to toxic plant products and other noxious compounds, which is why the mouth can begin rejecting a food before the stomach or intestine has been forced to absorb the lesson in a harsher way.

Cucurbits make that system unusually easy to read because the bitter warning comes from the same molecules driving the risk. In squash, zucchini, cucumbers, and gourds, abnormal bitterness points toward elevated cucurbitacins, the bitter triterpenoid defense compounds that cultivated edible varieties are normally bred to keep low. Extension guidance on toxic squash states that fruits with higher cucurbitacin levels can still look normal while tasting bitter, and clinical reviews of bitter bottle gourd poisoning describe the same chemistry from the medical side, with increased cucurbitacin levels turning the fruit bitter and producing gastrointestinal toxicity. The appearance stays friendly. The taste changes first.

That is why taste functions as an alarm rather than as a garnish on the meal. The eye can miss the problem because a bitter zucchini or gourd may still look fresh, hydrated, and edible. The knife can miss it because the flesh can still slice and cook like an ordinary vegetable. The tongue is often the first tissue that catches the plant's reasserted defense chemistry. If the bitterness is sharp, unusual, and out of character for the food, the plant is no longer presenting the eater with the mild cultivated tissue they expected. It is presenting a fruit whose deterrent chemistry has risen enough to be felt directly. Poison information and extension sources say to stop eating at that point because bitter cucurbits are the recognized signal condition for toxic squash syndrome.

People get into trouble when they reinterpret that warning as a culinary flaw instead of a biological one. They cook the bitterness down, season over it, dilute it into a dish, or in the case of bottle gourd, juice it and swallow a concentrated exposure quickly. The chemistry does not care that the eater hoped the bitterness meant rustic flavor or garden variability. Clinical reports of bitter bottle gourd poisoning and toxic squash poisoning describe abrupt nausea, vomiting, diarrhea, abdominal pain, and in severe cases bleeding, hypotension, or shock after ingestion of unusually bitter cucurbits. The mouth had already given the correct diagnosis. The gut pays when that alarm is overruled.

So taste matters here because it is one of the few defense signals still readable without a laboratory. A bitter taste in an ordinary squash is not merely unpleasantness sitting on top of edible flesh. It is the plant's deterrent chemistry reaching a level high enough for the sensory gate to catch it. Once that signal is ignored, the same tissue moves into the stomach, the intestine, and the blood with no additional courtesy warning. The eater had the useful information in the mouth. The bowel receives the consequences when that information is treated like flavor instead of defense.

The Difference Between Ordinary Produce and Abnormal Defense Expression

An ordinary zucchini, squash, or gourd is still plant tissue, but it is plant tissue that has been bred and stabilized so the edible fruit carries low enough cucurbitacin burden that the flesh behaves like food rather than like deterrent chemistry. That distinction matters because the cultivated fruit people expect to cook is not neutral by nature. It is the result of selection against bitterness in the part humans eat. Reviews of cucurbit bitterness describe domestication of edible cucurbits as a process that reduced cucurbitacin expression in fruit tissue while leaving the plant family's underlying defense system intact.

Abnormal defense expression begins when that selected balance fails. The fruit still looks like produce. The shape may remain familiar, the skin may remain smooth, the water content may remain high, and the flesh may still cut and cook normally. But the chemistry has shifted back toward a more defended state. In bitter Luffa and other cucurbits, metabolomic and transcriptomic work shows that bitter fruit contains markedly higher cucurbitacin levels and higher expression of the biosynthetic pathway behind them than non-bitter fruit. The plant has not turned into a different species. The edible fruit has simply moved away from the low-defense profile expected of the cultivated form.

That shift can happen for more than one reason. Extension guidance on toxic squash points to cross-pollination with ornamental gourds and seed-saving problems as practical routes by which strong bitterness can reappear in garden fruit. Research literature adds another route: stress. Studies in luffa and other cucurbits show that drought, temperature extremes, and related abiotic stress can activate cucurbitacin biosynthesis, which means the fruit can move chemically before it looks visibly abnormal. The outside remains marketable. The inside has begun reasserting a defense program the eater was not expecting.

That is the real divide between ordinary produce and abnormal defense expression. Ordinary produce still belongs to a defended plant family, but the fruit flesh has been kept within a range where bitterness stays low and toxic burden stays low. Abnormal defense expression means the fruit has slipped back toward the chemistry of deterrence. The mouth usually catches that first. The bitterness becomes sharp, unfamiliar, and out of proportion to what zucchini, summer squash, or bottle gourd should taste like when the fruit is acting like food rather than like a warning structure. Extension and toxicology sources both treat that bitterness as the practical sign that the fruit is no longer behaving like ordinary produce.

This is why appearance is not a reliable safeguard. A fruit can remain visually ordinary while its metabolic profile has moved into a more aggressive state. The eater expects water, mild carbohydrate, soft fiber, and a low-friction vegetable. The bowel receives bitter triterpenoid defense compounds instead. Once the flesh has shifted that far, the problem is no longer spoilage or flavor variation. It is that the cultivated edible tissue has begun expressing chemistry closer to the plant's ancestral defensive pattern than to the low-bitter profile the kitchen expects.

So ordinary produce and abnormal defense expression are not separated by category labels. They are separated by what the fruit is doing chemically. One behaves like selected edible flesh. The other behaves like cucurbit tissue that has tightened its chemical guard again. The shape on the cutting board may be the same. The digestive sequence is not.

Chapter 17

Other Natural Plant Toxins Worth Understanding

Some plant tissues do not defend themselves mainly with bitterness, crystals, or mineral traps. They defend themselves with light-reactive chemistry. Furanocoumarins, sometimes called furocoumarins, are one of the clearest examples. Chemically, they are coumarin compounds fused to a furan ring, which gives them a structure able to absorb ultraviolet A light, the longer-wave ultraviolet range that reaches the skin and shallow tissues. They are found in several ordinary food plants, especially in members of the citrus and parsley-carrot families, including grapefruit, limes, lemons, celery, and parsnip. WHO describes them as plant stress toxins that are released or increased under stress and physical damage, which already tells you what kind of tissue they belong to. They are not there to nourish the eater. They are there because the plant expects injury.

That tissue context matters because furanocoumarins are often concentrated where contact and damage are most likely to occur. Celery and parsnip are exposed stalk and root tissues that still have to survive microbial attack, bruising, and feeding. Citrus peel and outer fruit tissues sit at the plant-environment boundary and carry their own protective chemistry. Surveys of food plants have measured furanocoumarins in celery and parsnip, and broader food-chemistry work identifies phototoxic furanocoumarins in citrus species, parsley, celery, parsnip, and figs. The useful pattern is simple. These compounds tend to appear in tissues that need a harder outer chemistry than the pleasant public reputation of the food would suggest. The produce still looks ordinary. The plant has built a light-activated deterrent into it.

The most obvious damage pathway is phototoxicity. Once furanocoumarins contact skin and are then exposed to ultraviolet A light, they can react with cellular material and trigger phytophotodermatitis, a plant-light skin injury pattern marked by redness, burning, blistering, and later dark pigmentation. WHO identifies furanocoumarins as phototoxic compounds capable of causing severe skin reactions after sunlight exposure, and dermatology reviews point to citrus, celery, parsnip, and fig as common human sources of this reaction. This is why celery handlers, bartenders squeezing limes, and people working with parsnip or giant hogweed can end up with skin injury that looks chemical rather than allergic. The plant did not need thorns to punish contact. It used a molecule that waits for light to finish the job.

The same compound class can create a different burden after swallowing rather than handling. Grapefruit is the major food example because its furanocoumarins can inhibit cytochrome P450 3A4, usually shortened to CYP3A4, one of the main drug-metabolizing enzyme systems in the intestinal wall. That means the fruit can change first-pass metabolism, the early breakdown step that normally lowers how much of an oral drug enters the bloodstream. Reviews of grapefruit chemistry and drug interaction literature identify furanocoumarins as the main compounds responsible for this effect, and NCCIH notes that grapefruit juice can raise the blood levels of certain medicines through this mechanism. The fruit is still being sold as produce. The intestine is being asked to absorb a pharmacologically active exposure that can alter drug handling before the liver ever gets a chance to compensate.

That is why furanocoumarins belong in a chapter on other natural plant toxins worth understanding. They show two different ways plant chemistry can stop being nutritionally innocent. In one setting the compound stays on the surface, meets skin, and waits for sunlight. In another it enters the gut, meets the enzyme-rich wall of the small intestine, and changes what crosses into blood. Some of these compounds can also cause gastrointestinal problems in susceptible people, as WHO notes, but the larger lesson is structural. A celery stalk, a parsnip root, or a grapefruit can still be carrying a plant defense system that works through light activation, membrane contact, or enzyme interference rather than through the more familiar paths of bitterness or mineral binding. The food keeps the ordinary reputation. The tissue keeps the harder chemistry.

Psoralens and Photoactive Compounds

Some plant toxins do not do their damage by binding minerals, trapping enzymes, or poisoning the gut after swallowing. They wait for light. Psoralens are the clearest example. They belong to the broader furanocoumarin family, which means they are coumarin compounds fused to a furan ring, but the important part is not the name. The important part is that their structure absorbs ultraviolet A, the longer-wave ultraviolet light that reaches skin easily enough to turn simple plant contact into tissue injury. Reviews of phytophotodermatitis identify psoralens and related furanocoumarins as the key phototoxic agents in many plant exposures.

That chemistry makes sense in the tissues that carry it. Plants such as celery, parsnip, parsley, figs, limes, lemons, grapefruit, and other citrus fruits are not storing these compounds as nutrients for the eater. WHO describes furanocoumarins as stress toxins released or increased in response to plant stress and physical damage, which already places them in the defense category rather than the nourishment category. A cut celery stalk, bruised parsnip tissue, squeezed lime peel, or damaged citrus rind is not just leaking flavor. It may also be exposing a light-reactive defense chemistry the intact tissue had kept more contained.

Once psoralens reach skin and then meet ultraviolet A light, the mechanism becomes more specific. These molecules can intercalate, meaning slide into the space between DNA bases, and after ultraviolet A exposure they form covalent adducts with nucleic acids. Under continued exposure they can create cross-links, which means they tie strands of DNA together in a way the cell cannot tolerate cleanly. That is why the skin reaction can be so harsh. This is not ordinary irritation. It is photoactivated chemical injury. The resulting pattern, phytophotodermatitis, often begins with burning, redness, tenderness, or blistering and later leaves dark persistent pigmentation because the tissue has been damaged where plant compound and light overlapped.

This also explains why psoralens occupy a strange middle ground between toxin and drug. In one setting they are accidental plant defenses that punish contact. In another, the same chemistry is used deliberately in PUVA, psoralen plus ultraviolet A therapy, because the DNA-reactive and photoactive properties are strong enough to be used therapeutically against certain skin diseases. That medical use is not evidence of innocence. It proves potency. A compound chosen for controlled phototherapy is not a harmless flavor note when it arrives unintentionally on skin from lime juice, celery sap, or bruised parsnip tissue. The tissue changes. The compound activates. Light finishes the sequence.

So psoralens matter in this chapter because they show a different kind of plant warning system. The food or plant may still look fresh, edible, and familiar. The danger appears only after the tissue has been cut, squeezed, bruised, or handled and then exposed to sunlight. That makes these compounds easy to underestimate. The celery stalk looks like produce. The lime looks like garnish. The parsnip looks like a root vegetable. The skin receives a light-armed toxin whose damage is triggered only after contact has already happened.

Natural Nitrates and Nitrite Conversion in Context

A leafy green or beet is not carrying nitrate by accident. Nitrate is part of plant nitrogen handling. It moves through the plant as a nitrogen reserve and an intermediate in protein-building metabolism, which is why higher levels show up especially in fast-growing leafy tissues and some roots such as spinach, lettuce, beetroot, and celery. Food-source reviews estimate that most dietary nitrate in humans comes from vegetables, not from additives, and EFSA notes that leafy vegetables are among the highest natural accumulators. The plant is using nitrate as a workable nitrogen pool. The eater receives that chemistry in the same tissue that carries the vegetable's clean reputation.

Nitrate itself is the quieter molecule. The more reactive step is what happens after the body and the oral microbiome get hold of it. A significant fraction of absorbed nitrate is taken up by the salivary glands, concentrated back into saliva, and then reduced by nitrate-reducing bacteria on the tongue into nitrite. When that nitrite is swallowed, the acidic stomach can push part of it further toward nitric oxide and related reactive nitrogen chemistry. That is the useful side of the pathway people now talk about in vascular physiology, but the same sequence is also the reason nitrate cannot be dismissed as inert plant background. It is a precursor pool whose meaning depends on where it is converted, how much is present, and what other molecules are in the same digestive field.

The first danger lane is excess nitrite burden, not nitrate as an abstract number on a chart. Nitrite can oxidize hemoglobin into methemoglobin, a form that carries oxygen poorly. That is why methemoglobinemia, sometimes called blue baby syndrome, sits at the center of nitrate risk discussions. EFSA states that nitrate in leafy vegetables is not a health concern for most children, but it also notes that infants and young children consuming large amounts of high-nitrate spinach can reach exposures where a risk of methemoglobinemia cannot be excluded. The same statement adds two details that matter far more than most food tables ever show: bacterial gastrointestinal infection increases nitrate-to-nitrite conversion, and inappropriate storage of cooked leafy vegetables at room temperature can raise nitrite further. A pureed spinach meal left to sit is not the same physiological exposure as freshly cooked leaves on a plate.

The second danger lane is nitrosation. Nitrite can react with amines under acidic conditions and generate N-nitrosamines, a group of compounds that includes known carcinogens. That chemistry is not guaranteed every time nitrate-rich vegetables are eaten, and the food matrix matters, but the risk pathway is real enough that toxicology reviews keep returning to it. Reviews of nitrite chemistry describe the reaction with secondary amines as especially concerning because it can form carcinogenic nitrosamines, and human work has shown increased urinary N-nitrosodimethylamine, or NDMA, excretion when nitrate intake was paired with fish meals rich in nitrosatable precursors. The same nitrate molecule can therefore feed nitric-oxide biology in one context and nitrosating chemistry in another.

That is why "natural nitrates" have to be read in context rather than praised or condemned in one move. A spinach leaf, a beet, or a celery stalk is not identical to nitrate-contaminated well water, and ordinary vegetable intake is not identical to concentrated juice, stored puree, or repeated high-load feeding in a vulnerable infant. The source matters. The matrix matters. The co-traveling chemistry matters. Recent review literature has been moving in that direction, arguing that the food source moderates whether nitrate exposure leans more toward nitric-oxide generation or toward the more toxic side of nitrite and nitrosamine chemistry. But that moderation does not erase the burden. It only means the burden has to be judged where it is created, in the mouth, the stomach, the intestinal contents, the blood, and the host receiving the exposure.

So nitrates belong in this chapter because they show another way a plant compound can keep a wholesome public identity while still carrying a conditional toxic sequence inside it. The leaf stores nitrate as part of plant nitrogen metabolism. Oral bacteria turn some of it into nitrite. Acid pushes some of that nitrite further. In one body and one meal that chemistry may stay modest and uneventful. In another, especially with high exposure, poor storage, heavy pureeing, infection, or infant physiology, the same sequence can move toward methemoglobin formation and reduced oxygen handling. The plant kept the nitrogen reserve. The body inherits the conversion chemistry.

Salicylates and Amines in Sensitive Hosts

This is a narrower and less settled lane than oxalate, phytate, or cassava, but it still matters because the symptoms can be real even when the chemistry is harder to prove cleanly. The key point is that these reactions are usually framed as food chemical intolerance, meaning a non-immune, pharmacologic-type response to naturally occurring compounds rather than a classic immunoglobulin E, or IgE, food allergy. The symptom pattern is usually mixed rather than tidy. The same person may report urticaria, which is hives, angioedema, which is deeper tissue swelling, rhinitis, flushing, abdominal pain, or diarrhea after foods that do not fit a simple allergy story. Reviews of food chemical intolerance also emphasize that the evidence base is limited and that the true prevalence is unknown.

Salicylates are naturally occurring salicylic-acid-related compounds found in plant foods. They matter here not because they are proven universal toxins, but because in a subset of sensitive people they appear to behave more like recurrent pharmacologic exposures than like ordinary nutrients. The stronger modern evidence is still narrow. A 2025 systematic review and meta-analysis found low-certainty evidence linking salicylate intolerance to flare in atopic dermatitis, and the broader 2015 review concluded that some individuals may benefit from short-term removal of natural food chemicals, including salicylates, if the foods are later reintroduced to test whether the response was real. That is a much smaller claim than "salicylates are bad." It is a host claim. The same chemical load can pass quietly through one body and keep provoking skin, airway, or bowel symptoms in another.

Amines are a different chemical family. Here the most important food examples are biogenic amines, meaning small nitrogen-containing compounds such as histamine, tyramine, putrescine, and cadaverine that can accumulate in foods or be present as part of normal tissue chemistry. The current histamine-intolerance literature frames the problem as an imbalance between histamine exposure and histamine degradation, especially when diamine oxidase, or DAO, the main intestinal enzyme that degrades dietary histamine, is low or blocked. That model becomes more interesting because other amines can interfere with histamine breakdown in vitro, which means the host is not only dealing with histamine itself but with a broader amine field competing for the same degradative machinery. This does not prove that every person with headaches, flushing, itch, or bowel symptoms is reacting to food amines. It does show why the problem, when it exists, would be host-dependent and chemically cumulative rather than visually obvious from the plate.

The evidence on dietary amines is more conflicted than the evidence on oxalate or phytate, and that has to stay visible in the chapter. An older review of oral challenge studies concluded that the conclusive studies available at the time did not support a relation between ingestion of biogenic amines and food intolerance reactions. A more recent eczema-focused meta-analysis, by contrast, reported low-certainty evidence that histamine, amines, and salicylates may flare symptoms in a substantial subgroup of people with atopic dermatitis. The 2015 review sits between those positions. It describes the clinical suspicion as persistent, the mechanisms as poorly studied, and the quality of the dietary evidence as limited. That combination is exactly why this section belongs under "other toxins worth understanding" rather than under the stronger structural chapters. The chemistry is plausible. The host responses may be real. The certainty is lower and the subgroups matter more.

So the useful frame is not that fruits and vegetables rich in salicylates or amines are secretly poisoning everyone. The useful frame is that some hosts appear to react to these compounds as repeated chemical exposures rather than as neutral background components of food, and that the symptoms can involve skin, airway, gut, or vascular responses rather than one clean organ system. When that pattern is investigated, the literature supports short-term elimination followed by reintroduction or challenge, not indefinite ideology, because broad low-food-chemical diets can create nutritional deficiency if they are imposed carelessly. In the wrong host, the same meal keeps returning to the same mucosal surfaces, the same mediator systems, and the same degradative bottlenecks until itch, bowel urgency, flushing, or eczema flare stop looking random and start reading like repeated chemistry.

Why Some Compounds Matter Only in Subgroups While Others Matter at Population Scale

The difference begins with where the chemistry collides with human physiology. Some compounds strike a near-universal bottleneck. They enter the gut and run into machinery that works the same way in most people. Phytate is the clearest example. Its phosphate-rich structure binds zinc and iron in the intestinal lumen, the hollow interior of the gut where digestion and absorption are still unfolding, and that binding chemistry does not depend on a rare host trait to become relevant. If a meal is heavily built from cereals, legumes, nuts, or seeds and the phytate load is high enough, zinc absorption falls in predictable ways across populations because the mineral is being held in complexes the absorptive surface cannot recover easily. Reviews on zinc absorption and phytic acid keep returning to this point: high-phytate staple diets lower zinc bioavailability broadly, not just in a tiny sensitive minority.

Other burdens behave the same way at the level of mechanics rather than mineral chemistry. FODMAP carbohydrates, the fermentable oligosaccharides, disaccharides, monosaccharides, and polyols that remain poorly absorbed in many intestines, create osmotic pull and bacterial fermentation because of what the molecules are, not because of a rare immunologic defect. But here the scale shifts. The chemistry is broad. The symptom burden is not. Many people can absorb enough, dilute enough, or tolerate enough luminal expansion that the same retained carbohydrate does not turn into major distress. In people with irritable bowel syndrome, altered motility, or visceral hypersensitivity, meaning a bowel that feels stretch and gas pressure too strongly, the same carbohydrate burden becomes bloating, pain, urgency, or constipation much more reliably. The molecule is common. The clinical cost is concentrated in a subgroup whose bowel has less reserve.

That host dependence becomes even stronger with food chemicals such as salicylates, amines, and histamine-related exposures. These do not usually create a clear population-scale lesion the way phytate lowers zinc absorption in high-phytate staple diets. The evidence base is narrower, the mechanisms are less settled, and the reactions appear to depend much more on individual thresholds, degradation capacity, barrier behavior, mediator release, and symptom pattern. Recent review work on salicylate and amine intolerance in atopic dermatitis found only low-certainty evidence for a meaningful subgroup effect, and broader reviews of food chemical intolerance describe the field as clinically plausible but limited in prevalence data and mechanistic certainty. These compounds matter, but they matter through host susceptibility far more than through a universal digestive choke point.

Dose, frequency, and dietary role then decide whether a chemistry stays subgroup-specific or starts looking population-wide. A food chemical that appears only occasionally, in small amounts, or in foods that are not foundational may never rise above the threshold where most people notice it. A compound carried daily in staple grains, legumes, and seed foods can become a governing feature of mineral biology because the same binding sequence keeps returning meal after meal. A single onion may be harmless in one bowel and provocative in another. A diet structurally built on phytate-heavy staples forces the same zinc and iron losses through the same intestinal machinery often enough that the burden stops being anecdotal and becomes nutritional architecture. An occasional food and a foundational food are not the same biological decision.

So the dividing line is not whether a compound is natural, famous, or chemically active. The dividing line is where it acts, how universally that mechanism applies, and whether the host has to bring a special vulnerability for the burden to become visible. Phytate matters at population scale because it binds minerals in staple foods through a chemistry most intestines cannot simply outthink. FODMAPs sit in the middle, common molecules with subgroup-heavy symptom expression because pressure tolerance differs from bowel to bowel. Salicylates and amines matter further downstream in host-specific territory, where the same meal can move quietly through one body and keep returning to the same skin, airway, mast cell, or bowel sensitivity in another. The food may look the same on the plate. The physiology decides whether the chemistry becomes a broad public burden or a narrower recurrent problem in susceptible tissue.

How to Rank Toxins by Strength of Evidence and Frequency of Real-World Exposure

Do not rank plant toxins by how frightening they sound. Rank them the way food-risk assessment is actually done. The formal structure used by Codex, FAO, WHO, and related risk frameworks moves through hazard identification, hazard characterization, exposure assessment, and risk characterization. For this book, that can be compressed into two governing questions. First, how hard is the mechanism and human evidence. Second, how often does ordinary real-world eating create the exposure. A toxin that is dramatic but rare belongs in a different place from a compound that is less theatrical but enters common meals every day. FAO's risk-ranking guidance and WHO's dietary exposure framework both make that logic explicit. Relevance depends on public-health risk, which means hazard and exposure have to be judged together rather than separately.

The first axis is evidence strength. The strongest section-level compounds are the ones where the mechanism is clear, the human consequence is established, and the digestive or metabolic failure point is easy to show in tissue. Oxalate and phytate rank high here. Oxalate has a clean gut-to-kidney sequence, with dietary oxalate contributing to urinary oxalate burden and calcium oxalate stone risk, while phytic acid has strong evidence for reducing iron and zinc bioavailability in phytate-rich diets. FODMAPs also carry a strong mechanism, but they belong in a different subcategory because the chemistry is broad while the clinically significant symptom burden concentrates in susceptible bowels such as irritable bowel syndrome. At the weaker end sit salicylates and amines, where the literature still describes limited or low-certainty evidence and a much stronger dependence on subgroup response.

The second axis is exposure frequency. This is where many rankings fail. A severe toxin can matter less to the average reader than a less dramatic compound that appears in ordinary staple foods or common health foods every week. WHO notes that in a usual balanced diet many natural toxins remain below thresholds for acute and chronic toxicity, which means frequency and concentration determine whether a toxin stays theoretical or becomes physiologically relevant. That is why oxalates in spinach and nuts, phytate in cereals and legumes, and FODMAP burdens in common fruits, onions, garlic, and legumes deserve more chapter weight than their drama level alone would suggest. By contrast, cassava cyanogenic glycosides can produce acute poisoning and chronic neurologic disease, but the exposure is concentrated in cassava-dependent populations or in failed processing events. Cucurbitacins in bitter squash can be violent, but they are irregular. The chemistry is serious. The ordinary exposure is not common in the same way.

Once those two axes are held together, the ranking becomes much cleaner. The first tier in a book like this should be the compounds with strong mechanism and common exposure, especially when the burden can be repeated through staple foods or socially approved "healthy" foods. That puts oxalates and phytates near the top, with FODMAP burden close behind, though FODMAPs should be written as a high-frequency subgroup burden rather than a universal toxin chapter. The next tier is the compounds with strong mechanism but more conditional exposure. Glycoalkaloids belong there because potatoes are common but the toxic burden rises mainly in stressed, greened, or sprouting tubers, and EFSA did not identify evidence of repeated long-term health problems from ordinary potato glycoalkaloid intake in the general population. Furanocoumarins belong there too. Grapefruit and some celery- or citrus-related exposures are real and well established, but the burden is route-specific or drug-specific rather than a universal population-wide loss built into every meal. Cassava cyanogenic glycosides and bitter-cucurbit cucurbitacins sit in the high-hazard but lower-frequency tier. Salicylates and amines remain lower-priority chapters because the evidence is weaker and the host-dependence is stronger.

So the ranking rule for the manuscript should stay blunt. Put first the toxins and antinutrients that are mechanistically hard, common in ordinary foods, and capable of creating repeated loss in digestion, absorption, or excretion. Put next the compounds that are mechanistically serious but need stress, failed preparation, or a narrower exposure route to become dangerous. Put last the compounds that may matter, but mostly in subgroups and with weaker evidentiary support. That keeps the book organized by biological consequence instead of by spectacle. The reader needs the compounds that quietly win the exposure battle every day before they need the compounds that only occasionally make the news.

Part V

Endocrine and Metabolic Interference

Chapter 18

Goitrogens and the Thyroid

The thyroid does not use iodine as a loose nutrient drifting through blood. It pulls iodine into a very specific piece of tissue architecture. The gland is built from follicles, small spheres lined by thyrocytes, the epithelial cells that make thyroid hormone, around a central pool of colloid, the protein-rich material stored in the follicle lumen. Dietary iodine arrives in blood mainly as iodide, the charged form of iodine, and the thyrocyte pulls that iodide in across its basolateral membrane, the blood-facing side of the cell, through the sodium-iodide symporter, usually shortened to NIS, a transport protein that couples iodide entry to the sodium gradient maintained by the sodium-potassium pump. The gland does not passively receive iodine. It concentrates it.

Once iodide is inside the thyrocyte, the job is still only partly done. The iodine has to be moved across the apical side of the cell, the side facing the follicular lumen, into the colloid where hormone assembly occurs. At the same time the thyrocyte is producing thyroglobulin, a large protein that is secreted into that colloid and serves as the scaffold on which thyroid hormone will be built. Thyroglobulin by itself is only the storage framework. It does not become useful hormone until iodine is attached to specific tyrosine residues on that protein. This is why the follicle matters so much. The gland is not simply storing iodine. It is building a reaction chamber where iodine, protein scaffold, and oxidative enzymes meet in the same confined space.

The enzyme that turns iodide into hormonally useful iodine is thyroid peroxidase, usually shortened to TPO. TPO oxidizes iodide, meaning it converts it into a more reactive form, and then attaches that iodine to tyrosine residues on thyroglobulin. That attachment step is called organification, which in thyroid physiology means iodine is being fixed onto organic protein structure rather than remaining free iodide in solution. One iodine attached creates monoiodotyrosine, or MIT. Two iodines attached create diiodotyrosine, or DIT. The gland has now moved iodine out of the blood pool and into stored molecular intermediates inside the colloid.

The next step is coupling. TPO helps link one MIT and one DIT to form triiodothyronine, or T3, and two DIT residues to form thyroxine, or T4. These are not released immediately as free hormones. They remain attached to thyroglobulin and are stored in the colloid until the gland is signaled to mobilize them. When thyroid-stimulating hormone, or TSH, from the pituitary rises, the thyrocyte increases iodine uptake, organification, thyroglobulin handling, and hormone release. The cell then endocytoses, meaning pulls back in, portions of iodinated thyroglobulin from the colloid, digests the protein in lysosomes, and releases free T4 and T3 into blood. The thyroid is therefore not a gland that simply secretes iodine-derived hormone as soon as it is made. It stores hormone in protein-bound form first, then retrieves and frees it when stimulation demands it.

This is why iodine matters so much to thyroid biology and why goitrogens matter later in the chapter. The gland has to capture iodide, move it into the follicle, oxidize it, organify it onto thyroglobulin, couple iodotyrosines into T3 and T4, store those products, and then retrieve them on demand. A weakness at any one of those steps lowers hormone output or forces the gland into compensation. The thyroid does not need iodine in the abstract. It needs iodine delivered into this exact tissue sequence, inside this exact follicular architecture, or the gland is left trying to maintain metabolic command with too little usable raw material.

Why Cruciferous Vegetables Can Interfere With This Process

The interference begins before the thyroid ever sees the vegetable. Cruciferous plants, the Brassica family that includes cabbage, kale, broccoli, Brussels sprouts, cauliflower, collards, and related vegetables, store glucosinolates inside their tissues. Those molecules are comparatively quiet while the tissue is intact. Once the plant is cut, chewed, crushed, or blended, the cells rupture and glucosinolates meet myrosinase, the plant enzyme that breaks them down into smaller reactive products. The important point for the thyroid chapter is that the vegetable does not deliver one single "goitrogen." It delivers a tissue chemistry that can generate several different compounds after damage, and some of those compounds can interfere with the gland's use of iodine. Reviews of Brassica-thyroid interactions and EFSA's older glucosinolate assessment both describe this hydrolysis sequence and identify thiocyanate and goitrin among the thyroid-relevant products.

That matters because the thyroid's iodine sequence is narrow and stepwise. The gland has to pull iodide, the charged form of iodine, out of blood through the sodium-iodide symporter, or NIS, then move it into the follicular lumen, oxidize it through thyroid peroxidase, or TPO, and organify it onto thyroglobulin, the large protein scaffold on which thyroid hormone is built. The Office of Dietary Supplements notes that thyroid-stimulating hormone, or TSH, increases thyroidal iodine uptake and drives synthesis of T3 and T4, and that inadequate iodine leaves TSH elevated as the gland strains to trap more iodide. A compound does not have to destroy the thyroid to matter. It only has to narrow one of those steps enough that the gland has to compensate harder.

Cruciferous vegetables can interfere mainly in two ways. Thiocyanate competes with iodide uptake at the thyroid, which means it can make the gland less efficient at pulling iodide in through NIS. Goitrin, formed from the glucosinolate progoitrin, acts further downstream and is generally discussed as interfering with thyroid hormone synthesis rather than only with iodide transport. The mechanisms are related but not identical, and that distinction matters because it keeps the chapter out of vague "goitrogen" language and inside the gland's real chemistry. EFSA's glucosinolate assessment states this directly, describing thiocyanates as interfering with iodine uptake and oxazolidinethiones such as goitrin as interfering with synthesis of T3 and T4. Recent reviews of Brassica vegetables reach the same conclusion in updated form.

This is also why the burden is conditional instead of automatic. If iodine intake is adequate, the gland has more room to tolerate this interference. If iodine intake is weak, the same vegetable chemistry matters more because the thyroid is already operating with less substrate. The Office of Dietary Supplements says this plainly: goitrogens can exacerbate iodine deficiency. The stronger recent human review literature on Brassica vegetables also lands in that same place. Daily Brassica intake does not appear to harm thyroid function in iodine-replete adults in ordinary amounts, but the chemistry remains relevant where iodine status is low, intake is very high, or the host is already vulnerable. Human plasma and food-content work makes that point more specific by showing that some Brassicas, such as collards, Brussels sprouts, and some Russian kale, can provide substantially more goitrin than low-risk vegetables such as commercial broccoli or turnip tops. The plant family is one category. The thyroid burden is not uniform across the family.

Cooking changes the sequence because it alters the plant's own enzyme activity and the amount of active hydrolysis that happens before the food reaches the gut. That does not make the food chemically blank, but it does mean raw, heavily chopped, blended, or juiced crucifer intake is not the same exposure as cooked crucifer intake. The deeper point for the chapter is simpler than the diet arguments built around it. Cruciferous vegetables can interfere with thyroid iodine use because the plant stores glucosinolates in intact tissue, damage releases their breakdown chemistry, and some of the resulting compounds strike the thyroid at exactly the points where iodide must be trapped and hormone must be assembled. The vegetable keeps its clean reputation. The gland still has to complete the iodine sequence with less room for error.

Glucosinolates, Thiocyanates, and Goitrin

The crucifer does not carry one thyroid compound. It carries a storage system. Glucosinolates are sulfur-containing plant metabolites held inside intact Brassica tissue until the leaf, stalk, or floret is cut, chewed, blended, crushed, or otherwise broken open. While the plant cells remain intact, the chemistry is comparatively quiet. Once the tissue ruptures, glucosinolates meet myrosinase, the plant enzyme that hydrolyzes them, and the vegetable stops being only a source of fiber, folate, and vitamin C. It becomes a damaged sulfur-rich tissue generating breakdown products in real time. Reviews of Brassica vegetables and EFSA's glucosinolate assessment both describe this as the core sequence: stored glucosinolates first, then hydrolysis after tissue disruption, then a branching set of products depending on the precursor and conditions.

That branching matters because the thyroid burden does not come from "crucifers" in the abstract. It comes from specific hydrolysis products. Some glucosinolates yield isothiocyanates, the compounds more often discussed in chemoprotective or signaling language. Others move toward thiocyanate or toward goitrin, and those are the molecules that matter more for this chapter. The plant is not deciding whether to be good or bad. It is releasing a family of sulfur compounds from one damaged tissue system, and some members of that family are more relevant to thyroid physiology than others. The 2024 systematic review on Brassica vegetables and the EFSA review both emphasize that thyroid concern depends on the breakdown chemistry, not on the vegetable name alone.

Thiocyanate matters because it strikes the gland early in the iodine sequence. The thyroid has to pull iodide, the charged form of iodine, from blood into the thyrocyte, the hormone-producing thyroid cell, through the sodium-iodide symporter, or NIS. Thiocyanate competes at that transport step and makes iodide trapping less efficient. That is the simplest version of the interference. The gland is still being stimulated. The blood may still contain iodide. The transport lane into the thyroid has become more crowded. The Office of Dietary Supplements states that goitrogens can interfere with iodine uptake and can worsen iodine deficiency, and EFSA specifically identifies thiocyanate as the glucosinolate-derived compound that interferes with iodine uptake.

Goitrin strikes later and differently. It is produced mainly from progoitrin, one of the glucosinolates present in some Brassica vegetables, and it is generally discussed as interfering with thyroid hormone synthesis rather than only with iodide transport. That distinction matters because a gland can lose efficiency at the transport step, the organification step, or both. EFSA identifies oxazolidine-2-thiones such as goitrin as compounds that interfere with synthesis of triiodothyronine, or T3, and thyroxine, or T4, while later review literature keeps the same separation visible: thiocyanate crowds iodide uptake, goitrin pushes on hormone production itself. This is why "goitrogen" is too blunt a word if left undefined. The thyroid is not facing one vague antithyroid force. It is facing distinct compounds striking distinct steps in the same hormonal assembly line.

The useful conclusion is therefore narrower and more mechanistic than the usual food advice. Cruciferous vegetables store glucosinolates. Tissue damage releases myrosinase activity and hydrolysis products. Some of those products are relatively unimportant to the thyroid. Thiocyanate can compete with iodide uptake. Goitrin can interfere with hormone synthesis. The burden then depends on which Brassica tissue was eaten, how it was prepared, how much was eaten, and whether the host's iodine status leaves the gland room to compensate. That is why the same cabbage family can look harmless in one diet and more costly in another. The leaf keeps its wholesome reputation. The gland still has to complete the iodine sequence while sulfur breakdown products are pressing on the same machinery.

Raw-Heavy Intake, Low Iodine Status, and Thyroid Vulnerability

The thyroid does not experience a crucifer as a vegetable category. It experiences a damaged sulfur-rich plant tissue that has already begun changing its chemistry before absorption is finished. When crucifer tissue is chopped and eaten raw, more glucosinolate breakdown products survive into the meal than after cooking. That difference begins in the plant, not in the gland. Glucosinolates sit in intact Brassica tissue until cutting, chewing, shredding, juicing, or blending ruptures the cells and lets them meet myrosinase, the plant enzyme that hydrolyzes them. Once that happens, the meal is no longer carrying only stored glucosinolates. It is carrying the products of damaged crucifer tissue, including compounds that can matter to thyroid iodine handling. Human review literature on Brassica vegetables keeps this distinction visible, and it is one reason raw-heavy patterns deserve a different reading than ordinary cooked intake.

Low iodine status is what turns that chemistry from a manageable subtraction into a tighter endocrine problem. The gland has to pull iodide, the charged form of iodine, out of blood through the sodium-iodide symporter, or NIS, move it into the follicle, oxidize it through thyroid peroxidase, or TPO, and then fix it onto thyroglobulin, the large storage protein on which triiodothyronine and thyroxine are built. If iodine supply is already thin, the gland is working with reduced raw material before the vegetable chemistry ever arrives. The Office of Dietary Supplements states that low iodine intake raises thyroid-stimulating hormone, or TSH, as the pituitary tries to force harder iodide trapping and hormone synthesis, and it also notes that goitrogens can exacerbate iodine deficiency. A gland that already has to strain for iodide has less room to tolerate compounds that crowd or slow the same sequence.

That is where thyroid vulnerability becomes visible as tissue physiology rather than as food folklore. Thiocyanate competes with iodide uptake. Goitrin presses further downstream on hormone synthesis. In an iodine-replete person eating ordinary amounts of cooked Brassica vegetables, the 2024 systematic review found little evidence of clinically important thyroid harm from daily intake. In an iodine-thin host, the same interference lands on a gland already compensating. The gland has to trap harder, oxidize harder, and hold hormone output steady with less substrate and less margin. The plant chemistry has not changed. The host reserve has.

Raw-heavy intake matters because repetition changes the gland's daily workload even when each single serving looks harmless in public nutrition language. A single raw serving of bok choy, kale, or cabbage is one exposure. A daily pattern of large raw salads, shredded slaws, juices, or green smoothies made from Brassica tissue is another. The raw bok choy case remains useful here not because it proves that crucifers are broadly dangerous, but because it shows what happens when extreme repetitive raw exposure lands on susceptible physiology. The published case described myxedema coma, the most severe form of decompensated hypothyroidism, in an elderly woman after consuming about 1 to 1.5 kilograms of raw bok choy daily for months. That is not ordinary eating. It is exactly the kind of repetitive raw exposure that stops being a vegetable habit and becomes a gland problem.

So the burden belongs to a particular configuration, not to the cabbage family in the abstract. The tissue is damaged raw and often. More glucosinolate breakdown chemistry survives into the meal. The host brings low iodine status or reduced thyroid reserve. The gland is forced to complete the same iodide-trapping and hormone-building sequence with less substrate and more interference. In a well-supplied thyroid, ordinary Brassica intake usually stays below that threshold. In an iodine-poor or already strained thyroid, the same chopped raw leaf can keep returning to the same vulnerable machinery until compensation stops being quiet and starts becoming visible in slowing, cold intolerance, rising TSH, or more severe thyroid failure.

Why Context Matters but the Mechanism Is Real

The thyroid does not need a moral verdict on cruciferous vegetables. It needs enough iodide reaching the follicle, enough thyroid peroxidase, or TPO, activity at the apical surface, and enough intact hormone assembly on thyroglobulin to keep triiodothyronine and thyroxine output steady. That is why context matters. The same cabbage family chemistry can land on a gland with full iodine supply and wide reserve, or on a gland already trapping iodide hard under rising thyroid-stimulating hormone, or TSH, pressure. The mechanism does not change between those bodies. The room to compensate does. The Office of Dietary Supplements states plainly that goitrogens can interfere with thyroidal iodine uptake and can exacerbate iodine deficiency, which is exactly the condition that narrows the gland's margin before the vegetable chemistry even arrives.

That is also why the human literature does not justify a crude anti-crucifer conclusion. In iodine-replete adults eating ordinary amounts, the stronger recent review literature does not show clear clinically important thyroid harm from normal Brassica intake. The 2024 systematic review on Brassica vegetables and thyroid function concluded that daily consumption in iodine-sufficient individuals did not meaningfully alter thyroid function in the available human data. That finding matters because it keeps the chapter honest. A mechanism can be real without being dominant in every host at every dose. The gland can often absorb some interference and still hold output steady when substrate supply is adequate and exposure remains ordinary.

But that negative result does not erase the mechanism. It defines its range. Thiocyanate still competes with iodide uptake at the sodium-iodide symporter, or NIS. Goitrin still presses further downstream on hormone synthesis. EFSA's glucosinolate assessment states that thiocyanate interferes with iodine uptake and that oxazolidine-2-thiones such as goitrin interfere with thyroid hormone synthesis. Those are gland-level steps, not metaphors. The pathway is real even when the host can buffer it. Saying context matters should mean that dose, preparation, and iodine status determine whether the interference stays small or becomes biologically expensive. It should not mean the interference was imaginary all along.

The host variables that make the mechanism more visible are not mysterious. Raw repetitive intake matters because chopping, chewing, blending, or juicing crucifer tissue allows more glucosinolate breakdown chemistry to survive into the meal than cooking does. Low iodine status matters because the gland is already substrate-thin. Preexisting thyroid vulnerability matters because compensation is already narrower. The old raw bok choy case remains useful for that reason. It was not evidence that all crucifer intake is dangerous. It was evidence that extreme daily raw exposure can drive the chemistry far enough, in the wrong host, to contribute to catastrophic thyroid failure. At the other end of the scale, ordinary cooked Brassica intake in iodine-replete adults usually does not push the gland that far. Same plant family. Same basic chemistry. Different tissue reserve on the thyroid side, different delivery on the food side.

So context matters because the thyroid is a compensating organ, not because the plant chemistry is too weak to matter. The leaf is still storing glucosinolates. Tissue damage is still generating thyroid-relevant breakdown products. The gland is still trying to trap iodide and build hormone through a sequence that can be crowded or slowed. In one body the subtraction stays small. In another it keeps returning to the same follicular machinery until the cost stops being theoretical and starts showing up as rising TSH, slower hormone production, and a gland working harder to do the same job with less room.

Common Foods: Kale, Cabbage, Broccoli, Cauliflower, Brussels Sprouts

These are the foods that make the thyroid discussion confusing because they all sit under the same social label while their actual sulfur chemistry is not identical. Kale, cabbage, broccoli, cauliflower, and Brussels sprouts are all Brassica vegetables, which means they all store glucosinolates in their tissues and all can generate thyroid-relevant breakdown products once the cells are damaged. But the gland does not experience "Brassicas" in the abstract. It experiences whatever hydrolysis products the chopped leaf, floret, or bud actually delivers into the meal. The family resemblance is real. The burden is not uniform.

Kale is a good place to start because it often carries the cleanest public reputation. It is sold as a dark leafy staple, a smoothie ingredient, and a dense micronutrient food. But "kale" is already too broad a word for thyroid discussion. Human plasma and food-content work found that some Russian kale types carried enough goitrin to potentially matter to thyroid iodine handling, while commercial Brassica oleracea kales contained much lower goitrin levels and were considered minimal risk in that analysis. So the leaf category stays the same while the thyroid burden shifts with cultivar. A raw kale smoothie and a cooked commercial kale side dish are not automatically the same gland problem.

Cabbage belongs in the list because it is one of the oldest and most familiar crucifer staples, and it shows how repetition matters more than the family name alone. Raw cabbage tissue releases glucosinolate breakdown chemistry as soon as the leaf is shredded, chewed, or fermented. That does not make cabbage a universal thyroid toxin. It means the leaf is capable of contributing to iodide competition or hormone-synthesis interference under the wrong host conditions, especially when iodine status is thin and intake is repetitive. Cabbage is useful in the chapter because it is common enough to become habitual rather than occasional. The gland notices habits more than single meals.

Broccoli and cauliflower are often treated as if they settle the argument in a gentler direction, and in one sense they do. The stronger human review literature does not support broad thyroid alarm over ordinary intake of these foods in iodine-sufficient people. Broccoli is especially important because the same plasma-and-content study that found meaningful goitrin in some Russian kale and Brussels sprouts reported that commercial broccoli contained less than 10 micromoles of goitrin per 100-gram serving and could be considered minimal risk in that framework. That is a useful corrective. It keeps the mechanism real without flattening every crucifer into the same thyroid threat. Cauliflower belongs near broccoli in this section for the same practical reason: common, family-related, thyroid-relevant in principle, but not automatically a major gland burden in ordinary mixed diets with adequate iodine.

Brussels sprouts sit at the harder end of this short list. They are still ordinary produce, but they have shown up repeatedly in the literature as one of the more goitrin-relevant common Brassicas. The same food-content work found that Brussels sprouts contained enough goitrin to potentially decrease iodine uptake by the thyroid, placing them closer to the high-burden end of common crucifer intake than broccoli or commercial kale. That does not mean a serving of Brussels sprouts is a thyroid disaster. It means the gland is not meeting equal chemistry across the family, and repetitive intake from higher-goitrin foods deserves a different reading than repetitive intake from lower-goitrin ones.

So the useful way to read this list is not as a ban list and not as a reassurance list. It is a tissue-chemistry list. Kale can range from minimal concern to more meaningful goitrin burden depending on type. Cabbage matters because it is common and often eaten raw or fermented. Broccoli and cauliflower usually sit lower in thyroid concern under ordinary iodine-replete conditions. Brussels sprouts sit higher. The thyroid does not see "healthy vegetables." It sees damaged Brassica tissue delivering varying amounts of glucosinolate breakdown chemistry into a gland sequence that still has to trap iodide, oxidize it, and build hormone with whatever reserve the host has left.

Why "Healthy Vegetable" and "Thyroid-Friendly Food" Are Not Automatically the Same Thing

A vegetable earns the first label in public nutrition long before it earns the second one in the gland. Kale, cabbage, broccoli, cauliflower, and Brussels sprouts can all be nutrient-dense, fiber-rich, and chemically interesting foods while still asking the thyroid to complete hormone assembly under added interference. The thyroid does not care that the leaf is dark green, widely praised, or low in calories. It cares whether enough iodide reaches the follicle, whether thyroid peroxidase, or TPO, can keep oxidizing and organifying that iodide onto thyroglobulin, and whether triiodothyronine and thyroxine can still be built at the pace the body needs. The vegetable can keep the reputation. The gland still has to do the chemistry.

The conflict begins in the plant tissue itself. Cruciferous vegetables store glucosinolates inside intact cells. Once the tissue is chopped, chewed, shredded, blended, or juiced, those compounds meet myrosinase, the plant enzyme that hydrolyzes them into smaller sulfur-containing products. Some of those products are irrelevant to the thyroid. Some are not. Thiocyanate can compete with iodide uptake at the sodium-iodide symporter, or NIS, and goitrin can interfere further downstream with thyroid hormone synthesis. That is why the same vegetable can still be "healthy" in the broad nutritional sense and yet become less thyroid-friendly in a raw, repetitive, or high-load form. The phrase "healthy vegetable" describes the food category. "Thyroid-friendly" describes what that damaged tissue does once it reaches the gland's iodine sequence.

Context decides how much that interference costs. In iodine-sufficient adults eating ordinary mixed amounts of Brassica vegetables, the 2024 systematic review found no clear adverse thyroid effect from daily intake. That matters because it keeps the argument honest. The mechanism is real, but a well-supplied gland often has enough reserve to absorb modest interference without losing control of hormone output. The Office of Dietary Supplements makes the same distinction from the iodine side: goitrogens can exacerbate iodine deficiency, and the concern is mainly for people whose iodine intake is already weak, not for most iodine-replete adults. The same leaf therefore lands differently in different thyroids. A gland with margin can buffer the subtraction. A gland already short on substrate has to feel it.

This is also why the family name is too blunt. Broccoli is not Brussels sprouts in thyroid terms, and commercial kale is not every Russian kale or collard type. The 2016 goitrin and thiocyanate analysis found that some Brussels sprouts, collards, and certain Russian kale types contained enough goitrin to potentially reduce thyroid iodine uptake, while commercial broccoli and some other common Brassica vegetables fell much lower. So even inside the cabbage family, the gland is not receiving one uniform burden. The thyroid does not see a virtuous vegetable class. It sees varying amounts of damaged sulfur-rich tissue, varying goitrogen output, and whatever iodine reserve the host brought into the meal. That is why a "healthy vegetable" and a "thyroid-friendly food" are sometimes the same thing, sometimes not, and never automatically so.

Chapter 19

Plant Chemicals That Alter Drug and Hormone Handling

Grapefruit matters because the problem does not begin in the liver, in the prescription bottle, or in an abstract warning label. It begins in the fruit tissue. The pulp and juice carry furanocoumarins, a class of plant defense compounds concentrated enough to alter what the intestinal wall does with certain oral drugs before the drugs ever reach the rest of the body. FDA states that grapefruit and grapefruit juice can change how some medicines work and that the interaction is centered on the amount of CYP3A4 present in the intestine, the enzyme system that normally breaks down many drugs during first-pass handling in the gut wall.

That intestinal location is the whole reason grapefruit belongs in this chapter. A drug taken by mouth does not move straight from the stomach into the bloodstream unchanged. It first has to cross an epithelium, the sheet of cells lining the small intestine, that is rich in metabolic enzymes. CYP3A4 is one of the most important of those enzymes. It acts as a partial filter. Some of the swallowed drug is metabolized in that intestinal tissue before it ever reaches portal blood on the way to the liver. When grapefruit furanocoumarins inhibit that intestinal enzyme system, the filter thins. More parent drug survives the crossing. More drug reaches blood than the dose was meant to deliver under ordinary conditions.

The chemistry is not vague. Reviews of grapefruit interactions identify bergamottin and 6',7'-dihydroxybergamottin as important furanocoumarins behind the effect, and the interaction is not only competitive in the moment. These compounds can also drive loss of intestinal CYP3A4 protein, which means the bowel may remain less able to metabolize susceptible drugs even after the fruit is gone. The meal therefore does more than sit beside the drug in the stomach. It changes the enzyme capacity of the tissue the drug must cross.

That is why grapefruit is more revealing than many other food-drug warnings. It shows a fruit acting directly on the body's own handling machinery. The orange, the berry, or the apple may carry sugars, acids, and polyphenols without reliably changing drug metabolism at this level. Grapefruit carries a chemistry strong enough that FDA requires warnings for certain prescription and over-the-counter medicines because the result can be higher blood levels and greater risk of adverse effects. The fruit keeps the social identity of produce. The bowel becomes a pharmacology site.

The risk is selective, which is exactly what makes the mechanism easier to miss. Grapefruit does not interact meaningfully with every drug. It matters most for drugs that depend on intestinal CYP3A4 to limit how much parent compound reaches blood. If the drug does not rely much on that intestinal enzyme, the fruit may do very little. If the drug does, the same glass of juice can raise exposure enough that the intended dose is no longer the real dose the tissues receive. FDA's consumer guidance frames it this way: for some medicines, instead of being metabolized, more drug enters the blood and stays in the body longer.

So grapefruit is the primary case because it makes the chapter's larger point visible without needing any interpretive help. A plant compound stored in ordinary edible tissue reaches the small intestine, meets the enzyme-rich membrane the drug must cross, and changes what gets through. That is not nutrition in the narrow sense. It is plant chemistry altering human drug handling at the tissue boundary where absorption and metabolism are happening together.

Furanocoumarins and Intestinal Enzyme Inhibition

The grapefruit interaction begins in the enterocyte, the absorptive cell lining the small intestine, not in the bloodstream and not in the liver first. A swallowed drug has to cross that intestinal wall, and part of the wall's job is metabolic screening. Cytochrome P450 3A4, or CYP3A4, is one of the main enzymes carrying that load. It sits in the small-bowel epithelium and oxidizes many drug molecules during first-pass metabolism, the early metabolic loss that occurs before full systemic circulation is reached. FDA's grapefruit warning is built on exactly that tissue fact: some medicines normally lose part of their dose to intestinal CYP3A4 before they ever get past the gut wall.

Grapefruit does not block that screen through sugar, acid, or vitamin C. It does it through furanocoumarins, especially bergamottin and 6',7'-dihydroxybergamottin. These are citrus defense compounds, not incidental flavor notes, and the drug-interaction literature repeatedly identifies them as the main inhibitors behind the grapefruit effect. Reviews and mechanistic studies describe them as the major intestinal CYP3A4 inhibitors in grapefruit juice and show that they are strong enough to account for much of the increase in oral drug exposure seen with susceptible medicines.

The important part is how they inhibit. This is not only a brief competitive crowding of the enzyme surface. Furanocoumarins can act as mechanism-based inhibitors, sometimes described as suicide inhibitors, which means the enzyme begins processing the compound and in doing so is inactivated. Recent pharmacokinetic modeling and older human biopsy work both support that reading. Grapefruit juice lowers intestinal CYP3A4 activity in part by reducing functional enzyme protein in the small bowel, so the bowel wall does not simply face a temporary visitor at the binding site. It is left with less working CYP3A4 machinery for a period afterward.

Once that intestinal enzyme capacity falls, more parent drug crosses the membrane intact. That is the whole clinical consequence. The person swallows what looked like an ordinary dose, but the gut wall destroys less of it than expected, so more drug reaches blood than the prescription was calibrated to deliver under ordinary intestinal conditions. FDA explains the interaction in exactly those terms: instead of being metabolized in the small intestine, more drug enters the bloodstream and can stay in the body longer. This does not apply to every medicine. It matters mainly for drugs that rely meaningfully on intestinal CYP3A4 to limit how much of the oral dose escapes the bowel.

That is why grapefruit belongs in this chapter as more than a consumer warning. The fruit is carrying a plant-defense chemistry strong enough to alter the metabolic behavior of the intestinal epithelium itself. A food becomes a pharmacokinetic modifier, meaning it changes how much of a swallowed compound is absorbed and survives early metabolism. The drug label may still say one dose. The bowel may now be delivering another.

Cytochrome P450 3A4, Abbreviated CYP3A4, and First-Pass Metabolism

A swallowed drug does not move straight from the stomach into the bloodstream unchanged. It has to cross the wall of the small intestine first, and that wall is not a passive membrane. The absorptive cells, called enterocytes, carry enzymes that begin dismantling some oral drugs during absorption itself. Cytochrome P450 3A4, abbreviated CYP3A4, is one of the most important of those enzymes. It is highly relevant in the small intestine and is frequently implicated in human gut-wall metabolism of oral drugs.

That intestinal step is part of first-pass metabolism, which means presystemic metabolism, the fraction of an oral dose that is metabolized before full entry into the general circulation. People often hear that phrase and think only of the liver, but the intestine can make a substantial contribution before the drug ever reaches portal blood. Reviews of intestinal first-pass metabolism describe CYP3A4 substrates as drugs whose oral bioavailability can be lowered substantially by metabolism in the small intestine itself.

The consequence is simple. If intestinal CYP3A4 is active, some of the parent drug is oxidized and lost during transit through the bowel wall, so less unchanged drug reaches blood. If intestinal CYP3A4 is inhibited, that filter thins. More parent compound crosses intact. The dose on the label stays the same, but the delivered dose to tissue rises because the intestine destroyed less of it on the way through. FDA consumer guidance on grapefruit states this directly: instead of being metabolized in the small intestine, more drug may enter the bloodstream and remain in the body longer.

This is why CYP3A4 matters so much in food-drug interactions. Grapefruit furanocoumarins do not create a new drug. They change the intestinal handling of the drug already swallowed. For susceptible medicines, intestinal first-pass metabolism is part of what keeps systemic exposure within the intended range. Remove part of that intestinal metabolism and blood levels rise. FDA-approved labeling for several CYP3A4-sensitive oral drugs, including budesonide and nimodipine products, specifically warns that grapefruit juice inhibits CYP3A4 and can increase systemic exposure.

So CYP3A4 belongs in this chapter because it makes the tissue logic visible. The small intestine is not only absorbing. It is metabolizing at the same time. A fruit like grapefruit can alter that enzyme field, which means a plant compound in the lumen can change how much drug survives the crossing from bowel to blood. The food still looks like produce. The enterocyte is doing pharmacology.

Why a Fruit Can Raise Drug Exposure by Blocking Gut Wall Metabolism

A swallowed drug does not enter blood as soon as it leaves the stomach. It first moves through the small intestine, dissolves into the fluid inside the bowel, and then has to cross the intestinal epithelium, the sheet of absorptive cells lining the gut. Those cells are not passive. They are carrying cytochrome P450 3A4, abbreviated CYP3A4, an enzyme system that oxidizes many oral drugs while they are still trying to cross the bowel wall. This is part of first-pass metabolism, the early metabolic loss that happens before the dose ever becomes full systemic exposure. FDA describes grapefruit's interaction at exactly that intestinal step: many drugs are metabolized with the help of CYP3A4 in the small intestine, and grapefruit juice can block that action, allowing more drug to enter the blood and remain in the body longer.

The fruit does not do this through sugar, acid, or vitamin content. It does it through furanocoumarins, especially compounds such as bergamottin and 6',7'-dihydroxybergamottin, which are citrus defense molecules stored in the fruit tissue strongly enough to reach the gut wall in active form. Once they reach the enterocyte, the absorptive intestinal cell, they interfere with the CYP3A4 machinery the drug was supposed to encounter on the way through. Review literature describes these furanocoumarins as the principal drivers of the grapefruit interaction and shows that they can inactivate intestinal CYP3A4 in a mechanism-based way, meaning the enzyme is not merely crowded for a moment but functionally damaged during the interaction itself.

That is why the effect can be larger than people expect from a food. The prescription still says the same milligrams. The tablet or capsule still contains the same dose. But the intestinal wall destroys less of that dose than it was expected to destroy, so more unchanged parent drug crosses into portal blood, the blood draining from the intestine toward the liver, than the physician or label assumed under ordinary conditions. The fruit has not added drug. It has reduced intestinal loss. The dose on paper stays fixed while the delivered exposure rises. FDA puts the consequence in blunt terms: too much drug can end up in the body.

This is also why grapefruit does not interact meaningfully with every medicine. The fruit matters most when the swallowed drug depends on intestinal CYP3A4 to lower how much parent compound survives the crossing from bowel to blood. When that dependency is weak, grapefruit may do little. When it is strong, the same breakfast fruit can turn an ordinary oral dose into a much larger tissue exposure. That is the point worth keeping in the chapter. A fruit can still look nutritionally ordinary while carrying plant chemistry strong enough to thin the enzyme field in the bowel wall and let more drug through than the intestine was supposed to allow.

Why This Is a Direct Example of a Fruit Imposing Metabolic Burden

Grapefruit is one of the cleanest cases in the whole book because the burden does not need to be inferred from symptoms, mineral loss, or long-term epidemiology. The fruit reaches the small intestine carrying furanocoumarins, defense compounds built strongly enough to strike the enzyme field in the bowel wall itself. A swallowed drug dissolves into the fluid inside the intestine, reaches the enterocyte, the absorptive intestinal cell, and normally meets cytochrome P450 3A4, abbreviated CYP3A4, one of the gut wall enzymes that oxidizes part of the dose during absorption. FDA warns that grapefruit juice can block this intestinal CYP3A4 step for certain medicines, which means the fruit is acting directly on the body's own metabolic handling machinery rather than merely coexisting with it in the stomach.

That is already metabolic burden. The intestine is supposed to do work on the way from lumen to blood. It is supposed to break part of the drug down during first-pass metabolism, the early loss that occurs before full systemic circulation is reached. Grapefruit thins that filter. Reviews of the interaction identify bergamottin and 6',7'-dihydroxybergamottin as the key furanocoumarins, and mechanistic work shows that the effect is centered largely in the small bowel rather than only in the liver. The enterocyte loses part of its normal CYP3A4 activity, so less drug is destroyed while crossing the bowel wall. The label still says the same milligrams. The bowel delivers more parent compound than it was expected to deliver.

The burden is direct because the fruit changes the metabolic labor the tissue can perform. This is not a fruit that merely contains a chemically interesting phytochemical. It is a fruit that can inactivate intestinal CYP3A4 strongly enough that FDA requires warnings for certain prescription and over-the-counter drugs, and approved drug labeling specifically warns that grapefruit juice can raise systemic exposure by inhibiting gut mucosal CYP3A. Once that happens, the body has to absorb, distribute, and clear a larger drug load than intended. The fruit has not nourished the system. It has forced the system to handle a distorted dose.

The point lands even harder when the mechanism is kept at the membrane. The drug is trying to cross from bowel fluid into portal blood. The enterocyte is supposed to metabolize part of it on the way through. Grapefruit furanocoumarins interfere with that intestinal enzyme step and can do so in a mechanism-based way, which means the enzyme is not merely crowded briefly but functionally inactivated.

The gut wall then stops behaving like the metabolic barrier the dose was designed around. More drug gets through. More drug reaches blood unchanged. The liver and the rest of the body inherit a larger parent-drug burden because the fruit altered what the bowel wall did not destroy.

That is why grapefruit belongs here as a primary example of plant chemistry imposing metabolic burden. A fruit enters the bowel as food and leaves the bowel acting like a pharmacokinetic modifier, meaning it changes how much of a swallowed drug survives absorption and reaches the body. The reputation stays in the produce aisle. The burden appears in the enterocyte, in the portal blood, and then in the larger systemic exposure the tissues are forced to carry afterward.

The Broader Lesson That Plant Compounds Can Act Pharmacologically, Not Merely Nutritionally

The mistake is to assume that a plant compound enters the body as part of a food and therefore behaves only as food. The intestine does not make that assumption. It receives molecules one by one at the membrane. Some arrive as sugars, amino acids, fatty acids, minerals, and vitamins and are handled mainly as substrates or cofactors. Others arrive with enough structural force to act on enzymes, transporters, receptors, ion gradients, or membranes before they have done anything resembling nourishment. Grapefruit is the cleanest case because the fruit reaches the small bowel carrying furanocoumarins that strike cytochrome P450 3A4, abbreviated CYP3A4, in the intestinal wall and reduce first-pass drug metabolism there. The fruit is still being swallowed as produce. The enterocyte is being forced into altered drug handling.

Once that distinction is kept in view, a large amount of plant chemistry becomes easier to read. A compound does not stop being pharmacologically active because it came packaged inside a leaf, root, fruit, or seed. If it can inhibit an enzyme, it is acting pharmacologically. If it can compete at a transporter, it is acting pharmacologically. If it can change membrane permeability, alter signaling, or interfere with hormone synthesis, it is acting pharmacologically. Thiocyanate from damaged crucifer tissue crowds iodide uptake at the thyroid. Goitrin presses further into thyroid hormone synthesis. Psoralens and related furanocoumarins in citrus, celery, and parsnip can sit on skin and wait for ultraviolet A light to turn contact into tissue injury. These are not nutrient effects with a bit of side personality attached. They are tissue-level actions strong enough to change what the gland, the skin, or the bowel wall can do.

That is why the line between food and drug is much thinner in plants than nutrition language usually admits. The plant does not manufacture these compounds for human benefit. It manufactures them to control predation, regulate its own tissue chemistry, survive stress, and protect storage or reproductive structures. When those molecules enter the body, the body has to decide whether they will be absorbed, neutralized, excreted, or allowed to act at their target long enough to matter. Sometimes the target is the gut wall. Sometimes it is the thyroid. Sometimes it is the skin after light exposure. Sometimes it is the liver's downstream drug burden because the intestine failed to metabolize part of the swallowed dose. The same fruit can therefore provide water, carbohydrate, and vitamin C while also carrying a chemistry that changes drug exposure. The nutritional identity of the tissue does not erase the pharmacology of the compound inside it.

Dose, route, and host reserve decide how visible that pharmacology becomes. A small amount of a compound may pass below the threshold where the person notices anything. Repetition changes that. Concentration changes that. Juicing changes that. A vulnerable host changes that. Grapefruit matters most when a swallowed drug depends heavily on intestinal CYP3A4. Raw-heavy crucifer intake matters more when iodine reserve is thin and the thyroid is already trapping hard. Lime or celery contact matters more when the compound remains on skin and sunlight completes the reaction. The molecule is the same. What changes is how much of it reaches the target tissue, how often it returns there, and how much room that tissue has left to compensate.

That is the broader lesson the chapter needs to keep. Plant compounds cannot be judged only by nutrient tables because some of them are not behaving like nutrients at all. They are behaving like low-dose pharmacologic agents delivered inside ordinary food tissue. Sometimes the effect is mild. Sometimes it is conditional. Sometimes it is clinically important enough that regulators put warnings on drugs or toxicologists treat the food as a recognized poisoning risk. The produce aisle and the medicine cabinet are not the same place, but plant chemistry crosses that border easily. The food reaches the mouth as food. The molecule reaches the membrane as something more active than that.

Chapter 20

Liver Workload and Chemical Clearance

The intestine does not finish the chemical work of a meal. It hands that work forward. Blood leaving the gut does not flow randomly into the body. It enters the portal vein, the vessel that drains the stomach, intestine, pancreas, and spleen into the liver first. That routing is the point. The liver is positioned as the first large metabolic filter for what the bowel allowed across the membrane. Nutrients, plant defense compounds, microbial products, drugs, alcohol, and other absorbed chemicals arrive together in portal blood and strike hepatocytes, the main working cells of the liver, before the rest of the body has to carry them. Reviews of hepatic circulation and drug elimination describe the liver as the principal first-pass organ for material arriving from the gastrointestinal tract and emphasize that orally absorbed compounds are exposed to hepatic biotransformation before full systemic circulation is reached.

That first contact is not passive. A hepatocyte has to decide whether the absorbed compound can be used, stored, modified, packaged for bile, returned to blood, or made more water-soluble so the kidney can clear it. Drug-handling texts describe this as a sequence of uptake across the sinusoidal pole, meaning the blood-facing side of the hepatocyte, metabolism inside the cell, and then export either back to blood or across the canalicular pole into bile. The liver is therefore not only a detox organ in the popular sense. It is a sorting organ. Some molecules arrive and enter central metabolism. Some arrive and are rendered less active. Some are converted into more reactive intermediates first. Some are conjugated, meaning chemically linked to groups such as glucuronide, sulfate, glutathione, or amino acids so they can be carried out more safely. The absorbed compound is no longer just part of the meal. It has become liver workload.

The classic language for this work is phase I and phase II metabolism, but those terms matter only if the cell biology stays visible. Phase I usually means oxidation, reduction, or hydrolysis, chemical changes that expose or add a functional handle on the molecule. The cytochrome P450 system often does this work. Phase II usually means conjugation, where the liver attaches a polar group that makes the compound easier to retain in aqueous body fluids and easier to excrete. The important point is that the sequence does not always make a molecule gentler at the first step. A phase I reaction can create an intermediate that is more reactive than the parent compound and therefore more dangerous if the next step does not keep pace. Liver toxicology literature returns to this problem constantly. The liver protects the body by transforming xenobiotics, meaning foreign compounds, but the same transformation machinery can generate reactive metabolites that bind proteins, drain glutathione reserves, or damage membranes if the load is high enough or the host is vulnerable.

Where the transformed compound goes next matters just as much as how it was altered. Some products are sent into bile, the liver secretion that leaves through canaliculi and bile ducts into the intestine. Some are returned to blood for renal clearance. Some cycle between liver and gut through enterohepatic circulation, meaning the compound is secreted into bile, released into the intestine, reabsorbed, and sent back to the liver again. That cycling can prolong exposure and keep the same chemistry returning to the same tissues. StatPearls on bile secretion and broader bile reviews describe bile formation, canalicular export, and intestinal recirculation as central features of hepatic handling. A compound the liver has already worked on once may not be gone. It may come back. That is one reason plant chemicals and drugs can continue imposing burden after the meal itself has passed. The bowel delivered the first load. The liver modified it. Bile returned part of it to the gut.

The same chemistry keeps circulating until clearance finally outruns recirculation.

This is why the liver becomes such an important organ in a book about plant burden. The plant compound that survived digestion and crossed the intestinal wall is no longer only a gut event. It becomes a hepatic event the moment portal blood delivers it. A furanocoumarin, an alkaloid, an amine, an alcohol, a microbial endotoxin, or a reactive metabolite from an herbal extract all arrive at the same organ that must maintain lipid handling, glucose regulation, protein synthesis, bile production, and hormone metabolism at the same time. "Detox" is too soft a word for that. The liver has to keep the chemistry moving without letting it damage the cell that is doing the work. A meal or compound that repeatedly asks for oxidation, conjugation, glutathione use, transporter activity, and biliary export is not neutral just because the person does not feel symptoms immediately. The cost is being paid in hepatocyte chemistry first.

So the liver belongs here as the organ of chemical consequence after absorption. The intestine decides what gets in. The liver decides what form that absorbed chemistry will take next, whether it will be softened, activated, conjugated, recycled, or cleared. Some compounds pass through with little trouble. Some distort the whole workload because they arrive often, induce or inhibit enzymes, generate reactive intermediates, or keep returning through bile. The body may still call the item food, supplement, herb, medicine, or drink. The hepatocyte only sees a stream of absorbed chemicals it must transform fast enough that the rest of the body is not forced to carry them unchanged.

Why Detoxification Language Is Often Abused but Liver Workload Is Still Real

"Detox" gets abused because commercial language turns a real hepatic function into a vague moral promise. Juice fasts, powders, teas, and cleanses speak as if toxins are a single dirty substance floating through the body waiting to be flushed out by a branded ritual. That is not how the liver works. NCCIH notes that research on commercial detox and cleanse programs is sparse and low in quality, and some of these programs can be falsely advertised or unsafe. The problem with that language is not that the body never clears anything. The problem is that it replaces tissue physiology with a cartoon. The liver is not rinsing sludge out of the system. It is receiving a continuous stream of absorbed chemicals in portal blood and transforming them one by one under enzyme, transporter, and membrane constraints that have nothing to do with wellness marketing.

The workload itself is real and heavy. Blood leaving the stomach and intestine enters the portal circulation and reaches the liver before it reaches the rest of the body. Hepatocytes, the main working cells of the liver, sit inside that flow field and take up nutrients, drugs, microbial products, alcohol, plant compounds, and other xenobiotics, meaning foreign chemicals the body did not build as part of its own normal structure. StatPearls and liver cell biology reviews describe this arrangement clearly: hepatocytes have distinct blood-facing and bile-facing membranes, they filter and transform compounds arriving from the gut, and zone 3 hepatocytes near the central vein carry a large share of drug biotransformation. That is not a metaphorical burden. It is a constant biochemical load imposed on real cells with finite enzyme capacity, finite glutathione reserves, and finite tolerance for reactive intermediates.

This is where the language of phase I and phase II metabolism belongs, but only if the cell work stays visible. In phase I, enzymes often oxidize or otherwise modify a molecule so the liver can grab it more effectively or prepare it for the next step. In phase II, the hepatocyte conjugates it, meaning it attaches groups such as glucuronide, sulfate, or glutathione so the compound becomes easier to hold in water, move in blood, secrete into bile, or clear through the kidney. That sequence can protect the body, but it can also create trouble. A parent compound may become a more reactive intermediate before conjugation catches up. Reviews on xenobiotic metabolism and reactive metabolites make this point directly: hepatic metabolism can detoxify a compound or bioactivate it, and the balance between those two outcomes depends on dose, enzyme pattern, and host reserve. The liver does real chemical labor. The simplification is what is false.

That is why liver workload can rise without anyone feeling an immediate symptom. A compound absorbed from the bowel may require repeated oxidation, conjugation, transporter activity, and biliary export even if the person never experiences nausea, pain, or jaundice. Some of that chemistry then returns. Bile can carry conjugated material back into the intestine, where part of it may be deconjugated, reabsorbed, and sent through the portal vein again in enterohepatic circulation. The meal has passed. The compound has not. Hepatic handling is still going on because the liver must keep transforming, sorting, exporting, and sometimes rehandling the same chemistry until clearance finally outruns recirculation.

So the correction is simple. Commercial detox language deserves suspicion because it usually hides the actual physiology and sells a fantasy of easy cleansing. Liver workload deserves respect because it is one of the main reasons the rest of the body is not forced to carry every absorbed plant compound, drug, alcohol metabolite, and microbial product unchanged. The abuse is in the slogan. The workload is in the hepatocyte. Portal blood keeps arriving. Enzymes keep oxidizing. Conjugation keeps spending chemical resources. Bile and blood keep carrying the transformed products away. That work remains real even when the word wrapped around it has been cheapened.

Phase I and Phase II Handling in Simple Terms

The liver does not receive a swallowed compound as an idea. It receives it in portal blood, the blood draining from the stomach and intestine into the liver first, and that blood delivers the compound straight to the hepatocyte, the main working liver cell. By the time the molecule reaches that cell, the question is no longer whether it came from food, a plant extract, a drug, or alcohol metabolism. The question is whether the cell can use it as it is, or whether it has to change the molecule before the rest of the body can tolerate carrying it. Many compounds cannot move safely through the body in their original form. They are too lipid-soluble, meaning they dissolve too easily into membranes and not easily enough into watery body fluids, or too chemically reactive, or too awkward for direct clearance into bile or urine. That is where the language of Phase I and Phase II comes from. It is the liver's working sequence for taking absorbed chemistry and pushing it toward a form the body can finally move out.

Phase I is the first alteration step. The hepatocyte takes the incoming molecule and changes its surface enough to expose a reactive handle the cell can work with more easily afterward. Very often that means oxidation, a chemical step that adds or rearranges oxygen-containing structure through enzyme systems such as cytochrome P450. Sometimes it means reduction or hydrolysis instead, but the point stays the same. The liver is cutting into the original chemistry and reshaping it. This step can weaken the molecule, but it can also sharpen it. A compound that arrived in a relatively stable form can leave Phase I as a more reactive intermediate, which means the hepatocyte has not yet finished protecting the body. It has opened the molecule. Now the cell has to keep control of what it opened. That is why Phase I cannot be described honestly as simple detox. The liver may be moving the compound toward clearance, but it may also be generating a harder piece of chemistry on the way there.

That harder intermediate is where the danger in the sequence becomes easiest to see. If the cell cannot move quickly enough into the next handling step, the newly exposed chemistry can begin binding proteins, damaging membranes, stressing the mitochondria, the structures inside the cell that make much of its usable energy, or pulling too heavily on antioxidant defenses such as glutathione, a sulfur-rich molecule the liver uses to neutralize reactive compounds. The first alteration was necessary, but necessity does not make it gentle. A hepatocyte under repeated chemical traffic is constantly taking that risk. It keeps oxidizing, cutting, and exposing handles on compounds because unchanged clearance is often impossible, and every time it does that, it has to stay far enough ahead of the reactive intermediates it just created.

Phase II is usually the step that makes removal practical. Once the molecule has the right handle exposed, the liver attaches a larger, more water-friendly group to it. That attachment is called conjugation. Common conjugates include glucuronide, sulfate, and glutathione. The point of the attachment is physical, not rhetorical. The altered molecule now sits more comfortably in aqueous body fluids, clings less stubbornly to membranes, and can be pushed more easily toward bile or urine. In simple terms, Phase I opens the compound up. Phase II tags it for transport. The first step makes the liver able to grab it. The second step makes the body able to carry it out. When people say the liver "detoxifies," this is the real sequence they are usually trying and failing to describe. The hepatocyte takes a compound it cannot leave alone, cuts into it, survives the intermediate chemistry, fastens on a carry-out group, and then tries to move the altered molecule out before the work it is doing starts injuring the cell itself.

Why Repeated Exposure Matters More Than Isolated Contact

A single absorbed compound can pass through the liver as a brief piece of cell work. Portal blood, the blood draining from the stomach and intestine into the liver first, delivers that chemistry to the hepatocyte, the main working liver cell, and the cell begins doing what it always does with material it cannot simply leave unchanged. It oxidizes, reduces, hydrolyzes, conjugates, meaning it attaches a larger water-friendly group such as glucuronide, sulfate, or glutathione, and then pushes the altered compound back into blood or across the canalicular membrane into bile. One pass can stay quiet because the enzyme field still has room, the antioxidant reserve is still intact, and the transport machinery is not yet occupied by the same chemical traffic hour after hour. The molecule arrives, is altered, and leaves before the handling sequence has to reshape the cell around it.

Repeated exposure changes the same chemistry by changing the tissue that has to carry it. The hepatocyte does not experience those exposures as isolated tasks. The same chemistry keeps returning through the same portal route to the same cell. Phase I handling, the first alteration step, can generate reactive metabolites, intermediate compounds more chemically aggressive than the parent molecule. If the next step keeps pace, the cell survives the detour. If the same burden keeps returning, the hepatocyte has to keep generating those intermediates, keep neutralizing them, and keep spending glutathione, the sulfur-rich antioxidant used to quench reactive chemistry before it binds proteins, injures membranes, or reaches the mitochondria, the structures inside the cell that make much of its usable energy. The problem is no longer the existence of the compound alone. The problem is that the same cell has to keep opening the molecule, keep surviving what it just opened, and keep doing it again tomorrow.

The liver also adapts, and adaptation is still workload. Repeated xenobiotic exposure, xenobiotic meaning a foreign compound the body must handle rather than use as ordinary tissue fuel, can induce enzyme expression, change transporter density, and enlarge the biochemical apparatus devoted to chemical defense. Toxicologic reviews describe hepatic enzyme induction as an adaptive response associated with increased liver weight, altered gene expression, and structural change inside hepatocytes. That sounds protective because it is protective for a time. It is still a cost. A hepatocyte that keeps enlarging its chemical handling machinery is diverting structure and energy toward defense work instead of quieter metabolic housekeeping. The tissue may still look compensated from the outside while the cell is living in a different operating state underneath.

Some compounds make repetition even harder by refusing to leave cleanly after the first pass. The liver conjugates them, secretes them into bile, and sends them back into the intestine, where part of that chemistry can be deconjugated, reabsorbed, and delivered through the portal vein again. That cycling, called enterohepatic circulation, turns one swallowed exposure into repeated liver contact even before the next meal or dose arrives. The bowel hands the chemistry to the liver once. Bile hands part of it back. The same portal route fills again with the same burden. At that point isolated contact is over. The compound has become part of the liver's daily traffic, and the hepatocyte is no longer clearing a passing guest. It is working inside a stream that keeps returning to the same membrane, the same enzymes, and the same antioxidant reserve until clearance finally outruns recurrence.

What Happens When a Food Adds Little Nourishment but Still Adds Processing Demand

The digestive tract can finish a meal with very little to show for it and still deliver a substantial chemical workload to the liver. That is the bad trade. The food enters the mouth carrying a clean reputation, breaks apart in the stomach and small intestine, releases part of its chemistry into the lumen, the hollow interior of the gut where digestion is taking place, and then crosses the absorptive membrane in a form the body cannot use well enough to justify the handling cost. The intestine may recover little available mineral because the plant matrix trapped it. It may recover little useful protein because the tissue resisted cleavage or the seed chemistry blocked the enzymes meant to digest it. It may recover very little durable energy or structural material. The meal can still send alkaloids, polyphenols, sulfur compounds, amines, organic acids, fermentation byproducts, or other foreign chemistry into portal blood, the blood draining from the stomach and intestine into the liver first. At that point the question is no longer whether the food looked wholesome on paper. The question is what the hepatocyte, the main working liver cell, now has to do with what the bowel allowed across.

A hepatocyte does not receive that chemistry as a lifestyle choice. It receives it as workload. The cell pulls compounds in across its blood-facing membrane, sorts what can enter ordinary metabolism from what has to be altered first, and begins the transformation sequence people flatten into the word detox. Some molecules have to be oxidized, reduced, or hydrolyzed in Phase I, the first alteration step that exposes or creates a chemical handle the cell can work with more easily afterward. Some then have to be conjugated in Phase II, meaning the liver attaches glucuronide, sulfate, glutathione, or another water-friendly group so the compound can travel more safely in blood or be pushed out through bile or urine. That work spends oxygen, reducing power, enzyme capacity, transporter capacity, and antioxidant reserve even when the food that triggered it delivered very little retained biological value. The body can therefore lose the mineral, lose the protein yield, lose the clean energy return, and still pay for oxidation and conjugation as though something worthwhile had arrived.

The most deceptive foods in this category are often the ones that look light. They do not feel like burdens because they are not dense in the obvious way. They are not heavy roasts, thick sauces, or overtly intoxicating substances. They are leaves, juices, powders, teas, seed foods, concentrated plant extracts, or "healthy" staples that keep sending the liver chemistry to process while giving the tissues a weak return. The cell has to keep opening the molecule, keep neutralizing what that opening created, keep tagging it for export, and keep doing it fast enough that reactive intermediates do not start binding proteins, injuring membranes, or pulling too heavily on glutathione, the sulfur-rich antioxidant the liver uses to quench reactive chemistry before it damages the cell itself. A meal like that undernourishes at the same time it recruits defense work. The food keeps the reputation. The hepatocyte keeps the bill.

Repetition is what turns this from a biochemical annoyance into a tissue pattern. A single low-yield meal may pass quietly. The same low-yield chemistry arriving day after day is different. The same portal route fills again. The same enzyme field is used again. The same transporters have to push altered compounds into bile again. Some of that chemistry returns through enterohepatic circulation, meaning the liver secretes it into bile, the intestine receives it, part of it is reabsorbed, and portal blood brings it back to the liver again. At that point the food is no longer just failing to nourish generously. It is teaching the liver to spend itself on clearance. The person may still call the diet clean because the ingredients sound virtuous and the labels read well. The liver reads only what crossed, what had to be transformed, and how often the same cell had to do that work with little constructive return to justify it.

Burden Without Visible Poisoning as the Quiet Middle Ground of Plant-Food Physiology

The body does not need to collapse for a food to be costly. Most plant burdens never look like poisoning in the dramatic sense. There is no ambulance scene, no immediate neurologic crisis, no unmistakable meal-to-disaster sequence. The leaf, seed, tuber, or fruit enters the gut and instead begins a quieter kind of subtraction. Minerals are released and then trapped. Protein arrives and then resists cleavage. Carbohydrate stays in the lumen, the hollow interior of the bowel where digestion is taking place, long enough to pull water in and feed fermentation. Sulfur compounds from damaged crucifer tissue reach the thyroid sequence and make iodide handling less efficient. Oxalate reaches the kidney and becomes crystal pressure instead of nourishment. None of that has to announce itself as poison for the food to be biologically expensive. The chemistry can stay below the threshold of spectacle and still keep stealing from digestion, absorption, gland function, and clearance.

This is the middle ground most nutrition writing skips because it prefers cleaner categories. A food is presented as safe unless it causes acute toxicity, or it is presented as beneficial because it contains vitamins, minerals, fiber, antioxidants, or phytochemicals on a chart. The body works in a harsher register than that. It asks what digestion had to do to the tissue, what compounds were released when the tissue fractured, what stayed soluble, what bound calcium, zinc, or iron before those minerals reached the membrane, what slowed enzyme access, what crossed into portal blood, the blood draining from the intestine into the liver first, and what the liver and kidney were then forced to handle. A food can pass every social test of wholesomeness and still keep loading the intestine with interference and the organs of clearance with avoidable work. That is the quiet middle ground. The eater does not feel poisoned. The tissues still pay.

The gut usually sees the first version of that payment. A seed rich in phytate can keep zinc and iron in the bowel instead of letting them cross the absorptive surface. A high-oxalate leaf can make a calcium-rich meal behave like a calcium-poor one as soon as oxalate and calcium meet in intestinal fluid. A legume can carry respectable protein numbers and still send protein into the small intestine with protease inhibitors attached, forcing the pancreas and brush border enzymes to work against a defended storage tissue instead of a cooperative food. A fruit rich in poorly absorbed carbohydrates can leave water and fermentable residue in the bowel without causing anything dramatic enough to be called toxicity. The person may only feel bloating, bowel irregularity, heaviness, or a low-grade aversion to the food. But the symptom is only the readable part of the event. The more important part is that the meal yielded poorly while still demanding digestive work.

The burden can also move downstream without ever becoming theatrical. The intestine allows a compound across, and the body still gains nothing from having absorbed it. The liver has to oxidize it, conjugate it, export it into bile, or return it to blood for renal clearance. The kidney has to filter it, concentrate it, and keep it dissolved in urine without allowing it to precipitate into crystals. That is the second quiet zone of plant-food physiology. The food did not poison acutely, but it still turned part of the liver into a chemical work site and part of the kidney into an excretion problem. A compound that arrives often enough does not need to injure explosively. It only needs to keep returning through the same portal route to the same hepatocyte, the main working liver cell, or into the same urinary stream to the same renal tubule until the cost stops being episodic and becomes part of the organ's daily workload.

This is why the absence of visible poisoning proves so little. It proves only that the food stayed below the threshold of obvious crisis. It does not prove that the food nourished well, cleared easily, spared the thyroid, preserved mineral value, or left the kidney with nothing troublesome to do. The middle ground is where most defended plant tissue lives. The meal is tolerated. The body is underpaid. The chemistry stays quiet enough to keep its reputation and active enough to keep draining yield from the same digestive membranes, the same enzyme systems, the same glandular sequence, and the same clearance organs until the burden stops looking like a food choice and starts looking like the background physiology of the person eating it.

Part VI

The Kidney, Urine, and the Organ of Consequence

Chapter 21

The Kidney as a Filter of Failed Food Logic

The kidney is not judging the meal by reputation. It is judging the remainder. By the time chemistry reaches the nephron, the kidney's microscopic filtering unit, digestion is over, absorption is over, and the liver has already had its first chance to sort what the intestine allowed across. What arrives at the kidney is the fraction still dissolved in blood that the body must either keep or eliminate. Each nephron begins with the glomerulus, a tuft of capillaries under pressure that filters plasma water and small dissolved compounds into the tubular fluid, while larger proteins and blood cells are normally retained in the circulation. The tubule then reclaims what the body still wants and leaves behind what the body cannot justify carrying further. That is why the kidney exposes failed food logic so clearly. A compound that entered the body with little constructive value and survived long enough to reach the nephron has already lost the argument once. The bowel did not build with it. The liver did not fully neutralize or retain it. Now the kidney has to decide how to clear it.

This is where the difference between nourishment and burden becomes hard to hide. A useful nutrient is usually reclaimed. Glucose, amino acids, bicarbonate, electrolytes, and much of the filtered water are pulled back across the tubular epithelium because the body still has work for them. A failed compound keeps moving downstream in tubular fluid. The kidney may secrete even more of it into that fluid through the tubule, which means the nephron is not only filtering the blood but actively loading unwanted chemistry into the urine stream. Reviews of oxalate handling make this especially clear. With normal kidney function, oxalate is excreted mainly through the kidney by glomerular filtration and net tubular secretion, which means the nephron is not preserving it as a useful metabolite. It is moving it out. The compound has become urinary work.

That is why the kidney is the organ that reveals what the body could not use. It turns hidden nutritional failure into excretory pressure. A high-oxalate leaf can already fail in the gut by trapping calcium before absorption. If enough soluble oxalate still crosses into blood, the kidney inherits the second half of the problem. Now the nephron has to filter it, secrete part of it, concentrate it into a shrinking volume of water, and keep it dissolved under conditions that favor crystal formation. Calcium oxalate stones are the clearest expression of that failure because the same compound that added little value to the body becomes a major component of the solid the kidney could not keep in solution. NIDDK and kidney-stone reviews both treat calcium oxalate as a dominant stone chemistry and identify urinary oxalate as one of the main variables pushing that chemistry toward crystallization. The food may still carry a healthy public identity. The urine shows what the body was left trying to discard.

The nephron also strips away another common illusion. Elimination is not effortless. Tubular cells have to reclaim sodium, potassium, bicarbonate, glucose, amino acids, and water while the same fluid column is carrying metabolic waste, acids, plant-derived solutes, drug metabolites, and crystal-forming ions. Concentration makes that work harder because the kidney can only eliminate many compounds by pushing them into progressively smaller amounts of water. A solute that looked trivial in blood can become dangerous in urine once the water is pulled back and the concentration climbs. Stone-pathway reviews describe this shift through supersaturation, the state in which urine holds more dissolved crystal-forming material than it can keep stable in solution. The kidney does not create the bad food decision, but it is often the organ that has to finish paying for it.

So the kidney belongs in this chapter because it shows the last stage of a failed bargain. The plant compound or poorly handled food chemistry entered the mouth as something that looked edible, useful, or at least harmless. It reached the bowel and gave little back. It reached the liver and still required handling. It reached the kidney as dissolved remainder. At that point the nephron is no longer asking what the food contained. It is asking what must be filtered, what must be secreted, what can still be reclaimed, and what must leave as urine before it injures the tubule or crystallizes in the urinary tract. The body can call it food for as long as it wants. By the time the chemistry reaches the nephron, the useful fraction has already been reclaimed. What remains is the dissolved remainder the body still has to excrete without damaging the tubule or precipitating into crystals.

Filtration, Concentration, and Excretion as a Final Sorting Step

By the time blood reaches the glomerulus, the capillary tuft inside each nephron that begins urine formation, digestion is over, absorption is over, and the liver has already taken its first pass at the compounds the intestine allowed into blood. What enters the glomerular circulation is no longer a meal. It is plasma carrying the dissolved fraction the body still has to reclaim, transform, buffer, or discard. Small solutes and water are driven across the filtration barrier into Bowman's space, while larger proteins and blood cells are normally retained in the circulation. That first step is mechanical rather than nutritional. The glomerulus is not deciding what the food meant. It is sieving blood into a fluid the tubule can work on next.

The real sorting begins after filtration. The nephron does not leave the filtrate alone because the filtrate still contains too much that the body cannot afford to lose. Glucose, amino acids, bicarbonate, sodium, calcium, and most of the filtered water are pulled back across the tubular epithelium because they still have use. Other compounds are left in the lumen, the hollow interior of the tubule, precisely because the body does not want them returned. Some substances are added to that lumen deliberately through tubular secretion, which means the kidney is not only filtering unwanted chemistry from the blood but actively loading more of it into the forming urine. Reabsorption and secretion are therefore the kidney's second and harder cut. Filtration makes the first crude copy. The tubule edits it.

This is where failed food logic becomes visible. A useful nutrient is usually reclaimed because the body still wants it in circulation. A low-value compound that crossed the bowel wall and survived the liver does not win that argument in the nephron. It keeps moving. If the body has no structural, energetic, or signaling use for it, the tubule does not rescue it. Oxalate is the clean example because it can already fail earlier in the sequence by trapping calcium in the gut, then fail again in blood by arriving at the kidney as a solute the body still has to eliminate. Reviews of oxalate handling describe renal excretion as the major route of oxalate clearance, with both glomerular filtration and tubular handling contributing to how much finally appears in urine. The kidney is left clearing what digestion absorbed, the liver did not keep, and the body could not use.

Concentration is what turns that quiet remainder into risk. The kidney does not usually excrete many solutes by leaving them in a large pool of water. It does the opposite. It reclaims water aggressively and leaves the rejected chemistry behind in a shrinking fluid column. That strategy is efficient only while the solute remains dissolved. Once concentration rises far enough, the chemistry changes. A compound that was harmless enough in diluted plasma can become dangerous in tubular fluid and urine because the water has been pulled back and the solute is now crowded against other crystal-forming or irritating molecules. In stone disease this appears as supersaturation, the state in which urine contains more dissolved crystal-forming material than it can keep stably in solution. Higher calcium oxalate supersaturation tracks with greater stone risk, which is exactly what you would expect when concentration pushes the urine past what it can still hold safely.

Excretion therefore is not passive disposal. It is the final result of repeated selection under narrowing conditions. The nephron filters broadly, reclaims aggressively, secretes selectively, and then concentrates what remains until the body either gets the dissolved remainder out or loses control of the chemistry on the way. Some solutes leave quietly. Others keep dragging water with them, acidifying the stream, irritating the epithelium, or moving toward precipitation. The tubular cell has to survive that contact while still reclaiming sodium, bicarbonate, glucose, and water from the same flow. The kidney does not merely remove waste. It keeps narrowing the fluid until what still cannot be reclaimed is forced into a form that can leave as urine.

That is why filtration, concentration, and excretion belong in this book as a final sorting step rather than as an afterthought. A food can look nutritious at the level of label content, fail to build the body well in the intestine, add handling work in the liver, and still reach the nephron as dissolved burden. By the time the chemistry enters the final urine, the useful fraction has already been taken back. What remains is the part the kidney still has to push out without injuring the tubule or letting the solutes crystallize in the shrinking volume of water left behind.

When Food Compounds Become Urinary Burdens

A food compound becomes a urinary burden when it crosses the intestine, survives the liver, reaches the renal circulation, and still gives the body no reason to keep it. That is the shift. In the gut the question is absorption. In the liver the question is transformation. In the kidney the question becomes whether the compound can be excreted without damaging the tubule or crystallizing in the shrinking volume of water that will become urine. By the time blood reaches the glomerulus, the capillary tuft inside each nephron that begins filtration, digestion is over, absorption is over, and the liver has already taken its first pass at the compounds the intestine allowed into blood. What enters the nephron is the dissolved remainder the body still has to sort. Oxalate is the cleanest example because it contributes little or nothing constructive once absorbed and is cleared predominantly by the kidney through glomerular filtration and tubular secretion, which means the nephron is not trying to reclaim it as useful chemistry. It is trying to move it out.

That burden becomes more serious as the nephron keeps pulling water back. The filtered fluid entering the tubule still contains many solutes the body wants, so water, sodium, bicarbonate, glucose, amino acids, and other useful compounds are reclaimed along the way. What the body does not want is left behind in a smaller and smaller volume. This is where a dissolved food-derived compound stops looking trivial. A low concentration in plasma can become a high concentration in urine because the kidney has removed so much water around it. In stone disease that change becomes visible as supersaturation, the state in which urine contains more dissolved crystal-forming material than it can keep stably in solution. Oxalate reaches that point with calcium. Uric acid reaches it when urinary pH is low enough and the urine is concentrated enough that the acid stops staying dissolved. StatPearls on uric acid nephrolithiasis identifies persistently low urinary pH and low urine volume as major drivers, while renal physiology sources describe tubular secretion as one of the kidney's main ways of disposing of undesirable solutes such as uric acid and drug metabolites. The compound did not have to poison dramatically on the way in. It only had to remain useless long enough to become concentrated on the way out.

That is why the kidney is such a hard organ to fool with food reputation. A compound can arrive in a leaf, seed, tuber, or drink carrying a clean public identity and still end in urine as crystal pressure, acid load, or tubular work. Oxalate shows the full sequence best. In the bowel it can already lower calcium yield. In blood it remains a solute with no constructive role. In the kidney it is filtered, secreted, concentrated, and forced into a chemical environment where calcium oxalate can precipitate if the urine becomes too crowded. Kidney-stone reviews and NIDDK materials keep returning to this logic because it is the point at which the failed bargain becomes physical. The body absorbed the compound, but the kidney now has to keep it dissolved or let it become a crystal. That is not passive disposal. It is excretory work imposed by chemistry the body could not turn into tissue.

The same reasoning extends beyond stones. Drug metabolites, organic acids, sulfate from sulfur handling, and other low-value or foreign solutes can all become urinary burdens when the kidney has to filter them, sometimes secrete more of them into the tubular lumen, and then concentrate them enough that irritation, osmotic drag, or precipitation become possible. Renal physiology and renal function reviews describe the kidney's role in excreting waste products, toxins, drugs, and metabolites while maintaining volume and acid-base balance at the same time. That is the broader lesson the chapter needs. A food compound stops being a food question once the body has finished taking back the useful fraction. From that point forward the nephron is handling the dissolved remainder, and the quality of that handling determines whether the compound leaves quietly in urine or keeps returning as crystal injury, acidic urine, low-volume stress, or repeated tubular contact.

Why the Story of a Plant Food Does Not End at Absorption

Absorption is only the point where the body stops negotiating with the food in the lumen and starts negotiating with the chemistry in its own tissues. A compound crossing the intestinal membrane has not yet proven itself useful. It has only proven that it got through. The bowel can absorb sugar and still leave the pancreas, liver, and circulation to deal with the consequences of the dose. It can absorb oxalate and hand the kidney a crystal problem instead of a nutrient. It can absorb a plant alkaloid, a sulfur breakdown product, a furanocoumarin, or a biogenic amine and give the liver, thyroid, skin, nervous system, or vascular system a new burden to sort out. The membrane is not a finish line. It is the border crossing between digestive handling and tissue handling.

The first organ to inherit that chemistry is usually the liver because blood leaving the intestine enters the portal vein and reaches the liver before it reaches the rest of the body. At that point the plant compound is no longer just part of the meal. It is part of portal blood, the blood draining from the gut into the liver first, and the hepatocyte, the main working liver cell, has to decide what to do with it. Some molecules are simple enough to enter ordinary metabolism. Others have to be oxidized, reduced, hydrolyzed, conjugated, pushed into bile, or sent back into blood for renal clearance. A meal can therefore fail in a very specific way. It can give the intestine little worth keeping and still ask the liver to spend enzyme activity, glutathione, transporter work, and bile flow on chemistry the body did not get to keep as nourishment. The food leaves the plate as food and reaches the hepatocyte as workload.

Then the rest of the body has to live with whatever the liver did not fully neutralize or remove. The thyroid has to keep trapping iodide and building hormone while sulfur compounds from damaged Brassica tissue compete at the same sequence. The bowel wall itself can be changed by repeated exposure to compounds that inhibit enzymes, irritate membranes, or alter permeability. The skin can be injured by psoralens after plant contact and ultraviolet A light meet in the same tissue. A drug dose can be distorted because grapefruit furanocoumarins thinned the cytochrome P450 3A4, abbreviated CYP3A4, enzyme field in the intestinal wall before the drug ever reached blood in its intended form. Absorption did not solve the question in any of those cases. It moved the question downstream.

The kidney is often where the last answer appears because the body cannot keep a useless absorbed compound in circulation forever. Once the useful fraction has been reclaimed, burned, stored, or incorporated into tissue, the dissolved remainder reaches the nephron, the kidney's filtering unit, and has to leave in urine. That is where low-yield plant chemistry becomes physically visible. Oxalate becomes urinary oxalate. Uric acid becomes acidic concentrated urine and, under the wrong conditions, stone chemistry. Drug metabolites, organic acids, sulfate, ammonium, and other low-value solutes keep moving through tubular fluid while the kidney pulls water back around them. A compound that looked small in blood can become dangerous in urine because concentration changes what the chemistry can do. The body absorbed it. The kidney still has to survive excreting it.

Repetition is what makes this impossible to dismiss as a one-meal curiosity. A single exposure can stay quiet because the organs have reserve. The same chemistry returning every day is different. The same portal route fills again. The same hepatocyte keeps altering the same molecules. The same thyroid keeps handling the same interference. The same nephron keeps concentrating the same dissolved remainder. Once that happens, the story of the food is no longer in the produce aisle, the kitchen, or the nutrition table. It is in the tissues that had to absorb, transform, buffer, filter, secrete, and excrete what the plant delivered after the meal was already over.

The Kidney as the Organ That Pays for the Parts of the Meal the Body Must Get Rid Of

The kidney meets the meal at its most unforgiving stage. By the time blood reaches the glomerulus, the capillary tuft inside each nephron that begins filtration, the food has already passed through chewing, acid, enzymes, absorption, and the liver's first round of chemical handling. What remains in the circulation is no longer the meal as the eater imagined it. It is the dissolved fraction the body kept in blood long enough that the nephron now has to sort it. Water and small solutes are pushed through the filtration barrier into Bowman's space, the first collecting space of the nephron, while larger proteins and blood cells are held back. That first step is broad. It does not distinguish nourishment from burden. It simply moves a large part of the plasma water and its dissolved chemistry into a tubular stream the kidney can work on. The harder judgment comes after that, when the tubule begins taking back what the body still wants and leaving behind what the body can no longer justify carrying.

That reclamation is what makes the kidney such a clean organ of consequence. A useful compound is usually rescued. Glucose is pulled back. Amino acids are pulled back. Much of the sodium, bicarbonate, calcium, and water are pulled back. If the body still has a reason to keep the molecule, the tubule spends membrane transport, oxygen, and cellular work to reclaim it from the filtrate. The parts of the meal that added little value do not get that rescue. They stay in the tubular fluid, or the nephron secretes even more of them into that fluid from blood. A plant compound can therefore survive digestion, survive the liver's first pass, and still reach the kidney with no constructive role left to play. At that point the nephron is not evaluating the food's reputation, nutrient label, or cultural status. It is deciding whether the chemistry can be left in urine without injuring the tubule on the way out.

This is where food burden becomes physically visible. Oxalate is the cleanest example because once it has crossed the intestine and entered blood, the body does not turn it into tissue. The kidney filters it, secretes part of it, and then keeps pulling water back around it. The urine becomes more concentrated, which means the dissolved oxalate is now sharing a smaller fluid space with calcium and other solutes. If the concentration rises far enough, supersaturation develops, meaning the urine is holding more crystal-forming material than it can keep stably dissolved. That is when the chemistry stops being quiet. The dissolved remainder becomes a precipitation problem. The same sequence can happen with uric acid under acidic urinary conditions, or with other low-value solutes that drag osmotic load, acid load, or tubular irritation into the final urine. The kidney is not creating the burden. It is concentrating the parts of the meal the body took in but could not turn into anything worth keeping.

That is why the kidney pays for failed food logic more clearly than almost any other organ. A leaf can enter the mouth looking mineral-rich and leave the kidney as oxalate pressure. A fruit can look light and clean and still leave behind acids, metabolites, or drug-handling consequences the nephron must carry out in concentrated urine. A seed can nourish thinly and still contribute to the chemical traffic the liver and kidney have to clear. The body can absorb a compound without benefiting from it, and once that happens the nephron inherits the last stage of the problem. It has to filter the dissolved remainder, reclaim water around it, and push it out through a narrowing stream without letting the chemistry injure tubular cells, disturb acid-base handling, or crystallize into a more durable form of damage. The meal is over long before that point. The kidney is still paying for what the body could not use.

Chapter 22

Crystal Burden, Irritation, and Stone Vulnerability

Urine is supposed to carry dissolved waste out of the body without letting that waste become structure. That is the job. The kidney filters blood, reclaims water, sodium, bicarbonate, glucose, and other useful material, and leaves behind a smaller fluid volume carrying whatever chemistry still has to leave as urine. That shrinking matters because a dissolved compound can remain harmless in a large fluid space and become dangerous in a small one. Supersaturation is the point where the urine is holding more of a crystal-forming substance than it can comfortably keep dissolved. The easiest way to picture it is not as poison floating in water but as crowding inside solution. Calcium, oxalate, uric acid, phosphate, and other solutes can stay suspended while the fluid is dilute enough and the surrounding chemistry still favors dissolution. Pull enough water back, lower the pH in the wrong direction, or raise the concentration of one of the crystal partners high enough, and the dissolved state becomes unstable. The urine is no longer only carrying waste. It is carrying waste at the edge of becoming solid.

That edge is where crystal burden begins. A person does not feel supersaturation directly because it starts as a chemical condition, not as a stone large enough to notice. The urine simply reaches a state where dissolved ions are crowded enough that they begin finding each other and staying together. A tiny crystal nucleus forms. More calcium and oxalate, or more uric acid, deposit onto that first seed. Small crystals aggregate, meaning they begin sticking to one another instead of washing away separately, and the tubule or urinary space now has to carry particles instead of only dissolved solute. This is why the kidney pays for concentration so heavily. The organ saves water for the body by pulling fluid back, but that same efficiency pushes the rejected chemistry closer together. A compound the body could not use becomes a crystal risk only after it has been filtered, left behind, and concentrated hard enough that the dissolved state starts failing.

Once crystals appear, the problem is no longer only one of chemistry on paper. It becomes contact, abrasion, retention, and irritation inside real tissue. The tubular epithelium and urinary lining are now exposed to hard microscopic structures moving through spaces built for fluid. Some crystals pass. Some lodge. Some scrape, inflame, or seed further growth. That is why supersaturation matters more than the average person thinks. It is the quiet precondition for a solid burden. The body absorbed a compound it did not need, failed to reclaim it as useful material, concentrated it into urine, and then lost control of its physical state. A high-oxalate meal, low urine volume, acidic urine, excess calcium loss, or repeated delivery of the same dissolved burden can all push the kidney toward that point. The stone is late. Supersaturation is the earlier failure, when the urine stops being only a carrying fluid and starts becoming a place where rejected chemistry can turn into structure.

Calcium Oxalate as the Main Example

Calcium oxalate is the main example because it makes the whole sequence visible without any interpretive help. The compound begins as plant chemistry, not as a stone. Oxalate enters the body from food and from endogenous production, meaning oxalate the body makes through its own metabolism. If enough oxalate remains in soluble form in the gut, crosses the intestinal membrane, and survives into blood, the kidney becomes the organ that has to finish the mistake. Reviews of dietary oxalate and stone disease identify calcium oxalate as the dominant stone chemistry in human nephrolithiasis, and NIDDK's current stone guidance treats calcium oxalate as the central dietary stone problem, with oxalate-rich foods specifically singled out because they can raise urinary oxalate.

What makes calcium oxalate so useful as the model case is that the same molecule can fail the body twice. In the intestine, oxalate can already reduce nourishment by binding calcium and lowering how much free calcium remains available for absorption. If enough oxalate still reaches blood, the burden moves downstream into renal handling. The kidney filters it, tubular cells secrete part of it, water is pulled back around it, and the rejected chemistry is left in an ever smaller volume of fluid. Once calcium and oxalate are crowded together in urine strongly enough, supersaturation develops, meaning the urine is holding more dissolved crystal-forming material than it can keep stably in solution. At that point the chemistry is no longer only dissolved remainder. It is crystal risk.

That is where calcium oxalate stops being a food chemistry issue and becomes a physical burden inside the nephron. A crystal nucleus forms. More calcium and oxalate deposit onto it. Crystals enlarge, aggregate, and in some kidneys begin attaching to renal tissue rather than washing away cleanly. Reviews of stone mechanisms describe calcium oxalate as the most common stone type and emphasize that supersaturation, crystal growth, aggregation, and retention are the steps that turn dissolved urinary chemistry into stone disease. The kidney is no longer clearing only fluid. It is carrying a solid-forming burden through structures built for flow.

Calcium oxalate also reveals why concentration matters more than label content. A spinach leaf, an almond-heavy meal, or another oxalate-rich exposure may still look light, plant-based, and nutritionally respectable from the outside. The nephron does not see the reputation. It sees urinary oxalate, urinary calcium, urine volume, and the point at which those variables stop behaving safely together. NIDDK advises stone-formers to reduce high-oxalate foods and notes that enough calcium with meals can help because calcium in the gut lowers how much oxalate is later absorbed and excreted in urine. That is the same logic seen from the other end. The body is safer when the oxalate is trapped before blood ever carries it to the kidney.

So calcium oxalate is the main example because it shows the entire failed bargain in one line of physiology. The food gives little back in the gut, the body absorbs what it cannot use, and the kidney is left concentrating a dissolved remainder that can turn into crystal, abrasion, retention, and stone. By the time the chemistry becomes a calcium oxalate stone, the meal is long gone. The nephron is still carrying what the body could not turn into tissue and could not leave in solution.

Why Concentration, Hydration, Calcium Balance, and Oxalate Load All Matter

A calcium oxalate stone does not appear because one molecule behaved badly in isolation. It appears because several variables are being forced together in the same shrinking volume of urine. The kidney filters calcium. It filters oxalate. It then pulls water back because the body cannot afford to lose fluid carelessly. That concentration step is useful until it stops being safe. Once water is withdrawn far enough, the same calcium and oxalate that floated harmlessly enough in plasma are left crowded together in tubular fluid and urine. This is where supersaturation begins, the state in which urine contains more crystal-forming material than it can keep stably dissolved. The stone is late. The earlier failure is concentration outrunning solubility.

Hydration matters because urine volume changes that crowding directly. More water means the same dissolved oxalate and calcium are dispersed through a larger fluid space, which lowers the chance that they will find each other often enough and tightly enough to begin crystal formation. Less water means the opposite. The kidney still has to excrete the solute load, but now it has less fluid to hide it in. That is why low urine volume keeps showing up in stone prevention and stone recurrence guidance. The chemistry does not need to become more exotic. It only needs to become more concentrated.

Calcium balance matters for a reason that confuses people until the gut and kidney are kept in the same picture. Calcium in the intestine is protective against oxalate absorption because it binds oxalate there, before the oxalate can cross the intestinal wall and enter blood. A low-calcium diet sounds protective if the problem is called a calcium oxalate stone, but the physiology runs the other way. Reduce calcium too far and the gut leaves more oxalate free, which means more oxalate is absorbed, more oxalate reaches blood, and more oxalate finally reaches urine. NIDDK and nephrology reviews both make this point clearly. Enough calcium with meals lowers urinary oxalate burden by trapping oxalate upstream, where the kidney never has to see it.

Oxalate load matters because the kidney cannot turn oxalate into something useful once it has been absorbed. It has to clear it. A high-oxalate meal, repeated often enough, changes the chemistry of the urine even if the person never thinks of themselves as eating a "stone diet." Spinach, Swiss chard, beet greens, almonds, rhubarb, sweet potatoes, and similar foods can keep returning soluble oxalate to the intestine, and the fraction that escapes gut binding becomes renal work later. This is why calcium oxalate is such a harsh model of failed food logic. The meal can lower mineral yield in the gut first and still become crystal burden in the kidney later. The same molecule underperforms on the way in and injures on the way out.

So these four variables belong to one sequence, not four separate lifestyle tips. Oxalate load determines how much oxalate reaches the urine. Calcium balance in the gut determines how much of that load is stopped before absorption. Hydration determines how much fluid is left to carry the rejected chemistry out. Concentration determines whether the remaining calcium and oxalate stay dissolved or begin turning into structure. The kidney pays when all four drift in the wrong direction at once.

How Repeated High-Oxalate Intake Can Shift Urine Chemistry

A high-oxalate meal does not become a kidney problem the moment it is swallowed. The shift begins earlier, in the intestine, where oxalate enters the same fluid field as calcium and other minerals. If enough calcium is present in the gut, more oxalate is trapped there as poorly soluble calcium oxalate and leaves in stool. If less calcium is available, or if the oxalate load is simply high enough, more soluble oxalate stays free, crosses the intestinal wall, and enters blood. That is the first change that matters to the kidney. The meal has already failed once by letting more oxalate through than the body can use for anything constructive. Reviews of dietary oxalate handling describe the same sequence clearly, and NIDDK's current guidance for calcium oxalate stone prevention still points back to high-oxalate foods because dietary oxalate can raise the amount of oxalate that finally appears in urine.

Once that absorbed oxalate reaches the kidney, repetition changes the chemistry more than a single exposure does. The nephron filters oxalate and leaves the body to clear it mainly in urine. One high-oxalate meal may produce only a brief rise in urinary oxalate. Repeated intake changes the baseline traffic through the same route. More oxalate keeps arriving in the renal circulation, more oxalate keeps entering tubular fluid, and the same dissolved burden keeps being concentrated as water is pulled back. That is why newer human data continue to find that moderate and large oxalate loads increase urinary oxalate excretion and can even promote nanocrystalluria, the presence of tiny crystals in urine, before a person ever reaches the stage of a visible stone. The urine is no longer carrying the old chemistry. It has been shifted toward a more crowded oxalate state.

The next part of the shift is physical, not just numerical. Oxalate does not travel through urine alone. It travels beside calcium, and the kidney keeps withdrawing water around both. As urine volume falls, the same calcium and oxalate are forced into a smaller fluid space, and the risk of supersaturation, meaning urine holds more crystal-forming material than it can keep stably dissolved, begins to rise. High fluid intake pushes in the opposite direction by expanding the carrying volume. Adequate calcium intake with meals pushes upstream by lowering intestinal oxalate absorption before the kidney ever has to see it. This is why the usual stone-prevention advice is physiologically tighter than it looks. Hydration is not generic wellness advice. Calcium with meals is not a contradiction. Both are ways of keeping urinary oxalate and calcium from being crowded together under conditions that favor calcium oxalate crystallization.

So repeated high-oxalate intake shifts urine chemistry by changing what reaches the kidney, how often it returns, and how much dissolved room the kidney still has to carry it out safely. The bowel absorbs more soluble oxalate. The nephron filters more oxalate. The tubule concentrates that oxalate into a smaller fluid volume. Supersaturation rises. Crystal pressure rises with it. The meal may still look plant-based, light, or clean in the kitchen. In urine it has become a repeated calcium oxalate problem waiting for enough concentration and enough time to turn dissolved burden into structure.

Stone Formation as a Visible Endpoint of Plant Burden

A stone is late. The chemistry failed earlier. Long before a person feels flank pain or sees a crystal in a urine report, the body has already absorbed a compound it could not use, delivered it to the kidney, and concentrated it into a shrinking volume of fluid until the dissolved state began to break down. In calcium oxalate stone disease, the burden usually begins with oxalate entering the body from food or endogenous production, meaning oxalate made inside the body through normal metabolism, then reaching the nephron as a solute the kidney must clear rather than reclaim. Reviews of kidney stone mechanisms describe supersaturation of urine with calcium oxalate or other stone-forming salts as the key precondition for crystal formation, and calcium oxalate remains the dominant stone chemistry in human nephrolithiasis.

What makes the stone such a useful endpoint is that it turns an invisible dissolved burden into visible structure. Urine can carry calcium and oxalate quietly for a time. Then the concentration rises, the dissolved ions begin finding each other often enough to stay together, and a crystal nucleus forms. From there the sequence hardens. More calcium and oxalate deposit onto the same nucleus. Small crystals aggregate, meaning they begin sticking to one another instead of washing away separately. Retention becomes the next problem. A crystal that leaves in urine may remain a brief event. A crystal that adheres to renal tissue or lodges in a tubular space becomes a growth site. Reviews of stone pathophysiology make this progression explicit: supersaturation first, then nucleation, growth, aggregation, and retention.

This is why the stone should not be read as a random object that appeared one day in the kidney. It is the visible endpoint of repeated low-yield chemistry the body kept having to clear. A high-oxalate leaf can already fail the person in the gut by trapping calcium and lowering mineral value there. If enough soluble oxalate still crosses into blood, the kidney inherits the second half of the problem. The nephron filters it, may secrete more of it into tubular fluid, then pulls water back around it. The body has now taken in what it did not need and concentrated it under conditions that favor precipitation. What looked like a nutrition question at the plate has become a urine-chemistry question inside the kidney.

The visible stone matters because it exposes a pattern the body had been trying to manage silently. Higher urinary supersaturation of calcium oxalate tracks with greater likelihood of being a stone former, and stone growth itself tracks with that same chemistry. This is the point where plant burden stops being theoretical. The rejected chemistry has acquired mass, shape, friction, and the ability to injure tissue mechanically. The kidney is no longer only carrying dissolved remainder. It is carrying hard particulate matter through spaces built for fluid.

So stone formation belongs in this book as a visible endpoint, not because every plant burden ends in a stone, but because a stone shows the whole failed bargain in one object. The meal added little retained value, the body absorbed part of it anyway, the kidney was forced to concentrate the dissolved remainder, and the chemistry finally crossed from invisible load into structure. By the time the person notices the stone, the plant burden has already moved through gut, blood, nephron, and urine and hardened into something the body can no longer keep dissolved.

Why the Story of a Plant Food Does Not End at Absorption

Absorption only means the compound crossed the intestinal membrane. It does not mean the body wanted it, used it well, or was improved by taking it in. A plant food can release a molecule in the lumen, the hollow interior of the bowel where digestion is taking place, carry that molecule across the absorptive surface, and still leave the rest of the body with a burden instead of a gain. The intestine is only the first gate. Once a compound enters blood, the question changes. Now the liver has to decide whether the molecule can enter ordinary metabolism, whether it has to be oxidized or conjugated before the body can tolerate carrying it, or whether it should be pushed toward bile or urine as quickly as possible. The food may have looked nutrient-dense on the plate. The absorbed fraction can still arrive at the hepatocyte, the main working liver cell, as chemical work rather than as nourishment.

The kidney sees the next part of that argument. A compound that entered blood but gave the body little constructive value is eventually filtered at the glomerulus, the capillary tuft in each nephron that begins urine formation, then concentrated as water is pulled back around it.

This is where dissolved burden becomes physically dangerous. NIDDK notes that kidney stones are caused by high levels of calcium, oxalate, and phosphorus in the urine, and that these minerals are normally present in urine without causing trouble at lower levels. The problem is not mere presence. The problem is concentration strong enough to push the urine toward crystal formation. In oxalate-rich plant foods, the sequence is especially unforgiving. Oxalate can already reduce calcium availability in the gut, then reach the kidney as a solute the body still has to excrete, and finally become part of calcium oxalate crystal chemistry in urine.

That is why absorption is not a victory. A high-oxalate leaf can fail twice. It can lower calcium yield in the intestine first and still raise urinary oxalate burden later. NIDDK's current stone guidance still advises people prone to calcium oxalate stones to reduce high-oxalate foods, and current prevention reviews continue to note that higher dietary calcium lowers stone risk partly by binding oxalate in the gut before it can be absorbed and reach urine. The body is safer when that chemistry is stopped upstream. Once it crosses into blood, the kidney has to carry the rest of the burden in a shrinking volume of water.

The same logic applies beyond oxalate. Plant foods can test dense in minerals and still deliver those minerals poorly because phytate and oxalate reduce bioavailability before or during absorption. Reviews of plant-food bioavailability and phytochemical-mineral interactions describe phytate and oxalate as factors that reduce the efficiency of mineral absorption from vegetables, grains, legumes, nuts, and seeds. That means a food can cross the line from promising to costly without ever producing visible poisoning. It enters the intestine carrying both nutrients and opposition, gives the body a thin return, and still hands the liver and kidney enough dissolved remainder to keep processing and excreting afterward. A label can count what the food contained. The body has to live with what the food released, what it let through, and what the kidney still has to push out at the end.

Chapter 23

Sensitive Hosts and High-Risk Physiology

The oxalate problem changes completely when fat is not being absorbed well. In an ordinary meal, calcium in the intestinal lumen, the hollow interior of the bowel where digestion is taking place, can bind part of the oxalate load there and keep it in the gut as insoluble calcium oxalate rather than letting it cross into blood. Fat malabsorption scrambles that arrangement. Unabsorbed fatty acids stay in the bowel, and calcium begins binding those fatty acids instead, forming calcium-fatty acid soaps. The calcium is still present in the meal, but it is no longer available to trap oxalate. More oxalate stays free in soluble form, and soluble oxalate is the fraction much more able to cross the intestinal wall and become a renal burden later. Reviews of enteric hyperoxaluria, the state of excessive oxalate absorption from the intestine, describe this as the central mechanism linking fat malabsorption to increased urinary oxalate.

That is only the first part of the shift. The bowel itself becomes easier for oxalate to cross. Unabsorbed bile acids and fatty acids reaching the colon can increase colonic permeability, meaning the barrier becomes more permissive to oxalate movement than it would be under quieter digestive conditions. The result is a double loss. Calcium is diverted away from oxalate binding, and the bowel wall becomes a better entry route for the oxalate left behind. Human and review literature on enteric hyperoxaluria keeps returning to exactly that sequence in Crohn's disease, pancreatic insufficiency, short-bowel states, and malabsorptive bariatric surgery. The food may still look like spinach, nuts, sweet potatoes, or another ordinary oxalate exposure. The host has changed the terms of absorption so the same meal now delivers a larger oxalate burden into blood.

This is why a person with fat malabsorption does not meet a high-oxalate food on the same terms as a person with intact fat handling. The bowel is no longer simply choosing whether to absorb oxalate. It is being forced into a different mineral economy. Calcium is tied up in fat soaps. More free oxalate remains in solution. More oxalate reaches the nephron, the kidney's filtering unit, and the kidney then has to excrete that oxalate in urine, where it can drive calcium oxalate supersaturation and crystal formation. StatPearls and renal crystal disease reviews describe enteric hyperoxaluria in exactly those terms: steatorrhea, meaning fat-rich stool from fat malabsorption, sequesters intestinal calcium and leaves more oxalate available for gastrointestinal absorption, pushing urinary oxalate upward.

That is why this section belongs under sensitive hosts and high-risk physiology rather than under the ordinary oxalate chapter alone. The food did not become more toxic on the plate. The host became more permissive to the toxin-like part of the food chemistry. A low-calcium meal, a fatty malabsorptive state, or repeated high-oxalate intake can all push in the same direction, but fat malabsorption is the cleaner demonstration because it changes the gut chemistry at the exact point where oxalate is either trapped safely in the bowel or allowed into the body. Once that shift happens, the intestine stops being only a site of undernourishment and becomes the place where a renal burden is created meal after meal.

Bowel Disease, Microbiome Disruption, and Altered Handling

The same high-oxalate food does not enter every bowel on equal terms. A healthy intestine can still absorb too much oxalate under the wrong diet, but a diseased or disrupted bowel changes the chemistry before the meal has even left the lumen, the hollow interior of the gut where digestion is taking place. Inflammatory bowel disease, ileal resection, short bowel states, pancreatic insufficiency, celiac-related malabsorption, and bariatric surgery all matter here for the same reason. They can leave more fat and bile acids unabsorbed, more calcium tied up in fatty acid soaps, more mucosal permeability, meaning an easier crossing route through the bowel wall, and more oxalate left free in soluble form. Reviews of enteric hyperoxaluria, the state of excessive oxalate absorption from the intestine, keep returning to this sequence because it is the core route by which bowel disease turns an ordinary oxalate exposure into a larger renal burden.

The first shift is chemical. In a quieter bowel, calcium in the intestinal contents can bind part of the oxalate load and leave it behind as insoluble calcium oxalate in stool. In a malabsorbing bowel, unabsorbed fatty acids seize that calcium first. The mineral is still present in the meal, but it is no longer available to trap oxalate. Bile salts and free fatty acids add a second injury by making the colonic surface more permissive to oxalate passage. Older colonic transport work showed that bile salts and fatty acids increase colonic oxalate absorption through a nonspecific change in mucosal permeability, and modern enteric hyperoxaluria reviews still cite that same mechanism as central. The bowel has not merely become inflamed. It has become a better entry route for chemistry the body does not want.

The microbiome changes the same equation from another side. Some gut bacteria degrade oxalate in the intestinal lumen, which means they destroy part of the load before the bowel can absorb it. Oxalobacter formigenes is the best known example because it uses oxalate as a carbon source and has repeatedly been linked with lower urinary oxalate and lower stone risk. When that organism is missing, or when antibiotic exposure and broader microbiome disruption reduce oxalate-degrading capacity, more of the dietary oxalate burden is left intact in the bowel fluid. That does not mean one bacterium governs the whole disease, but it does mean the host is not absorbing oxalate from a sterile tube. The microbiome is part of the gate. Change the gate and the same food sends a different load into blood.

This is why bowel disease and microbiome disruption are not side notes in oxalate physiology. They alter the handling sequence at the exact place where the body either leaves oxalate behind or allows it through. The intestine binds less of it, degrades less of it, and in diseased states often leaks more of it. The kidney then inherits that change as hyperoxaluria, meaning excessive urinary oxalate excretion, with all the downstream consequences that follow from concentrating oxalate in a shrinking urine volume beside calcium. The stone may appear later. The altered handling began in the bowel.

That is what makes these hosts high-risk. The food did not become chemically stranger on the plate. The intestine became easier to exploit. A spinach meal, an almond-heavy snack, or another oxalate-rich exposure enters a bowel where calcium is being diverted, bile acids are irritating the surface, microbial degradation is thinner, and the membrane is less selective than it should be. Under those conditions the same meal stops behaving like a dietary choice and starts behaving like a repeated oxalate-delivery system aimed straight at the nephron.

Reduced Kidney Function and Lower Toxin Clearance

The kidney can protect the body from a large solute burden only while enough working nephron remains. Each nephron, the kidney's microscopic filtering and reclamation unit, begins with a glomerulus, the capillary tuft that filters plasma water and small dissolved compounds, then continues through a tubule that takes useful material back and leaves the rest for excretion. NIDDK describes the kidney that way for a reason. Filtration alone is not enough. The nephron has to filter, reclaim, secrete, and concentrate in sequence. When kidney function falls, that whole sequence narrows. Less blood is cleared per unit time, fewer dissolved compounds are filtered, and the tubular system has less reserve to carry waste out while still holding on to water, bicarbonate, sodium, glucose, amino acids, and other chemistry the body needs to keep. What reaches the kidney in blood is no longer just passing through a strong sorting organ. It is reaching a smaller working surface with less room to compensate.

That reduction is easiest to see in estimated glomerular filtration rate, or eGFR, the clinical estimate of how much blood the kidneys filter each minute. Chronic kidney disease is defined in part by an eGFR below 60 $mL/min/1.73\ m^2$ for three months or more, and kidney failure sits below 15. Those numbers matter because they mark a falling clearance field, not just an abnormal lab value. As filtration falls, compounds that would once have left quietly in urine begin staying in blood longer. The kidney still has to clear acids, nitrogenous waste, drug metabolites, plant-derived solutes, organic acids, sulfate, uric acid, oxalate, and countless smaller molecules, but it is doing that work with reduced throughput and reduced nephron reserve. The same absorbed burden that a healthy kidney could dilute, secrete, and excrete with little consequence can become retention, concentration stress, and urinary difficulty once filtration falls.

This is why lower kidney function changes the meaning of the same meal or compound. A high-oxalate exposure, a drug with renally cleared metabolites, a sulfur load, or a stream of low-value solutes from repeated plant chemical exposure no longer lands in a kidney with broad excretory margin. The nephron has less capacity to filter the load forward and less margin to keep the rejected chemistry dissolved as water is pulled back. Retention then begins to show itself through the chemistry the body could once clear more easily. StatPearls describes uremia as the clinical condition that develops with declining renal function, marked by retention of waste products, metabolic abnormalities, electrolyte disturbance, and physiologic change. The phrase is blunt, but the tissue meaning is more exact. Blood is now carrying solutes the nephron could not remove fast enough. The body is no longer living on what it used from the meal alone. It is also living with what the kidney failed to clear.

That is why reduced kidney function belongs in a chapter on sensitive hosts and high-risk physiology. The food did not become more aggressive on the plate. The excretory margin became thinner in the body. A plant compound that once would have passed as minor urinary work can become persistent dissolved burden. A stone-forming solute can spend longer in the nephron. A drug metabolite can remain in circulation longer than intended. A fluid volume that once diluted the chemistry well can now be harder to maintain. The kidney does not need a dramatic poison to get into trouble. It only needs a steady stream of chemistry arriving at a filtering system with less remaining power to move that chemistry out.

Thyroid Vulnerability

The thyroid becomes vulnerable when a gland that already has to work hard is given less iodine, less reserve, or more interference and is still expected to hold the same metabolic pace. That is the condition this book keeps returning to. A plant food does not need to destroy the thyroid outright to matter. It only needs to press on one of the narrow steps the gland depends on every day. The thyrocyte, the hormone-producing thyroid cell, has to pull iodide, the charged form of iodine, out of blood through the sodium-iodide symporter, abbreviated NIS. It then has to move that iodide to the follicular lumen, oxidize it through thyroid peroxidase, abbreviated TPO, and attach it to thyroglobulin, the large protein scaffold on which thyroid hormone is built. A gland with good iodine supply and broad reserve can absorb some friction in that sequence. A gland already running close to the edge cannot. That is where vulnerability begins. The book's point is not that cruciferous vegetables or other plant foods are universally thyroid-toxic. The point is that a defended plant can still add interference to a gland whose working margin is already thin.

This is why the same food can belong to two different biological stories. In a robust host with adequate iodine, good protein status, and enough gland reserve, ordinary Brassica intake may remain a small subtraction the thyroid can cover quietly. In a host living on low iodine, repeated raw crucifer intake, or preexisting gland strain, the subtraction lands differently. Thiocyanate crowds iodide uptake. Goitrin presses further downstream on hormone synthesis. The vegetable still carries fiber, folate, and a clean nutritional reputation. The gland sees a damaged sulfur-rich plant tissue delivering compounds that make iodide trapping and hormone assembly less efficient. That is the book's frame in miniature. The food can keep the reputation while the organ inherits the cost. Thyroid vulnerability is what makes that cost visible. The person is no longer meeting the vegetable only as food. They are meeting it as plant chemistry landing on a gland with too little room left.

The symptoms that appear later are downstream proof that the thyroid could not keep absorbing the subtraction forever. Temperature drops. Pulse slows. Bowel movement slows. Skin dries. Hair thins. Thinking becomes heavier. Energy flattens. The body looks vaguely underpowered because thyroid hormone sets tempo across too many tissues for failure to stay local. But those symptoms are late. The earlier event was simpler. The gland kept being asked to complete the same iodine sequence while the host supplied too little raw material or too much interference. That is why thyroid vulnerability belongs in this book. It is the point where defended plant chemistry stops being an abstract feature of food and starts becoming expensive in a specific organ whose margin was already too narrow to tolerate repeated friction.

Irritable Bowel States and Fermentation Sensitivity

An irritable bowel is not just a bowel that complains more. It is a bowel that turns ordinary digestive residue into a larger physiological event. The meal enters the stomach, leaves into the small intestine, and whatever carbohydrate escapes clean absorption keeps moving forward into a lumen, the hollow interior of the bowel, that is already more reactive to stretch, water shifts, and chemical contact than it should be. Fermentation means microbes breaking down carbohydrate the human small intestine did not finish. In a quiet bowel, some of that can remain modest. In an irritable bowel state, including irritable bowel syndrome, or IBS, the same retained carbohydrate becomes a bigger problem because gas production, luminal expansion, and altered motility are no longer being absorbed by a system with much reserve. The bowel does not simply contain the residue. It feels it, reacts to it, and moves differently because of it.

This is where the plant side of the book matters again. A food does not have to poison acutely to become expensive in this host. It only needs to leave behind enough poorly absorbed carbohydrate, resistant structure, or fermentable substrate that the colon inherits more work than the small intestine cleared. Onions, garlic, apples, pears, legumes, and other plant foods rich in FODMAPs, fermentable oligosaccharides, disaccharides, monosaccharides, and polyols, are the cleanest examples because they can leave water in the bowel by osmosis, meaning dissolved particles hold water around themselves, and then feed microbial fermentation further downstream. The same meal therefore creates two kinds of pressure. It increases fluid volume first. Then it increases gas. In a resilient host, that may remain tolerable. In an irritable bowel, it becomes distension, cramping, visible bloating, urgent stool, constipation, or unstable alternation between the two. The food still looks like fruit, vegetable, legume, or healthy fiber. The colon receives a swelling fermentable burden inside a tube already too easy to provoke.

The sensitivity is not only psychological and it is not only microbial. The bowel wall itself changes the meaning of the same chemistry. Visceral hypersensitivity, meaning exaggerated sensory response to stretch or pressure inside the gut, is one part of the problem. Altered motility is another. The intestine may segment, spasm, stall, or rush the contents forward in ways that make retained carbohydrate feel worse than the same load would feel in a steadier bowel. A person with an irritable bowel state therefore does not meet a fermentable plant food on equal terms with a more resilient host. The gas may be the same gas. The pressure may be felt more intensely. The transit pattern may be less stable. The meal did not become more innocent because the symptom is common. The bowel became less able to carry the consequence quietly.

That is why this belongs in a book about plant burden rather than in a chapter on "food sensitivity" in the vague sense. The plant food is still doing real mechanical work in the lumen. It is still leaving residue that holds water, feeds microbes, and expands volume. The difference is that a sensitive bowel turns that residue into a larger symptom event at a lower threshold. A high-fiber plant meal that is socially praised for regularity can become a lumen full of wet fermenting substrate. A fruit that is light on the plate can become a pressure problem in the colon. A legume that looks protein-rich can reach the large bowel as bacterial fuel after delivering less amino acid value upstream than the label implied. The bowel is not overreacting in some mysterious way. It is revealing what the meal became after absorption failed to finish the job.

This is the pattern the chapter needs to keep visible. An irritable bowel state does not create new plant chemistry. It removes margin. The same fermentable carbohydrates keep returning to the same lumen, the same microbes, the same sensory nerves, and the same unstable motility pattern until the food stops behaving like ordinary produce and starts behaving like recurrent intraluminal pressure. The person may only say that certain fruits, vegetables, or legumes do not agree with them. The physiology is harsher and more exact than that. The bowel is being asked to carry water, gas, stretch, and residue from plant food it did not finish cleanly enough to turn into a low-friction meal.

Why the Same Food Is Not the Same Event in Every Body

A food does not arrive in an empty system. It arrives in a host with a particular stomach acid output, enzyme reserve, bile flow, intestinal surface, microbial pattern, thyroid margin, liver workload, renal clearance capacity, and tolerance for pressure, stretch, and chemical contact. That is why the same spinach, almond flour, kale smoothie, onion, bean, zucchini, or grapefruit can produce different biological results in different people without the food itself changing identity on the plate. The meal enters one body with enough calcium in the gut to trap part of its oxalate and another body with fat malabsorption tying that calcium up in fatty acid soaps. It enters one thyroid with broad iodine reserve and another thyroid already trapping hard under rising thyroid-stimulating hormone, or TSH, pressure. It enters one bowel that clears fermentable carbohydrate quietly and another bowel that turns the same residue into gas, water retention, distension, and pain because the lumen, the hollow interior of the bowel, is already easy to provoke. The chemistry is the same. The tissue receiving it is not.

This is why host context matters without turning the mechanism into something vague. The plant does not become innocent just because one person tolerates it. The plant does not become universally dangerous just because another person reacts to it. Oxalate still binds calcium. Phytate still chelates zinc and iron. Thiocyanate still crowds iodide uptake at the thyroid. Furanocoumarins in grapefruit still inhibit cytochrome P450 3A4, abbreviated CYP3A4, in the intestinal wall. FODMAPs, fermentable oligosaccharides, disaccharides, monosaccharides, and polyols, still hold water in the bowel and feed fermentation if they escape absorption. What changes from body to body is not whether the chemistry exists. What changes is how much room the host has to absorb the subtraction, neutralize the interference, or clear the burden without symptoms or tissue cost.

Some differences begin in the gut itself. A person with intact fat handling meets oxalate under one set of mineral conditions. A person with fat malabsorption meets the same oxalate with more free fatty acids in the bowel, more calcium tied up, more soluble oxalate left available for absorption, and more urinary oxalate later. A person with a calm colon can carry a moderate fermentation load with little distress. A person with visceral hypersensitivity, meaning the bowel senses stretch and pressure too strongly, can feel the same gas burden as cramping, bloating, and urgency. A person with enough dietary iodine and low repetitive crucifer exposure can tolerate ordinary Brassica intake without much thyroid consequence. A person with low iodine intake, heavy raw Brassica intake, or reduced thyroid reserve is meeting the same sulfur chemistry with less room for error. These are not different opinions about food. They are different tissue conditions meeting the same food chemistry.

The liver and kidney widen the difference further. A plant compound absorbed from the bowel enters portal blood, the blood draining from the intestine into the liver first, and reaches the hepatocyte, the main working liver cell, as chemical work. A robust liver may oxidize, conjugate, and export that chemistry quietly. A liver already carrying repeated alcohol exposure, drug traffic, reactive metabolite burden, or poor glutathione reserve is receiving the same compound into a different biochemical environment. The kidney works the same way. One nephron can filter, concentrate, and excrete a solute without obvious consequence because urine volume is good, oxalate load is modest, and crystal inhibition still holds. Another kidney, with lower urine volume, lower clearance margin, or more repeated oxalate delivery, meets the same solute as supersaturation, crystal pressure, and irritation in the tubule. A plant burden that stays invisible in one body can become renal work in another because the organs of clearance are not starting from the same place.

That is why the same food is not the same event in every body. The food brings the chemistry. The host supplies the margin. A robust host can hide some of the cost by compensating well. A vulnerable host exposes the cost sooner because the gland, bowel, liver, or kidney has less reserve to spend. The contradiction people think they are seeing is usually no contradiction at all. One body still had room. The other did not.

Part VII

Fruit Is Not Exempt

Chapter 24

The Chemical Problem with Fruit

Fruit keeps a kind of immunity that other plant foods do not. A bitter seed is allowed to look suspicious. A bean can be discussed as hard to digest. A potato can be warned about when it greens or sprouts. Fruit is granted innocence almost automatically. That protection begins in the tissue itself. Fruit flesh is soft, wet, sweet, fragrant, brightly colored, and easy to chew. It does not announce defense the way a tough hull, a bitter leaf, or an astringent skin does. The mouth receives sugar, water, acid, aroma, and yield. Those traits are real. They are also exactly the traits most likely to hide the rest of the chemistry. The flesh feels like permission, so the food is judged before digestion has done anything to it.

That matters because fruit is still plant tissue, not dissolved nutrition. The sugars are real, but so are the acids, the poorly absorbed carbohydrates, the salicylates and amines in susceptible hosts, the polyphenols in skins and seeds, the furanocoumarins in certain citrus tissues, the sorbitol and fructose load in some varieties, and the defended reproductive structures sitting inside or beside the edible flesh. The public usually judges fruit by the outer tissue alone, by sweetness, vitamin content, color, and the idea of freshness. The body has to judge the whole structure after chewing, acid, enzymes, absorption, microbial fermentation, liver handling, and renal clearance are finished. A fruit can therefore look light and clean at the level of reputation while still delivering osmotic load to the bowel, histamine-like or salicylate burden to a sensitive host, drug-handling interference to the intestinal wall, or a repeated sugar load to a system already struggling with regulation.

Fruit also benefits from a nutritional framing that rarely asks the hard downstream questions. The conversation stops at what the fruit contains. Vitamin C. Potassium. Polyphenols. Fiber. Water. That way of talking is unusually flattering because fruit often does contain attractive compounds while asking the body to handle them inside a matrix that is metabolically or chemically less innocent than the label suggests. A fruit high in fructose and sorbitol can still be called wholesome even if the small intestine leaves part of that sugar load behind to pull water into the bowel and feed fermentation in the colon. A citrus fruit can still be called healthy while its furanocoumarins alter cytochrome P450 3A4, abbreviated CYP3A4, in the intestinal wall and change drug exposure. A berry or grape skin can still be praised for polyphenols while the same binding chemistry has real consequences for mineral handling and gut contact. The food keeps the reputation because its positive chemistry is counted first and its opposing chemistry is treated as secondary even when the body experiences both at once.

The reproductive logic of fruit also helps protect its image because people confuse edibility of the flesh with safety of the whole structure. Fruit is built around dispersal. The outer tissue may soften and sweeten precisely because the plant benefits from that part being eaten at the right stage. The seed, pit, or kernel can remain chemically guarded at the same time. That is why apricot flesh and apricot kernel do not belong to the same biological story, and why apple flesh and apple seeds do not carry the same burden. But even when the flesh itself is the intended edible tissue, it is still not neutral. It is still carrying whatever sugars, acids, fermentable residues, amines, salicylates, or phototoxic compounds the plant kept in that tissue. Fruit's reputation is protected because the plant made the invitation visible and kept much of the conflict hidden in chemistry that sounds benign until the digestive or metabolic sequence is followed all the way through.

There is also a moral protection around fruit that keeps people from reading symptoms accurately. If a bean produces gas, people are willing to say the bean may be the problem. If an onion produces bloating, the onion is allowed to be questioned. If fruit produces loose stool, distension, flushing, itching, reflux, or unstable blood sugar handling in a particular host, the person is often told the problem must lie elsewhere because fruit has already been assigned a clean category. That is one reason fruit deserves a dedicated chapter. Its reputation is not only nutritional. It is cultural and almost untouchable. The tissue arrives with a presumption of virtue strong enough that many people will reinterpret their own physiology before they reinterpret the food.

So fruit's reputation is unusually protected because the plant made the invitation easy to see and modern nutrition kept repeating the invitation after the chemistry should have complicated it. Sweetness protects it. Freshness protects it. Bright color protects it. Vitamin language protects it. The body does not protect it that way. The bowel still has to absorb the sugars cleanly, the liver still has to handle what crosses, the drug-metabolizing enzymes in the intestinal wall can still be altered by certain fruit compounds, and the kidney still has to excrete what the body could not use. Fruit remains one of the easiest plant tissues to romanticize because it feels least defended at first bite. That is exactly why its chemical problems are so easy to overlook.

Sugar, Acids, Polyols, Seeds, Skins, and Defensive Compounds

Fruit is usually discussed as if its chemistry begins and ends with sugar. That is the first simplification that has to go. The flesh of a fruit is not a syrup packet wrapped in color. It is a layered plant tissue carrying sugars, organic acids, water, fiber, aroma compounds, polyols in some species, pigments, phenolics, and whatever defensive chemistry the plant left in the skin, around the seed, or in the flesh itself. The sweetness is real, but the sweetness is only one fraction of the event. Once the tissue is chewed and ruptured, fructose, glucose, sorbitol, malic acid, citric acid, salicylates, amines, tannins, seed oils, seed inhibitors, and other smaller compounds all stop being part of an abstract fruit identity and begin mixing in the lumen, the hollow interior of the gut where digestion is taking place. That is why fruit is so easy to misread. The mouth notices sweetness first. The intestine has to deal with the whole chemical assembly afterward.

The sugar itself does not behave as one thing. Glucose and fructose do not cross the intestinal membrane through the same route, and fruits that carry a heavier fructose burden or a meaningful amount of sorbitol can become a bowel problem in ways that sweeter starchy foods do not. Sorbitol, a sugar alcohol found in fruits such as apples, pears, peaches, and some stone fruits, is absorbed slowly and incompletely, which means part of it can stay in the bowel, hold water there by osmosis, and then move into the colon as fermentation substrate. Fructose can do the same when the transport capacity of the small intestine is exceeded. The fruit can therefore look light and hydrating on the plate while becoming luminal water retention, distension, gas, and altered transit in the bowel. The same tissue that looked simple at the level of taste becomes a more complicated mechanical problem once the sugars are judged by absorption instead of by sweetness.

The acids matter too because they change what kind of fruit the body is actually receiving. A fruit rich in organic acids is not only delivering carbohydrate. It is delivering a low-pH tissue whose acids can affect oral tolerance, gastric handling, and symptom generation in a sensitive host. Citric acid, malic acid, and other fruit acids help create the sharpness people call freshness, but freshness is a sensory word, not a physiological verdict. Acidity can irritate an already inflamed upper gut, worsen reflux in a susceptible person, and change how the fruit is tolerated when large amounts are eaten without much buffering protein or fat. Then there are the skins and seeds. Fruit skin is often where part of the phenolic and defensive chemistry concentrates because the outside of the fruit still has to meet light, insects, fungi, and damage. The seed has an even harder job. It is not expendable tissue. It is reproductive tissue, and reproductive tissue is rarely surrendered without chemical resistance. That is why fruit can carry a soft, edible flesh around a core that is harder, more astringent, more inhibitor-rich, or even cyanogenic in some species. The sweetness of the flesh does not clear the chemistry of the rest of the structure.

This is where defensive compounds stop sounding exotic and start sounding ordinary. A citrus fruit can carry furanocoumarins strongly enough to alter gut wall drug metabolism. A grape skin or berry skin can carry polyphenol chemistry that sounds protective in public language and still behaves as protein-binding or mineral-interfering chemistry in the gut. A stone fruit can carry sorbitol, fructose, acids, and defended seed tissue in the same biological package. A pomegranate can offer sugars in the flesh and tannin-rich astringency around the seed and membrane. Fruit keeps its reputation because these chemistries are scattered across different layers of the tissue and because the first bite is usually more pleasant than the deeper handling sequence. The bowel does not receive "an apple" or "a peach" in the cultural sense. It receives dissolved sugars, incompletely absorbed polyols, acids, skin compounds, and whatever smaller plant molecules that tissue released when it was broken open.

That is the chemical problem with fruit in its plainest form. The tissue is built to attract and to defend at the same time. The attraction is visible. The defense is quieter. Sugar invites intake. Polyols can stay behind and ferment. Acids can sharpen tolerance or irritation depending on the host. Skins can carry a harder chemistry than the flesh they surround. Seeds can remain chemically guarded even when the fruit around them is edible. A person judging fruit by sweetness, vitamin content, and freshness will miss most of that. The body does not miss it. The body has to absorb the sugars cleanly, tolerate the acids, leave the defended seed chemistry out if possible, and clear whatever crossed into blood without adding more burden than the meal was worth.

Sweet Taste as a Marketing Shield

Sweetness hides chemistry better than almost any other sensory trait in food. The mouth meets sugar first, and sugar changes the whole moral reading of the tissue before digestion has had any chance to expose what else came with it. A sweet fruit is read as light, clean, energizing, hydrating, and naturally safe almost on contact. That reaction is understandable. Sweet taste usually signals available carbohydrate, and the body is built to recognize that quickly. But in fruit, sweetness does more than signal sugar. It covers the rest of the structure. Fructose, glucose, sorbitol, malic acid, citric acid, amines, salicylates, skin polyphenols, seed chemistry, and, in some fruits, compounds that can alter drug handling or provoke bowel symptoms all arrive inside the same tissue. The sweetness does not remove them. It makes them easier to ignore.

That is why sweet taste works so well as a marketing shield. It lets the fruit be judged at the sensory entrance instead of at the physiological exit. The person tastes sweetness and assumes nourishment, even when the small intestine may absorb the sugars unevenly, leave some of the fructose or polyols behind, and turn the remainder into osmotic load and fermentation further down. A fruit can therefore look metabolically gentle in the mouth and behave as a bowel burden later. The same shield protects the food from harder questions about dose, context, and host tolerance. A sugary fruit eaten occasionally by a healthy person with steady glucose handling, good bowel reserve, and no relevant sensitivities is one event. A high-fruit pattern built into smoothies, juices, dried fruit, snacks, and repeated "healthy" eating is another. Sweetness makes those two exposures feel similar even when the metabolic and digestive consequences are not.

The shield becomes even stronger because sweetness is culturally fused to the language of nature. Candy has to defend itself. Fruit is defended by the fact that its sugar arrived in plant tissue. That distinction can matter in some contexts, but it is also used too carelessly. The body still has to absorb the sugar, buffer the acid load, tolerate the skin chemistry, leave the seed chemistry out if possible, and process whatever smaller compounds crossed into blood after the meal. A grapefruit can be sweet and still inhibit intestinal drug metabolism. An apple can be sweet and still deliver sorbitol and fructose in a form that some bowels do not clear cleanly. A dried fruit can look concentrated and wholesome at the same time while delivering a far denser sugar load than the fresh tissue it came from. Sweetness makes these contradictions hard to see because it encourages the eater to classify the food before the rest of the physiology has spoken.

This is one reason fruit keeps such a protected reputation in modern nutrition. Sweet taste helps the food cross the first threshold of trust so easily that later problems are often blamed on the host rather than on the chemistry of the meal. Blood sugar swings, bowel urgency, bloating, flushing, reflux, histamine-like symptoms, and unstable appetite after fruit are often treated as strange exceptions because the sweetness made the food feel self-justifying from the beginning. But sweetness is only one layer of the tissue. It is not the whole argument. A sweet fruit can still be acidic, poorly tolerated, fermentation-prone, drug-interacting, or chemically defended in its skins and seeds. The sweet taste got the food into a protected category. The intestine, liver, and kidney still have to deal with everything sweetness did not mention.

That is the deeper problem. Sweetness does not only make fruit attractive. It makes the tissue look simpler than it is. It narrows attention to carbohydrate reward and hides the competing chemistry in the same bite. The fruit keeps the innocent sensory profile. The body still has to process the full plant structure that sweetness helped sell.

Why Fruit Can Still Create Gut, Metabolic, Dental, or Pharmacologic Burden

Fruit is protected by sweetness and water, but the body does not meet sweetness and water alone. It meets sugar, organic acids, polyols, skins, seeds, and whatever smaller defense compounds the tissue kept in place while the fruit was still on the plant. That means one fruit can create several different burdens at once depending on the host and the route of contact. In the bowel, the problem is often incomplete handling of fructose or polyols, sugar alcohols such as sorbitol, which can remain in the lumen, the hollow interior of the intestine, hold water there by osmosis, and then move into the colon as fermentation substrate. That is why apples, pears, stone fruits, and other fruits can look light on the plate and still become gas, distension, urgency, or unstable transit in a sensitive bowel. The sugar did not disappear because it came in fruit tissue. The intestine still had to absorb it cleanly.

The metabolic burden begins when the sugars are absorbed but still exceed what the host handles well. A fruit does not need to be candy to push blood sugar and hepatic workload in a direction that matters. The liver still receives fructose-rich portal blood first, still has to phosphorylate and sort that sugar load, and still has to decide whether it will be burned, stored, converted into glycogen, or pushed toward fat synthesis under the host's existing metabolic conditions. A resilient host can absorb a modest fruit load quietly. A person already struggling with unstable glucose control, high-fruit grazing, juices, dried fruit, or repeated sweet exposures is meeting the same tissue under different conditions. The fruit keeps the halo of "natural sugar." The liver still has to process the dose it was given.

The dental burden follows a different route because the fruit does not need to cross the intestine to matter. Teeth are exposed in the mouth first. Fruit sugars feed oral bacteria, which then generate acids that demineralize enamel, and the fruit's own acids can also contribute directly to dental erosion, the chemical loss of tooth structure not caused by bacterial acids. NIDCR explains the caries sequence plainly: bacteria use sugars in food to make acids that attack enamel. Broader oral-health reviews add the second half of the problem by noting that dietary acids from juice and fresh fruit can contribute to erosion as well, especially with frequent exposure. That means fruit can challenge the tooth two ways at once. It can supply fermentable sugar to plaque bacteria and deliver intrinsic acid directly to the enamel surface. Sweetness and freshness do not protect the tooth from either sequence.

The pharmacologic burden is clearest in grapefruit because grapefruit carries furanocoumarins, plant defense compounds that can inhibit cytochrome P450 3A4, abbreviated CYP3A4, in the intestinal wall. That changes first-pass metabolism, the early metabolic loss of some oral drugs as they cross the gut wall, and allows more parent drug to reach the bloodstream than the dose was meant to deliver under ordinary conditions. FDA's grapefruit warning and multiple grapefruit interaction reviews describe this mechanism directly. The fruit is still being eaten as produce. The enterocyte, the absorptive intestinal cell, is being forced into altered drug handling. That is pharmacology, not nutrition.

This is why fruit cannot be judged only by vitamin content, color, or the social safety conferred by sweetness. The same tissue can leave fermentable residue in the bowel, send a high sugar load through portal blood to the liver, strip enamel through repeated sugar-and-acid exposure in the mouth, or alter drug exposure at the intestinal membrane through furanocoumarin chemistry. None of those pathways requires fruit to stop being fruit. They only require the reader to follow the tissue all the way from bite to membrane to organ consequence instead of stopping at the first pleasant sensation.

Whole Fruit Versus Juice Versus Dried Fruit as Different Exposures

A whole fruit is not the same physiological event as its juice, and neither is the same event as the dried version. The difference begins in the structure before any sugar reaches blood. Whole fruit still carries its water inside intact plant cells, still asks for chewing, still moves through the stomach as hydrated tissue, and still brings fiber and cell-wall resistance into the digestive sequence. Juice breaks much of that structure open before the mouth ever sees it. The sugars are no longer riding inside the same intact matrix, the fiber burden is markedly lower, and the fluid reaches the gut as a faster carbohydrate exposure. WHO's sugar guidance treats the sugars in fruit juice as free sugars, which means they behave differently from sugars enclosed in intact fruit tissue. Reviews comparing whole fruit with 100% fruit juice also describe whole fruit as producing greater satiety, partly because the solid tissue slows gastric handling and keeps more of the original matrix intact.

That structural change matters in the bowel and in appetite. A whole apple, orange, or mango still has to be bitten, fractured, mixed with saliva, and reduced by gastric and intestinal handling before the sugars are liberated completely. Juice has already outsourced much of that work to processing. The intestine receives a faster sugar field in a larger fluid volume and with less friction from intact fiber. The person can therefore drink the equivalent of several fruits in minutes without the same mechanical stopping points that whole fruit creates. That is one reason whole fruit and juice do not produce the same satiety pattern. The 2025 review comparing whole fruit and 100% fruit juice reported greater fullness and delayed gastric emptying with whole fruit, and a controlled trial comparing fresh and dried mango found the fresh fruit performed better for satiety and postprandial glucose control than the dried form. The food category stays "fruit." The absorbed dose and the speed of delivery do not.

Dried fruit changes the exposure in a different direction. Water is removed, volume shrinks, and the sugar load is compressed into a much smaller piece of food. The chemistry is not gentler because the fruit is smaller. It is denser. A handful of dried fruit can carry the sugar of several servings of fresh fruit with far less chewing volume, far less gastric bulk, and a much easier path to repeated eating. The smaller physical size also makes it easier to treat the food as a snack rather than as a full serving of fruit tissue. That matters for blood sugar, for total dose, and for the bowel in sensitive people, because the same fructose and polyol load can now be delivered in a tighter package and in larger practical amounts. Fresh fruit at least forces some water, bulk, and stopping points into the event. Drying strips much of that protection away even when some fiber remains.

The mouth sees another difference. Juice changes the dental exposure because sugars and acids are delivered directly to the teeth in fluid form, without the same chewing pattern and without much of the original fruit structure. Dried fruit changes it again because the sugars are concentrated and the food can remain in contact with the teeth longer. The evidence on 100% fruit juice and dental outcomes is not fully settled, but systematic review data show enough concern in adults that tooth erosion and caries cannot be dismissed casually, and broader oral-health guidance remains clear that sugars feed acid-producing oral bacteria while acidic beverages can add direct erosive pressure to enamel. Whole fruit is not automatically harmless to teeth, but it is still a different oral exposure from juice and from sticky concentrated dried fruit. The same fruit has become three different physiological problems once the matrix is left intact, destroyed into liquid, or concentrated by drying.

Chapter 25

Sugar Delivery, Fructose Load, and Intestinal Overrun

Fructose does not have the broad absorptive freedom that glucose has. The small intestine has to move fructose across the apical membrane of the enterocyte, the absorptive intestinal cell, mainly through GLUT5, the fructose transporter most closely tied to this step, while GLUT2 can contribute under some conditions as well. That matters because fructose absorption is not only a question of how much sugar is in the fruit. It is a question of how much transporter capacity the small intestine has available at that moment, how quickly the fruit is emptied into the bowel, and what else arrived in the same meal. Review literature describes fructose absorption in exactly those terms, with GLUT5 as the key transporter and intestinal fructose handling limited enough that excessive fructose can remain unabsorbed.

That limit is why fructose can behave well in one meal and poorly in another. A modest amount of fructose inside intact fruit tissue, eaten slowly and alongside other food, may be absorbed cleanly enough that little reaches the colon. Push the dose higher, deliver it faster, or send it in a form that overwhelms intestinal handling, and the sugar stops behaving like simple nourishment. More fructose stays in the lumen, the hollow interior of the small intestine where digestion and absorption are taking place. Once it stays there, it begins pulling water toward itself and moving downstream as unfinished carbohydrate. Recent review literature still describes GLUT5 as a comparatively low-capacity system and notes that excess dietary fructose can overload absorption and produce malabsorption.

This is also why glucose changes the story. Fructose is often handled better when glucose arrives with it, which helps explain why the same absolute fructose load does not behave identically across all fruits or all processed foods. Review sources note that fructose uptake is optimized in the presence of glucose and that fructose given in isolation is more likely to produce gastrointestinal discomfort because more of it escapes clean small-intestinal absorption. The intestine is not reading sweetness in the abstract. It is dealing with transporter traffic, luminal concentration, and the actual molecular mix that reached the membrane.

Once fructose escapes the small intestine, the problem changes organs. The colon inherits it. Bacteria ferment it. Gas rises. Water stays in the bowel. Pressure builds inside a tube that may already be easy to provoke. That is why fructose limits matter so much in a book about plant burden. The fruit can still look light, hydrating, and wholesome on the plate while the bowel is dealing with retained sugar, osmotic load, fermentation, and altered transit after absorption failed to finish the job. Fructose malabsorption is described in the literature as a common digestive disorder, and the symptoms that follow are the expected ones for carbohydrate that stayed in the bowel too long rather than crossing the membrane cleanly.

What Happens When Fructose Exceeds Absorptive Capacity

Fructose becomes a bowel problem at the membrane before it becomes a symptom in the room. The small intestine has to move fructose across the apical surface of the enterocyte, the absorptive intestinal cell, mainly through GLUT5, the transporter most closely tied to fructose uptake, with GLUT2 contributing under some conditions. That system is narrower than people assume. It does not give fructose the same broad clearance glucose enjoys. When the fructose load stays modest enough, enough transporter capacity is available, and the meal arrives in a slower, more buffered form, the sugar can move through the small bowel with little residue left behind. Push the load higher, send it in faster, or deliver it in a form that outruns that transporter field, and the sugar begins staying in the lumen, the hollow interior of the bowel where absorption was supposed to finish the job.

Once fructose stays in the lumen, the whole event changes character. It is no longer behaving like absorbed fuel. It is behaving like dissolved residue. Water is pulled toward it by osmosis, which means the bowel holds more fluid around the unabsorbed sugar instead of clearing it forward as a low-friction meal. That extra water increases luminal volume before the colon has even entered the story. Then the residue moves on, and the colon inherits carbohydrate the small intestine failed to take care of. Bacteria ferment it quickly. Gas rises. Pressure rises with it. Motility changes because the bowel now has to move a wetter, more distending load through a tube that may or may not tolerate that stretch well. Review literature on fructose malabsorption keeps returning to exactly this sequence: retained fructose increases osmotic load, provides substrate for rapid bacterial fermentation, and shifts bowel function through the chemistry of what stayed behind.

That is why the same fruit, juice, or sweetened food can feel trivial in one body and disruptive in another. The fructose did not become more sugar. The small intestine simply did not clear it fast enough. If the person already has an irritable bowel, altered motility, or greater sensitivity to luminal stretch, the same retained fructose becomes visible sooner because the colon and small bowel have less room to absorb the pressure quietly. The symptoms are the expected ones for unfinished carbohydrate trapped in the tube too long: bloating, abdominal discomfort, excess gas, loose stool, and sometimes unstable bowel rhythm rather than one clean pattern. The fruit or sweet exposure still looks light on the plate. The bowel is carrying water and fermentation instead of a fully absorbed sugar load.

The important point for this chapter is that fructose overrun is not a moral story about sugar. It is a structural story about a membrane limit. The small bowel has a finite ability to move fructose out of the lumen. When the load outruns that ability, the sugar stops behaving like quiet nourishment and starts behaving like osmotic and fermentative burden. A whole fruit may keep that burden lower because the matrix slows delivery. Juice, dried fruit, sweetened foods, and repeated high-fructose exposures make the intestine face a denser or faster wave of the same chemistry. The food keeps the sweetness. The bowel is left with the unfinished work.

Osmotic Pull and Fermentation

Fructose that fails to cross the small-intestinal membrane does not sit quietly in the bowel waiting to be ignored. It changes the physical state of the meal. The sugar remains in the lumen, the hollow interior of the intestine where digestion and absorption are supposed to finish, and dissolved sugar holds water there by osmosis, meaning water moves toward the area with more dissolved particles. That is the first shift. The small bowel begins carrying a wetter, heavier, more distending column of contents than it was meant to carry after a simple fruit meal. Review literature on fructose malabsorption describes this directly: unabsorbed fructose creates an osmotic load in the intestine before the colon has even had its chance to ferment the remainder.

That early water retention matters because the bowel is a tube, not a chemistry set sitting on a shelf. More water in the lumen means more volume. More volume means more wall stretch, more pressure, and faster delivery of unfinished carbohydrate into the distal bowel. In a resilient intestine that may remain modest. In a bowel already easy to provoke, the fluid shift alone can begin the symptom sequence before much gas has formed. MRI and clinical review work on FODMAP physiology makes this point clearly: poorly absorbed carbohydrates draw water into the small intestine and can generate symptoms before colonic fermentation becomes the dominant event.

The second shift begins when that retained fructose reaches the colon. The small intestine failed to clear it, so the microbiota inherit it. Bacteria ferment the sugar rapidly and produce gases, especially hydrogen, along with short-chain fatty acids and other fermentation products. At that point the bowel is no longer dealing only with excess fluid. It is dealing with expanding gas inside the same confined lumen. Review articles on fructose malabsorption and irritable bowel syndrome describe that sequence in blunt terms: exceed absorptive capacity, leave fructose behind, then let bacterial fermentation convert that residue into gas and abdominal symptoms.

This is why fructose overrun feels larger than the sugar load sounds on paper. The symptom is not "a little extra carbohydrate." The symptom is a bowel carrying water first and gas second. The lumen distends. The wall stretches. Motility changes because the intestine has to move a fluid-rich, fermenting burden through tissue that may already be sensitive to pressure. Diarrhea is one possible result because osmotic water retention and faster transit can move together. Constipation can still appear in some hosts when gas and altered motility interact differently. Bloating, pain, audible bowel activity, and unstable stool pattern are the expected mechanical consequences of sugar that stayed in the tube too long.

That is why osmotic pull and fermentation belong together in this chapter. They are not two separate theories about why fruit can bother the gut. They are two stages of the same failed handling sequence. First the small intestine leaves fructose behind and water follows it. Then the colon receives the unfinished sugar and microbes turn it into gas. A fruit can still look hydrating, refreshing, and light at the level of taste while the bowel is carrying retained water, retained residue, and fermentation pressure because the absorptive limit was crossed before the eater ever had reason to suspect the meal would become a problem.

Juice as Concentrated Delivery Without Much Structural Resistance

A whole fruit still makes the body work through tissue. The cells have to be broken, the fiber still occupies space, the water is still held inside structure, and the sugars are still arriving inside a plant matrix that slows how quickly the small intestine sees the full load. Juice changes that before the first sip is swallowed. Pressing, crushing, and filtering have already done much of the structural destruction. Much of the fiber is lost, the sugars are no longer enclosed in the same intact cellular architecture, and the liquid reaches the stomach as a fast carbohydrate exposure with very little physical resistance left to slow delivery. That difference is important enough that the World Health Organization counts sugars in fruit juice as free sugars, not as sugars enclosed within intact whole fruit tissue. Review literature on whole fruit versus 100% fruit juice also describes juice processing as reducing fiber and converting the fruit's intrinsic sugars into a more rapidly delivered form.

That loss of structure changes what the gut has to handle. A whole orange or apple still has to be chewed and fractured in the mouth, held in the stomach as solid food, and emptied forward in a way that is partly controlled by the bulk and viscosity of the tissue. Juice has almost none of that friction. It leaves the stomach faster, reaches the small bowel faster, and presents the sugars in a form that can be absorbed in a denser wave. Recent review work describes whole fruit as producing greater satiety than 100% fruit juice, and broader physiology reviews note that juice speeds gastric emptying and reduces satiety compared with whole fruit because the structure that would have slowed delivery has already been dismantled. The fruit is still being judged socially as fruit. The intestine is receiving a much easier sugar load.

That is why juice changes the metabolic event even when no table sugar was added. The issue is not only what sugars are present. The issue is how fast they are delivered, how little chewing and gastric resistance stand in the way, and how easy it becomes to consume the equivalent of several fruits in minutes. A person is unlikely to chew through the same quantity of intact fruit as quickly as they can drink it. That difference in pace matters because satiety arrives later when the tissue barrier has already been removed, and the liver receives a faster portal sugar wave from the bowel. Whole fruit and juice can therefore begin from the same plant but arrive at the absorptive membrane as different physiological exposures. Drying creates another version of the same problem by removing water and compressing the sugar dose into a smaller volume, but juice is the cleaner example because the structure is destroyed while the fluid load makes overconsumption easier rather than harder.

This is the real reason juice belongs in a chapter on fructose load and intestinal overrun rather than in a sentimental discussion of fruit serving equivalence. The body does not absorb "a serving of fruit" in the abstract. It absorbs whatever the processing left behind. Whole fruit still imposes chewing, bulk, and slower release. Juice delivers sugars with much less structural resistance, much less fiber, and a much easier path to large repeated intake. The produce identity stays the same. The delivery system does not.

Fruit Tolerance as Dose-Dependent and Host-Dependent

A fruit is not one fixed event. The tissue may be the same, the sweetness may be the same, and the public reputation may be the same, but the biological result still changes with dose and with the body receiving it. The first limit sits in the small intestine. Fructose does not have unlimited clearance there. It depends mainly on GLUT5, the fructose transporter at the apical surface of the enterocyte, the absorptive intestinal cell, and that transport capacity can be exceeded. Reviews of fructose absorption describe this directly and note that excess fructose can remain unabsorbed when intake outruns small-bowel handling. That is why one piece of fruit and three glasses of juice are not the same bowel event, and why whole fruit, juice, and dried fruit are not interchangeable exposures even when they came from the same plant. The dose changes how much sugar reaches the membrane at once, how quickly it arrives, and how much unfinished carbohydrate is left behind in the lumen, the hollow interior of the bowel where absorption was supposed to finish the job.

The host changes the same event from another side. A resilient bowel may absorb enough fructose, disperse enough of the luminal load, and tolerate enough downstream fermentation that the fruit remains uneventful. A sensitive bowel does not have the same margin. In irritable bowel syndrome, or IBS, fructose malabsorption is more clinically visible because retained fructose pulls water into the bowel by osmosis and then reaches the colon as microbial substrate, where fermentation raises gas, pressure, and wall stretch. Recent IBS and low-FODMAP reviews show that higher-FODMAP diets increase breath hydrogen and symptom burden, and fructose malabsorption continues to track with symptom improvement in susceptible patients when the fructose burden is lowered. The fruit did not become more sugary in one body than another. The bowel simply had less room to absorb the same subtraction quietly.

That same dose-and-host logic extends beyond the gut. A modest whole-fruit exposure in a person with good metabolic reserve is one portal blood event. Repeated fruit grazing, juice intake, dried fruit, or larger fructose loads in a host already struggling with glucose control, liver fat handling, or appetite regulation is another. Review literature on dietary fructose and metabolism keeps pointing back to context here as well: the metabolic consequence depends on dose, background diet, and host state rather than on the word fruit alone. Fruit tolerance therefore is not a moral category and it is not a fixed identity of the food. It is the point where the fructose load, the speed of delivery, the food matrix, the bowel's absorptive reserve, and the host's metabolic margin either stay within tolerance or outrun it. The same fruit can remain a small carbohydrate event in one body and become luminal water retention, fermentation pressure, or excess portal sugar delivery in another because the tissue stayed the same while the margin did not.

Why the Body Judges a Glass of Juice Differently Than a Piece of Fruit

A piece of fruit still makes the body deal with tissue. The teeth have to break cell walls, the stomach has to hold and grind a hydrated solid, and the small intestine receives sugars that are still arriving inside a partly intact plant matrix rather than as a free-running liquid load. A glass of juice arrives after much of that work has already been done outside the body. Pressing, crushing, filtering, and separation have already ruptured the cells, released the sugars, and removed much of the fiber and bulk that would have slowed delivery. The fruit may share the same botanical origin, but the body is not receiving the same object. One is a broken plant fluid with dissolved sugars moving quickly through the gut. The other is still a fruit.

That structural difference changes the first minutes of the digestive sequence. A whole orange, apple, or mango occupies space in the stomach as food mass. It takes chewing time, swallowing time, and gastric work before the sugars are fully liberated and passed forward. Juice does not ask for much of that. It empties faster, reaches the small bowel faster, and presents its carbohydrate load in a form that is easier to absorb quickly and easier to overconsume without mechanical resistance. The body therefore judges the two exposures differently because the stomach and small intestine are seeing different rates of sugar delivery, different fiber burden, different satiety signals, and different degrees of tissue resistance. The label may still say fruit. The gut is no longer meeting fruit in the same form.

The sugar handling changes with that loss of structure. Fructose and glucose arriving from whole fruit still move through a slower physical event. The same sugars arriving in juice reach the absorptive surface in a denser wave and with much less friction. That matters because the small intestine does not have unlimited capacity to clear fructose cleanly, and because the liver receives portal blood, the blood draining from the intestine into the liver first, at the speed the bowel delivers it. A whole fruit spreads that work out more. Juice compresses it. The difference is not sentimental and it is not mainly about whether the sugar is natural. The difference is that one exposure still contains brakes. The other has already had many of its brakes removed.

Satiety changes for the same reason. A whole fruit occupies the mouth longer, stretches the stomach more, and forces the eater through a slower physical sequence before the sugars are fully available. Juice slips past much of that. The person can drink the equivalent of several pieces of fruit before the body has much chance to object through fullness. That is why whole fruit and juice do not produce the same appetite response even when they came from the same produce bin. The body is not counting servings the way a nutrition chart does. It is reading volume, texture, chewing time, gastric emptying, and the rate at which carbohydrate reaches the bowel wall and then the liver.

This is why the body judges a glass of juice differently than a piece of fruit. Whole fruit still behaves like tissue. Juice behaves more like rapid sugar delivery wearing the identity of fruit. The difference begins in the mouth, widens in the stomach, sharpens at the intestinal membrane, and continues in portal blood on the way to the liver. The fruit kept the reputation. Processing changed the event.

Chapter 26

Fruit Acids, Polyols, Seeds, and Peel Chemistry

The mouth meets the acid before the intestine ever sees the sugar. Fruit enters as a wet plant tissue carrying water, fructose, glucose, aroma compounds, pigments, and organic acids dissolved through the flesh and juice. Those acids are part of the fruit's structure, not a decorative flavor note laid on top afterward. Citric acid, malic acid, tartaric acid, and other smaller acids help keep the tissue sharp, bright, and microbiologically less hospitable while the fruit is still on the plant. Once the tissue is chewed, that same chemistry spreads across enamel, dentin if any root surface is exposed, the tongue, the inner cheek, the gums, and the already thin irritated surfaces of a sensitive mouth. The first event is not metabolic. It is local chemical contact.

That contact matters because the mouth is built around mineral and membrane surfaces, and acid changes both. Tooth enamel is a mineral surface rich in hydroxyapatite, a calcium phosphate crystal. Drop the pH low enough at that surface and the crystal begins giving mineral back to the fluid around it. Saliva can buffer some of that and can return calcium and phosphate later, but repeated acid contact keeps shifting the balance the wrong way. This is why fruit can participate in dental wear without looking like candy. The issue is not only sugar feeding oral bacteria later. The issue is that the fruit arrives already acidic and can begin softening enamel directly while the sugars remain in the mouth long enough to feed acid-producing bacteria afterward. The sweet reputation hides the first half of the damage. The acid was working before the bacteria even got their turn.

The soft tissues of the mouth have their own version of the same problem. A resilient oral mucosa can tolerate a fair amount of acidity without much complaint. A mouth already dealing with dryness, reflux, mouth breathing, mechanical irritation, orthodontic hardware, broken sleep, nutrient deficiency, or chronic inflammatory stress is different. Acid fruit in that setting can sting, burn, redden the tongue, aggravate the corners of the lips, and make small erosions or ulcer-prone tissue feel raw out of proportion to what the person expects from "healthy food." The fruit did not become poison. The local tissue simply had less margin. A pineapple wedge, a glass of orange juice, or repeated bites of berries can therefore act less like refreshing produce and more like recurring acid exposure landing on a surface that is already too easy to injure.

This is also why form matters. Whole fruit still asks for chewing, slower release, and mixing with saliva. Juice is harsher because the acid is delivered as fluid over a wider surface with much less structural resistance. Sipping extends the contact time. Swishing makes it worse. Dried fruit changes the event again by concentrating sugars while often remaining in contact with the teeth longer, which gives bacterial acid production more time even if the intrinsic acid profile differs from juice. A person may therefore tolerate a piece of melon easily, feel a sharp sting from citrus, and notice their teeth feel rough or sensitive after frequent juice intake, not because the body is inconsistent, but because the oral surfaces are meeting different acid density, different contact time, and different opportunities for salivary recovery.

That is the point this section needs to keep. Fruit acidity is easy to excuse because it travels with freshness, brightness, and sweetness. The mouth does not judge it by those words. It judges it by pH, contact time, salivary buffering, enamel exposure, and tissue resilience. A fruit can still carry vitamins, water, and attractive flavor while imposing repeated acid contact on mineral and mucosal surfaces that have to survive every exposure. The pleasant taste does not cancel the local chemistry. It only makes the chemistry easier to underestimate until the teeth start losing shine, the mouth starts stinging, or the same "healthy" fruit keeps landing like irritation instead of refreshment.

Polyols in Selected Fruits

Some fruits do not deliver all of their sweetness as glucose or fructose. They also carry polyols, sugar alcohols that taste sweet enough to disappear into the general idea of fruit sugar but behave very differently in the bowel. Sorbitol is the main one that matters here. Apples, pears, peaches, plums, prunes, cherries, apricots, nectarines, and some related fruits can carry enough sorbitol that the fruit stops being only a sugar food and becomes a transport problem in the small intestine. Sorbitol is absorbed slowly and incompletely. That is the whole issue. The molecule does not clear the small bowel with the same ease as a more straightforward carbohydrate load, so part of it can remain in the lumen, the hollow interior of the bowel where absorption is supposed to be finishing the meal. Once it stays behind, the fruit is no longer being judged by sweetness. It is being judged by what the membrane failed to move across.

That retained polyol changes the bowel physically before the colon has even had its turn. Sorbitol is osmotically active, which means it holds water in the intestinal contents by attracting fluid toward the area with more dissolved particles. The small intestine is now carrying a wetter and more distending load than the eater expected from a piece of fruit. Then the residue moves forward. The colon inherits what the small intestine did not clear, bacteria ferment it, gas begins to accumulate, and the fruit that looked refreshing on the plate becomes pressure inside a tube. This is why certain fruits can produce bloating, loose stool, urgency, cramping, or unstable bowel rhythm out of proportion to how innocent they looked at first bite. The problem is not that the fruit was sweet. The problem is that part of the sweetness arrived in a form the bowel handles poorly.

Pears are a clean example because they often carry both fructose and sorbitol in a combination that makes the small intestine's job harder, not easier. Apples can do the same. Stone fruits push in the same direction. A peach, plum, apricot, or cherry is still being sold as fruit, still being praised for freshness and plant nutrients, while the bowel is being asked to absorb a carbohydrate mixture that can leave residue behind and then convert that residue into water retention and fermentation. Dried fruit often worsens the problem because the polyol load is now compressed into a smaller volume and can be eaten quickly without the bulk and water that whole fresh fruit would have imposed. A few prunes are one event. A larger handful taken as a "healthy snack" is another. The tissue changed. The dose changed. The bowel receives the result.

This is why polyols belong in a chapter on the chemical problem with fruit rather than in a side note about digestive sensitivity. A fruit can still carry vitamins, pigments, and attractive public language while also delivering sorbitol in a quantity large enough to overrun absorption in the wrong host. The chemistry does not need to be exotic. It only needs to stay in the bowel long enough to matter mechanically. In a resilient intestine, modest amounts may pass with little consequence. In an irritable bowel, in a person eating larger portions, or in someone using dried fruit or fruit-heavy smoothies repeatedly, the same sorbitol-bearing fruit stops behaving like a light food and starts behaving like retained carbohydrate that the bowel has to dilute, ferment, and force forward.

That is the pattern worth keeping. Selected fruits do not cause trouble because fruit is secretly poison. They cause trouble because some of them package part of their carbohydrate load in a form the small intestine clears poorly. The mouth notices sweetness. The bowel notices the sugar alcohol that stayed behind.

Seed and Pit Compounds as Protective Chemistry

A fruit can afford to sweeten the flesh long before it can afford to surrender the seed. That is the structural divide that keeps getting lost when people talk about fruit as though the whole thing belongs to one biological category. The soft outer tissue is allowed to become wet, fragrant, brightly colored, and easy to chew because that part can serve dispersal. The seed, pit, or kernel has a different job. It has to keep embryonic tissue, stored energy, and future growth potential intact long enough to survive the animal that ate the fruit or the environment that damaged it. So the chemistry hardens as you move inward. The flesh can invite. The reproductive core has to resist. That is why so many seeds and pits carry tougher shells, astringent surfaces, bitter notes, enzyme inhibitors, tannins, dense oils, or in some species outright cyanogenic chemistry, meaning compounds that can release cyanide after the tissue is broken and digested.

That protection is not decorative. It is built into the tissue because the seed is the part the plant cannot cheaply lose. A swallowed whole seed may pass with much of that chemistry still contained because the protective structure did its job. Crack the seed, grind it, chew it thoroughly, or turn it into flour, paste, powder, or extract, and the whole event changes. The compartment breaks. Water enters. Enzymes gain access. Digestive fluid reaches chemistry the intact seed was built to hide. In apricot kernels and other stone fruit seeds, amygdalin, a cyanogenic glycoside, stays comparatively quiet while the tissue is intact and becomes far more relevant once the kernel is crushed and digested. The same logic holds more broadly even when cyanide is not part of the story. The plant stored the vulnerable biology in a defended package. The person defeats the package and then expects the chemistry to remain harmless.

That is why seeds and pits so often create a false impression of nutritional promise. They can test dense in minerals, oils, polyphenols, or protein because they are concentrated tissues by design. Concentration is the whole reason the plant protects them so aggressively. A seed is not a loose scrap of plant matter. It is a compressed survival structure. Once the laboratory crushes it, the numbers can look impressive. Once the mouth or grinder crushes it, the intestine inherits the same defensive chemistry the plant attached to that density in the first place. A kernel can therefore look rich on paper while still bringing bitterness, tannin binding, inhibitor burden, or cyanogenic risk into the digestive sequence. The density is real. The resistance is just as real.

Fruit culture keeps hiding this because it encourages people to judge the whole fruit by the sweetness of the flesh. The peach tastes pleasant, so the pit begins to feel adjacent to food. The apple is wholesome, so the seeds feel like harmless details. The apricot is soft and sweet, so the kernel is easily romanticized as an intensified version of the fruit instead of what it actually is, which is protected reproductive tissue with a different chemical job. This is one reason whole-fruit language becomes sloppy so quickly. The flesh and the seed do not belong to the same physiological story. One tissue is built to be handled. The other is built to survive handling. Once that distinction is ignored, people begin grinding, blending, pressing, chewing, and concentrating the most chemically guarded part of the fruit while still talking as though they are only dealing with fruit.

The body reads that mistake more clearly than the eater does. The mouth notices bitterness or astringency. The stomach and small intestine meet tissue that was never designed to dissolve generously into human nourishment. The liver may inherit compounds that now need transformation and clearance. The kidney may later see the dissolved remainder of chemistry that crossed the intestinal wall and gave little back. That is the protective logic of seeds and pits in plain form. The fruit invites intake at the surface. The reproductive core keeps its guard underneath, and the closer a person moves toward eating that core as food, the more directly they are negotiating with plant protection rather than with plant nourishment.

Why Peeling, Deseeding, or Avoiding Certain Fruits Can Reduce Burden in Sensitive People

A sensitive person does not need a different category of food. They often only need less of the part of the plant doing the most chemical work. Fruit is not one uniform edible substance. The flesh, the peel, the membrane, the seed, the pit, and the juice-sac all carry different chemistry because they are different tissues with different jobs. The outer surface has to meet sunlight, insects, fungi, and abrasion. The seed has to protect the next generation. The flesh can sweeten and soften while those other tissues keep a harder profile. That is why peeling, deseeding, or avoiding certain fruits can reduce burden without changing the entire diet. The person is not becoming irrational or fragile. They are reducing contact with the parts of the fruit most likely to concentrate acidity, bitterness, astringency, salicylate burden, polyphenol binding chemistry, or defended reproductive tissue the gut was never meant to process generously.

The peel matters first because the peel is often where the fruit keeps part of its boundary chemistry. That outer layer can hold more acids, more phenolic compounds, more waxes, more residues from handling or storage, and in some fruits more of the smaller molecules that make a sensitive mouth, stomach, or bowel react harder than the sweet flesh alone would predict. A person with oral irritation, reflux, upper-gut sensitivity, or a bowel that reacts strongly to chemical contact may tolerate the inner flesh better once the peel is removed because the fruit reaching the mouth and stomach is no longer the same tissue. The person did not change. The exposure changed. The first bite is now meeting less of the plant's surface-defense chemistry and more of the part built to be eaten.

The seed and pit matter for a harder reason. Reproductive tissue is usually more chemically guarded than the flesh around it because the plant can afford to lose pulp more easily than it can afford to lose the embryo and stored reserves inside the core. That is why seeds and pits can carry bitterness, astringency, enzyme inhibitors, dense oils, or in some fruits cyanogenic glycosides, compounds that can release cyanide after the tissue is broken and digested. A whole seed may pass with much of that chemistry still contained. Crush it, chew it thoroughly, blend it, or grind it, and the protection has already failed before digestion even begins. Deseeding therefore is not cosmetic in a sensitive host. It can remove the most defended part of the fruit from the digestive sequence entirely. The sweet flesh may still behave like food. The core was never offering the same bargain.

Avoidance matters when the burden is built into the flesh itself or when the person's margin is already too narrow to negotiate even the edible part well. A bowel that handles fructose or sorbitol poorly may still overrun on apples, pears, stone fruits, or dried fruit even after peeling. A mouth or stomach that reacts to acid may still be irritated by citrus or pineapple even if the peel and seed are gone. A person with salicylate or amine sensitivity may find that certain fruits keep provoking flushing, itch, bowel symptoms, or oral discomfort because the relevant chemistry is not confined to the skin. In that setting avoidance is not a defeat. It is a way of stopping repeated contact with a tissue the body keeps underpaying for. The fruit may still look healthy in public language. The host keeps showing that the net result is friction rather than nourishment.

That is the practical lesson. Sensitive people often improve not because they rejected fruit in some ideological way, but because they changed which part of the fruit they were asking their body to process and how often they were asking for it. Peeling removes part of the boundary chemistry. Deseeding removes part of the reproductive defense. Avoidance removes the whole exposure when the flesh itself keeps overrunning tolerance. The body does not reward the reputation of the fruit. It responds to the tissue actually chewed, the compounds actually released, the sugars actually absorbed or left behind, and the chemistry the gut, liver, and kidney still have to carry after the pleasant taste is gone.

How Fruit Chemistry Changes With Ripeness and Processing

A fruit is not chemically fixed while it sits on the counter. The tissue keeps moving. As ripening advances, starch is converted into simpler sugars, organic acids shift downward in many fruits, aroma compounds expand, pigments deepen, and the cell wall begins to loosen. The fruit that was once hard, sharp, and resistant becomes softer, sweeter, wetter, and easier to eat quickly. Those sensory changes are the readable surface of a structural change inside the flesh. Ripening reviews describe the same sequence across many fruits: rising sugar concentration, changing acid balance, and progressive softening as the wall architecture is dismantled.

The wall loosening is one of the most important changes because it alters how much physical resistance still stands between the eater and the sugar load. Pectin, one of the main structural polysaccharides in fruit cell walls, is modified, solubilized, and broken down during ripening, and that loss of structure is a major part of why ripe fruit yields so easily in the mouth. The flesh ruptures faster, juice escapes faster, and the sugars are liberated with less chewing and less gastric work than the firmer version of the same fruit demanded earlier. Fruit-softening work keeps returning to this point. The pleasant softness of ripe fruit is the same structural change that makes its sugars easier to deliver.

The acid profile shifts alongside the texture. In many fruits the sugar-to-acid ratio rises as ripening progresses, which is why the fruit tastes less sharp and more immediately rewarding when fully ripe or overripe. The tissue is not only sweeter. It is less buffered by the earlier acid edge that once slowed intake and made the fruit feel more resistant. A greener fruit can therefore check appetite partly through firmness and acidity, while a riper fruit can become easier to overeat because the resistance has been stripped out of both the structure and the taste balance. Ripening literature describes this increase in sugar-to-acid ratio as one of the central changes in palatability.

Processing pushes the same dismantling further because the tissue arrives partly broken before the body ever touches it. Juicing crushes the cells, releases the sugars into fluid, removes much of the original bulk and fiber, and leaves the intestine receiving a faster carbohydrate wave with much less structural drag. The World Health Organization treats sugars in fruit juice as free sugars, not as sugars enclosed within intact fruit tissue, and recent comparisons of whole fruit with fruit juice describe the same practical result: less fiber, less satiety, and a different rate of delivery to the gut. The fruit keeps its name. The matrix no longer asks the same work from the mouth, stomach, or small bowel.

Drying changes the exposure in another direction. Water leaves, the tissue shrinks, sugars and acids are concentrated into a smaller mass, and the eater can take in the equivalent of several pieces of fruit in a handful. The fruit has not become sweeter by adding sugar. It has become denser because the water that once diluted the sugar and occupied gastric space has been removed. Reviews of dried fruit make that concentration plain: water loss compresses sugars, acids, and other soluble components into a much smaller serving volume. A greener fruit, a ripe fruit, a glass of juice, and a handful of dried fruit can all come from the same plant. The bowel, liver, and appetite system are not receiving the same event.

Why "Natural Dessert" Does Not Settle the Physiological Question

Calling fruit a natural dessert answers the social question and leaves the biological one untouched. Dessert is a cultural category. The body does not absorb categories. It receives a plant tissue carrying fructose, glucose, organic acids, polyols in some species, water, fiber, peel chemistry, seed-adjacent chemistry, and whatever smaller compounds were released when the flesh was crushed in the mouth and mixed into the stomach contents. Sweetness makes the tissue feel settled before digestion has done anything with it. That is the trap. A sweet taste can make a food feel self-justifying while the small intestine is still deciding whether the sugars will cross cleanly, whether some of the fructose will remain in the lumen, the hollow interior of the bowel, and whether the liver will receive a modest portal sugar load or a larger one than the tissue structure should have allowed. "Natural dessert" only says the fruit feels pleasant at the level of taste. It says nothing about what the tissue becomes after the membrane has to deal with it.

The physiology begins changing as soon as structure changes. Whole fruit still imposes chewing, gastric bulk, slower release, and at least some resistance from intact or partly intact cell walls. Juice removes much of that resistance before the body has a chance to use it. Dried fruit removes water and compresses the same sugar load into a much smaller mass. A ripe fruit softens, releases juice more easily, and presents its sugars with less mechanical friction than the firmer version of the same fruit would have imposed earlier. The produce identity stays stable while the delivery system changes underneath it. That is one reason the dessert frame fails. It makes a ripe mango, a glass of orange juice, a handful of dried dates, and a whole apple sound like variations of one innocent category when the bowel and liver are receiving very different rates, volumes, and densities of sugar.

The intestine does not read sweetness as innocence. It reads transport load. Fructose still has to cross the apical surface of the enterocyte, the absorptive intestinal cell, through a transporter system that can be overrun. If the dose outruns that capacity, the retained sugar holds water in the bowel by osmosis and then moves into the colon as fermentation substrate. A fruit can therefore look light at the fork and become distension, gas, urgency, or unstable transit further down because the membrane did not finish the job cleanly. Even when the sugars do cross, the body still has to handle what crossed. Portal blood reaches the liver first, not the muscles, not the myth of "natural energy." The hepatocyte receives the sugar load and has to sort it in real time. The fruit does not get a pass because it came wrapped in peel.

The phrase also hides dose. A dessert is usually understood as small and occasional, but fruit often escapes that limit because the word fruit already carries permission. One bowl becomes two. One smoothie becomes several pieces of fruit with the structure destroyed. One snack of dried fruit becomes the equivalent of multiple servings compressed into a handful. The body does not care that the sugars were natural. It cares how much arrived, how fast they arrived, what fiber and water were still slowing them, and whether the host had enough metabolic and digestive reserve to absorb the load quietly. A piece of fruit after a mixed meal is one event. Repeated fruit grazing, juice, dried fruit, and sweet ripe fruit used as a standing source of comfort are another. The label dessert is too weak to carry that distinction.

That is the real problem with calling fruit natural dessert. The phrase ends the discussion where the body begins it. It treats sweetness as an answer when sweetness is only the invitation. The physiology still has to judge the tissue by absorption, fermentation, portal delivery, dental acid contact, bowel tolerance, and whatever smaller plant compounds came with the sugar. The fruit may remain socially innocent all the way through the meal. The body still has to decide whether the same sweet tissue behaved like a modest food, a rapid sugar delivery system, a fermentation burden, or a repeated exposure that was easier to praise than to process.

Chapter 27

Grapefruit, Star Fruit, and Other Fruits with Special Risks

Grapefruit is one of the clearest fruits in the book because the problem is not hidden behind nutrient charts, vague symptom language, or long chains of speculation. The fruit reaches the small intestine carrying furanocoumarins, plant defense compounds strong enough to change what the gut wall does with certain oral drugs. A swallowed drug does not move straight from the stomach into the bloodstream unchanged. It dissolves into the fluid inside the bowel, reaches the intestinal epithelium, the absorptive cell layer lining the small intestine, and then has to cross that membrane while the cells in the wall are still metabolizing part of the dose. FDA states that grapefruit and grapefruit juice can interfere with this step by affecting cytochrome P450 3A4, abbreviated CYP3A4, an enzyme present in the small intestine that normally breaks down many medicines before they reach the rest of the body.

That is what makes grapefruit a pharmacologic fruit rather than merely a nutritious one. The tissue is still fruit tissue. It still carries water, acids, sugar, and vitamin C. But the bowel is also receiving bergamottin and 6',7'-dihydroxybergamottin, two of the major grapefruit furanocoumarins repeatedly identified in the interaction literature as important inhibitors of intestinal CYP3A4. The enterocyte, the absorptive intestinal cell, is supposed to metabolize part of the drug load during first-pass metabolism, the early metabolic loss that happens before full systemic circulation is reached. Grapefruit weakens that intestinal filter. Less drug is destroyed at the gut wall. More unchanged parent compound crosses into portal blood and then into the wider circulation than the dose was meant to deliver under ordinary conditions.

The effect is not a polite nutritional side note. It is real pharmacology at the membrane. Human and mechanistic work show that grapefruit furanocoumarins can do more than crowd the enzyme briefly. They can inactivate intestinal CYP3A4 strongly enough that the bowel wall is left with less working enzyme afterward. That is why the fruit can keep changing drug handling beyond the first swallow. FDA's consumer guidance puts the practical consequence plainly: instead of being metabolized in the small intestine, more of the drug may enter the blood and stay in the body longer. The fruit has not added milligrams to the tablet. It has thinned the gut's own metabolic filter and raised the delivered exposure.

This does not happen with every medicine, which is one reason the fruit keeps its harmless reputation so easily. The effect becomes important mainly when the drug depends meaningfully on intestinal CYP3A4 to limit how much of the oral dose survives the crossing from bowel to blood. When that dependency is weak, grapefruit may do very little. When it is strong, the same breakfast fruit can turn an ordinary prescribed dose into a much larger tissue exposure. The produce identity stays intact. The gut wall has already turned the fruit into a pharmacokinetic modifier, meaning a food that changes how much swallowed drug survives absorption and reaches the body.

Star Fruit in Kidney Vulnerability

Star fruit is one of the clearest cases where a fruit stops behaving like produce and starts behaving like a direct hazard in a vulnerable host. The flesh looks watery, bright, acidic, and ordinary. The chemistry is not ordinary once renal reserve is thin. Reviews of star fruit toxicity identify two main burdens in the fruit, oxalate and caramboxin, and kidney organizations now warn people with kidney disease to avoid it because reduced renal function can turn what looks like a simple fruit exposure into neurotoxicity and nephrotoxicity.

The kidney vulnerability begins with clearance. A person with chronic kidney disease does not move dissolved burdens out of blood with the same margin as a person with intact renal function. That matters here because caramboxin is a neurotoxin cleared by the kidney, and oxalate adds a second burden through crystal-forming chemistry. When renal excretion falls, the fruit is no longer being handled as a modest dietary exposure. The retained toxin and the retained oxalate stay in the body longer, and the consequences widen from bowel discomfort into hiccups, vomiting, confusion, agitation, seizures, and in severe cases death. The National Kidney Foundation warns about exactly this pattern, and nephrology reviews describe star fruit intoxication in kidney disease as a condition where impaired excretion lets the neurotoxic chemistry accumulate instead of leave quietly in urine.

The oxalate side makes the same fruit even harder on the kidney. Star fruit is rich enough in oxalate that it can contribute to acute oxalate nephropathy, meaning sudden kidney injury caused by oxalate crystal deposition in the tubules. That matters most in people with reduced kidney function, but the literature also contains reports of acute kidney injury in previously healthy people after large star fruit exposures, especially when the fruit or juice was taken on an empty stomach or in a dehydrated state. In that host the fruit is no longer only a neurotoxin problem. It is also a tubule and urine-chemistry problem, with oxalate moving from dissolved load into crystal injury.

This is why star fruit belongs in a chapter on special risks rather than in the ordinary fruit discussion. The fruit does not need to be spoiled, processed strangely, or eaten as a supplement to become dangerous. It only needs to land in a body with too little renal clearance to move the chemistry out. A person with chronic kidney disease meets star fruit under completely different physiological conditions than a person with broad renal reserve. The same slice of fruit can remain uneventful in one host and become retained neurotoxin plus oxalate burden in another because the kidney is no longer able to filter, secrete, and excrete the load with enough margin to protect the rest of the body.

That is the form of vulnerability this book has been building toward. The food did not become chemically stranger on the plate. The host lost the ability to clear what the fruit was already carrying. Once that happens, sweetness, freshness, and produce status stop mattering. The bowel absorbs the chemistry, blood carries it, the kidney fails to clear it fast enough, and the nervous system and renal tubule inherit the cost.

Why Rare Cases Still Matter Because They Reveal the Principle Clearly

A rare case is useful when it strips the system down to its moving parts. Ordinary exposures are messy. The dose is smaller, the host has more reserve, the symptoms are softer, and the chemistry can hide inside a reputation the food has already earned. Rare cases remove some of that camouflage. A kidney-vulnerable patient eats star fruit and suddenly the fruit stops looking like produce and starts showing its real chemistry. A patient on the wrong medication drinks grapefruit juice and the fruit stops looking like breakfast and starts acting on the enzyme field in the gut wall. A person chews raw apricot kernels and the pleasant outer fruit no longer protects the seed chemistry from scrutiny. A bitter zucchini makes someone vomit and the softness of squash flesh no longer hides the deterrent compounds in the tissue. These are not the exposures that tell you what every person will feel after every bite. They are the exposures that show the plant principle with less noise around it.

That is why rarity does not make the case biologically trivial. It often makes the mechanism easier to see. Grapefruit reveals that a fruit can carry furanocoumarins strong enough to inhibit intestinal cytochrome P450 3A4, abbreviated CYP3A4, and raise exposure to susceptible oral drugs. Star fruit reveals that a fruit can carry oxalate and caramboxin strongly enough that reduced renal clearance turns an ordinary slice of fruit into neurotoxicity and nephrotoxicity. Raw apricot kernels reveal that the edible sweetness of fruit flesh tells you almost nothing about the chemistry of the reproductive tissue inside it, where amygdalin can release cyanide after chewing or grinding. Bitter squash reveals that cultivated softness and familiar shape do not erase the underlying ability of cucurbit tissue to re-express cucurbitacins and become acutely toxic when the defensive chemistry rises high enough. The case may be uncommon. The structure is ordinary.

A rare case also helps separate two questions people usually confuse. One question is how often a food creates a major clinical event in the general population. The other is what kind of tissue the food actually is and what compounds it is capable of delivering under the right conditions. Those are not the same question. Star fruit toxicity is rare in the broad population and still highly revealing because it shows what happens when a fruit carrying renal and neurotoxic chemistry lands in a host with too little kidney reserve. Grapefruit interactions are selective rather than universal and still highly revealing because they show that plant compounds can act pharmacologically at the intestinal membrane instead of merely nutritionally in the bloodstream. Rare cases do not prove that every exposure is catastrophic. They prove that the public reading of the food was incomplete.

This is the book's real use for them. A rare case is not there to frighten the reader into treating every fruit or vegetable as a poison. It is there to keep the reader from trusting reputation more than mechanism. The dramatic case shows the same law the quieter cases follow. Plant tissue can be edible and still chemically defended. A compound can be natural and still alter enzymes, injure membranes, release cyanide, or overload a vulnerable clearance system. A host can look healthy enough until one ordinary-looking food lands on the wrong weak point and makes the hidden chemistry impossible to ignore. Once that happens, the lesson is no longer limited to the rare case itself. The same principle has to be carried back into the more common foods and the more common exposures, where the burden is smaller, slower, and easier to romanticize, but built from the same kind of plant logic.

The Difference Between Population Advice and High-Risk Physiology

Population advice is built for the body that still has margin. It assumes a stomach that acidifies adequately, a pancreas that releases enzymes on time, a small intestine that absorbs with reasonable efficiency, a liver that still has broad metabolic reserve, a thyroid that can trap iodide without much friction, and kidneys that can filter and concentrate urine without carrying the same dissolved burden for too long. That is what makes population advice useful and also what makes it blunt. It is trying to describe what most people can usually tolerate without immediate visible trouble. It is not trying to describe what happens when the same food lands in a bowel with fat malabsorption, a thyroid running on thin iodine supply, a kidney with reduced clearance, or an enterocyte, the absorptive intestinal cell, already forced to process a drug the gut wall is supposed to metabolize before it reaches blood.

Once the physiology changes, the food changes with it even though the plate looks the same. A population guideline can call spinach nutrient-dense because many people will never develop an obvious stone after eating it occasionally. That does not change the oxalate chemistry in a host with fat malabsorption, higher intestinal oxalate absorption, and a kidney already concentrating a larger urinary load. A population guideline can treat cruciferous vegetables as broadly healthful because, in iodine-replete people eating ordinary amounts, the thyroid usually absorbs the subtraction quietly. That does not change what thiocyanate and goitrin do in a gland already trapping hard under rising thyroid-stimulating hormone, or TSH, pressure. A population guideline can place fruit inside a protected category because most people do not collapse after eating it. That does not change what fructose, sorbitol, acids, furanocoumarins, or seed chemistry do in the host whose bowel, drug handling, or oral tissues have less room to absorb the same exposure.

High-risk physiology begins where reserve narrows. The same plant tissue now meets a membrane, gland, tubule, or enzyme field already working too close to its limit. In an irritable bowel, poorly absorbed carbohydrate becomes luminal water retention, gas, and wall stretch at a lower dose because the bowel is easier to provoke. In fat malabsorption, calcium is pulled into fatty acid soaps, more oxalate stays free, and the same high-oxalate food delivers more renal burden downstream. In reduced kidney function, a fruit such as star fruit no longer behaves like a modest produce exposure because the chemistry remains in blood longer and the nephron, the kidney's filtering unit, has less power to move it out. In a patient taking a CYP3A4-sensitive drug, grapefruit is no longer breakfast in the ordinary sense. It is a fruit carrying furanocoumarins strong enough to thin the intestinal metabolic filter and raise systemic drug exposure. None of those cases contradict population advice. They expose its boundary.

This is why the book cannot stop at majority experience. Majority experience is useful for broad guidance, but it hides the exact places where defended plant chemistry becomes expensive. The bowel does not care that the public health statement was written for the median host. The thyroid does not care that crucifers are usually tolerated in iodine-sufficient people. The kidney does not care that only some people form stones. The liver does not care that most people call a fruit or vegetable natural and clean. Each organ receives the actual compounds crossing the membrane and has to process them with the reserve available in that body, not in the statistical average. A food can therefore remain acceptable at population scale and still be the wrong food for a host whose margin is gone.

That distinction has to stay hard all the way through the book. Population advice tells you what many bodies can usually carry without obvious breakdown. High-risk physiology tells you where the same food starts costing more than it returns because the host no longer has enough digestive, endocrine, hepatic, or renal room to keep the chemistry quiet. The plate may look identical in both cases. The outcome changes because one body still has reserve and the other is already paying for the meal in the gut wall, the follicle, the hepatocyte, or the concentrating urine long before symptoms become dramatic enough for the public categories to notice.

Fruit as a Category That Includes Both Low-Risk and High-Consequence Cases

Fruit is one of the easiest categories to flatten because the public sees sweetness first and biology second. The word sounds singular. The tissues are not singular. A ripe melon, a handful of blueberries, a glass of grapefruit juice, a serving of dried apricots, a bitter star fruit in a patient with kidney disease, and an apricot kernel do not belong to the same physiological class simply because they all sit under the word fruit. One may be a modest hydrated sugar exposure in an intact matrix. Another may be a concentrated fructose load delivered with little structural resistance. Another may alter drug handling at the intestinal wall. Another may carry enough oxalate and neurotoxic chemistry that a reduced-clearance kidney cannot move it out safely. Another may keep the edible flesh sweet while the reproductive core stays chemically guarded. The category is broad because the plant structures inside it are broad. The body has to sort fruit by tissue, dose, host, and consequence, not by the innocence of the label.

At the lower-risk end sit fruits whose chemistry, dose, and delivery often remain modest enough that a resilient host can absorb them without much downstream cost. Intact whole fruit still imposes chewing, gastric bulk, slower sugar release, and at least some structural drag from cell walls, water, and fiber. A person with good bowel reserve, stable glucose handling, broad hepatic capacity, and normal renal clearance can often meet that exposure quietly. The fruit is still plant tissue. It still carries sugars, acids, and smaller compounds. But the load may remain small enough and slow enough that the intestine clears it, the liver handles it, and the kidney never has to concentrate a meaningful burden from it. That is real. It also tells only one part of the story.

The higher-consequence cases reveal the other part. Grapefruit shows that a fruit can act pharmacologically by carrying furanocoumarins into the small intestine strongly enough to inhibit cytochrome P450 3A4 at the gut wall and raise exposure to certain oral drugs. Star fruit shows that a fruit can become dangerous when renal reserve is too thin to clear oxalate and caramboxin safely. Apples, pears, prunes, and some stone fruits show that a fruit can remain socially gentle while delivering sorbitol and fructose in a form that some small intestines do not clear cleanly, leaving the bowel with retained water and fermentation. Citrus shows that fruit can challenge teeth and oral tissues through acid contact before the sugars have even been absorbed. Apricot kernels and similar reproductive tissues show that the sweetness of the flesh says very little about the chemistry of the seed inside it. These are not exceptions that weaken the category. They expose what the category was hiding.

That is why fruit has to be judged on a gradient of burden instead of in one moral block. The real questions are always the same. How fast is the sugar delivered. How much structural resistance is still intact. Does the fruit carry polyols that stay in the lumen. Does the peel or seed hold a harder chemistry than the flesh. Does the host have enough bowel, thyroid, hepatic, renal, or pharmacologic margin to absorb the exposure quietly. A piece of intact fruit after a mixed meal is one event. Juice is another. Dried fruit is another. Grapefruit during certain drug regimens is another. Star fruit in reduced kidney function is another. The produce aisle groups them together. The organs do not.

So fruit belongs in the book as a category with both low-risk and high-consequence cases because that is the honest shape of the physiology. Some fruits, in some forms, in some hosts, stay modest enough that the body clears them with little friction. Some become bowel burden, acid burden, drug-handling interference, renal burden, or direct risk in a vulnerable host. The mistake is not enjoying fruit. The mistake is assuming the category settles the question before the tissue, the host, and the downstream organ work have been seen clearly.

Part VIII

Preparation, Dose, and Exposure Pattern

Chapter 28

Why Preparation Changes the Biological Event

Preparation changes the food before the body ever gets a vote. A raw plant tissue is not the same biological event as that same tissue peeled, soaked, boiled, fermented, pressure cooked, or sprouted, because each step changes what remains enclosed, what is released, what is destroyed, what is leached out, and what digestion will finally have to handle. The plant came with structure, water content, enzyme systems, storage compounds, mineral-binding compounds, and defense molecules arranged in a specific way. Preparation disturbs that arrangement. A knife can remove the outer tissues where some bitter compounds, pesticide residues, waxes, fibers, glycoalkaloids, and other protective chemistry tend to concentrate. Water can enter a seed or legume and begin dissolving smaller compounds out of it. Heat can denature proteins, soften cell walls, gelatinize starch, and shut down plant enzymes that would otherwise remain active in the meal. Fermentation can let microbes begin doing the chemical damage to the plant matrix before the intestine has to. Sprouting can turn a dry defended storage tissue into a tissue already spending its own reserves. These are not culinary details sitting outside physiology. They are upstream changes in what the gut will actually meet.

Peeling is the bluntest version of that change. It removes surface tissue, and surface tissue is often chemically harder than the flesh underneath it because the surface is where the plant meets light, insects, fungi, and mechanical injury. A peeled potato and an unpeeled stressed potato are not the same glycoalkaloid exposure. A peeled fruit and a whole fruit with the skin intact are not the same acid, phenolic, wax, or residue exposure. A peeled cucumber, apple, or pear may be easier on a sensitive mouth, stomach, or bowel not because peeling makes the food innocent, but because the first layer of contact chemistry has been physically cut away. The same logic applies to deseeding. Once the core, pit, membrane, or seed is removed, the digestive tract is no longer being asked to process the most guarded reproductive tissue in the structure. A person may say the food is "better tolerated" after peeling or deseeding. The more exact statement is that the digestive sequence is now meeting less of the plant's outer defense and less of its reproductive defense at the same time.

Soaking changes a different part of the problem. It does not usually destroy the structure fully, but it changes water movement and solubility inside the tissue. A dry seed, grain, or legume is a compact storage organ built to stay stable. Once soaked, that stability begins to soften. Water enters. Some small soluble compounds leave. Some enzyme systems begin to wake up. In legumes and grains, soaking can lower part of the burden of smaller water-soluble compounds and begin shifting the tissue away from a dry protected reserve toward something more chemically open. But soaking has limits. It does not erase the seed's storage logic. It does not reliably dismantle phytate the way fermentation or sprouting can. It does not guarantee that lectins, protease inhibitors, saponins, or other burdens have been reduced enough to make the food low-friction. It simply changes the first terms of contact. The seed becomes less rigid, less dry, and in some cases less chemically concentrated in the water-soluble fraction. The body still has to finish the rest.

Boiling and pressure cooking change the event more aggressively because heat alters proteins and structure in ways water alone cannot. A raw bean is still carrying active lectins and protease inhibitors in a form close enough to the original plant defense that the bowel can be punished quickly if the tissue is undercooked. Boiling denatures those proteins, meaning their folded structure unravels enough that the toxic or inhibitory function weakens. Starch granules also hydrate and gelatinize, which makes them more accessible to digestive enzymes. Fibrous tissues soften. Cell walls lose rigidity. Pressure cooking pushes the same transformations further by raising temperature and forcing water deeper into the structure. This is why a raw or lightly cooked kidney bean is one physiological event and a fully pressure-cooked bean is another. The plant tissue has already been chemically damaged before the pancreas, brush border, and colon receive it. That does not mean the burden disappears. A cooked legume can still carry phytate, fermentable carbohydrate, residual saponins, and storage-tissue resistance. But the bowel is no longer facing the same active lectin load or the same rigid starch-protein matrix it would have faced in the undercooked state.

Fermentation and sprouting go further because they do not only soften or denature. They begin spending the plant's own reserves. Fermentation lets microbes cut into the matrix before the human intestine has to do all the work. They acidify the food, consume part of the carbohydrate, change the redox environment, break down some smaller compounds, and in some cases supply enzymes the plant did not provide in sufficient amount on its own. Sprouting changes the seed from protected storage tissue into early growth tissue. The seed begins mobilizing phosphorus, minerals, and carbohydrate because it is trying to build a seedling. That matters nutritionally because part of what made the dry seed burdensome was its refusal to surrender stored material cheaply. Once germination begins, the seed itself starts dismantling some of that locked architecture. Phytase activity can rise. Storage compounds begin to break down. The same grain or legume is no longer chemically identical to the dry form from which it came. Again, this is not magic. Fermentation and sprouting reduce burden by moving the plant out of stillness and into biochemical turnover. The food becomes easier because the tissue stopped defending its reserves so completely.

The practical point is harder than most food language wants it to be. Preparation can reduce burden, sometimes dramatically, and still fail to make a food truly low-cost in a sensitive host. A peeled food may still carry fructose or acids in the flesh. A soaked grain may still lock up minerals. A boiled green may still carry oxalate. A pressure-cooked bean may still ferment heavily in an irritable bowel. A fermented vegetable may still be rich in amines or acids that some people handle poorly.

Preparation changes the biological event because it changes the plant before the body receives it. But the body still has to judge the result by net yield. What was removed. What was weakened. What was made more soluble. What was made easier to digest. What still crossed into blood. What still reached the liver, thyroid, kidney, or colon as burden. Preparation is not a moral cleansing ritual. It is a way of reducing how much raw plant logic survives into the meal.

What These Methods Physically and Chemically Reduce

Preparation reduces burden by changing what part of the plant the body is forced to negotiate with. A raw plant food still arrives as defended tissue. The skin is still intact, the storage proteins are still folded in their original shape, the starch granules are still packed, the cell walls are still holding much of the structure together, the seed still treats its phosphorus and minerals as reserves for germination rather than as gifts for the eater, and the smaller defensive compounds are still distributed through water, oil, membrane, peel, and storage compartments in the pattern the plant built. Once peeling, soaking, boiling, fermenting, pressure cooking, or sprouting begin, that pattern starts to break. Surface tissue can be removed. Water can enter and dissolve smaller molecules out. Heat can denature proteins, meaning it can distort their folded structure until they stop acting as active inhibitors or lectins. Starch can swell and gelatinize, which means the crystalline packing loosens and digestive enzymes gain access more easily. Fermentation can acidify, predigest, and partially dismantle the matrix before the intestine has to. Sprouting can shift a seed from guarded storage into active self-use. The food is no longer the same object by the time it reaches the mouth.

Peeling is the most literal reduction because it cuts away tissue. It removes part of the fruit skin, tuber surface, seed coat, or leaf edge that was doing boundary work for the plant. That often means less wax, less surface bitterness, less astringent peel chemistry, less glycoalkaloid burden in stressed potatoes, less fibrous outer resistance, and less of the smaller compounds that concentrate where the plant expected sunlight, fungi, insects, and abrasion. The body then meets more of the inner flesh and less of the boundary chemistry. A peeled apple and a whole apple are not the same acid and phenolic exposure. A deeply peeled greened potato and a whole greened potato are not the same glycoalkaloid event. The knife changes the chemistry by changing the tissue field the gut will actually see.

Soaking reduces a different class of burden. Water enters the dry structure and starts dissolving out what is soluble enough to leave. Some oligosaccharides, smaller bitter compounds, part of the saponin burden in certain foods, some tannin-related compounds, and part of the free surface chemistry can move into the soaking water and be discarded with it. The seed or grain also softens because hydration weakens the dry compact arrangement that made the raw tissue harder to digest in the first place. Water penetration alone does not fully unlock the food, but it lowers the first layer of resistance. The gut receives a wetter, more open matrix and, in some cases, less of the small water-soluble chemistry that would otherwise have entered the meal unchanged.

Boiling and pressure cooking reduce burden by forcing heat and water into the tissue together. Heat denatures lectins and protease inhibitors, meaning compounds that were active enough to bind gut surfaces or interfere with protein digestion lose much of that activity when their structure is disrupted. Pressure cooking drives the same change harder because the temperature rises above ordinary boiling and water is forced deeper into dense storage tissue. Starch granules hydrate and swell. Cell walls soften. Fibrous structure loses some of its rigidity. Some soluble compounds also leach into the cooking water, which is one reason boiling can lower part of the oxalate load in certain greens and tubers. The reduction is mixed. Some burdens are destroyed. Some are dissolved out. Some are merely softened enough that digestion can get a better grip on the tissue than it could before.

Fermentation reduces burden by letting microbes begin the digestive work outside the body. Carbohydrates are partially consumed. Acids are produced. The pH shifts. Enzymes from microbes and from the plant itself can break into structures the human intestine would otherwise have to fight through alone. This can lower part of the sugar load, reduce part of the phytate burden by activating or supplying phytase, alter protein structure, and change how tightly the matrix still holds minerals and starch. The food becomes chemically older before it is eaten. Some of the stored reserve has already been spent. Some of the resistance has already been weakened. The intestine inherits a tissue that has been partially opened instead of one still sealed in its original defensive arrangement.

Sprouting pushes that opening further because the plant begins digesting itself. A dry seed is a vault. A sprouting seed is a vault being emptied. The moment germination begins, stored starch, phosphorus, and protein are no longer being guarded only for future use. They are being mobilized for immediate plant growth. Enzymes rise. Phytate begins to break down. Some storage proteins are altered. The whole tissue shifts from static reserve into active metabolic turnover. That does not make the seed innocent, but it does reduce the extent to which the eater is facing untouched storage chemistry. The seed has started spending what it once refused to surrender.

These methods therefore reduce burden in three main ways at once. They remove defended tissue physically, they destroy or weaken active compounds chemically, and they open dense structure so digestion is not forced to do all the damage itself. What they do not guarantee is full safety or full nourishment. A boiled leaf can still carry oxalate. A soaked seed can still hold minerals in a low-yield form. A fermented food can still carry acids, amines, or host-specific burdens. Preparation changes the biological event by subtracting some of the plant's resistance before the body has to meet it. The useful question is never whether the food was prepared in some traditional or virtuous sense. The useful question is what the preparation actually removed, what it denatured, what it leached out, what it opened, and what still remained for the gut, liver, thyroid, kidney, and colon to handle afterward.

Oxalate Reduction Through Boiling

Boiling changes the oxalate problem by changing where the oxalate is allowed to stay. A high-oxalate leaf or tuber enters the pot carrying both soluble oxalate, the fraction dissolved enough to move through water easily, and insoluble oxalate, the fraction already tied up more tightly, often with calcium, and therefore less mobile. Once the tissue is cut, submerged, and heated, part of the soluble fraction leaves the plant and enters the cooking water. That is the real mechanism. Boiling does not neutralize oxalate in some abstract way. It gives the water access to the fraction of oxalate willing to travel. Studies on spinach and other vegetables repeatedly show the same pattern: boiling reduces oxalate mainly by leaching the soluble fraction out of the food and into the discarded water.

The reduction can be substantial because the soluble fraction is the part most relevant to absorption and later urinary burden. In the 2005 vegetable study by Chai and Liebman, boiling reduced soluble oxalate by roughly 30% to 87%, with stronger effects than steaming. Other cooking studies and food-chemistry reviews report the same general direction. Total oxalate may fall, but the more important shift is often in the soluble component, because that is the fraction more able to remain free in the gut, bind calcium from the meal, or cross the intestinal wall if it stays unbound. Boiling therefore changes the biological event upstream. The eater is no longer meeting the same ratio of mobile oxalate to trapped oxalate that existed in the raw tissue.

This is why boiling helps more than dry cooking methods. Steaming can reduce oxalate too, but less aggressively, because the water contact is weaker and the soluble oxalate has less room to leave the food. Baking can even concentrate oxalate in practical terms if water is lost from the tissue while the oxalate largely stays behind. Boiling gives the plant chemistry somewhere to go. The water becomes the sink for the burden. That only works if the water is discarded. Keep the boiling liquid in the soup, sauce, or puree, and much of the oxalate the plant released is still in the meal, only redistributed into the fluid instead of held inside the leaf or tuber.

The reduction is real, but it is not rescue. Insoluble oxalate is harder to move, which means a boiled high-oxalate food can still remain a meaningful oxalate exposure after cooking. Some studies even report that the proportion of insoluble oxalate in the remaining food can rise after boiling because the soluble fraction has been stripped away more effectively than the insoluble fraction. Spinach is still spinach after boiling. Swiss chard is still Swiss chard. The food may become less oxalate-dense in the soluble sense and still remain a poor choice for someone with severe oxalate sensitivity, enteric hyperoxaluria, or recurrent calcium oxalate stone vulnerability.

Boiling also asks for a trade. Water does not only pull oxalate out. It can pull water-soluble vitamins and other small compounds out with it. That does not erase the value of boiling. It simply puts the method back where it belongs, inside a real physiological tradeoff instead of inside a food myth. Boiling a high-oxalate green can reduce the part of the chemistry most likely to bind minerals in the gut and raise urinary oxalate later. It can also lower part of the vitamin return from the same tissue. The useful question is not whether boiling is virtuous. The useful question is whether the reduction in soluble oxalate changes the food enough to improve the net biological result for the host eating it. In a person burdened by oxalate, boiling can move the food in the right direction. It does not turn a chemically difficult plant into an automatically low-burden one.

Lectin and Protease Inhibitor Reduction Through Proper Heat

A raw bean is still carrying active protein defenses. The starch may be the part people think they are eating, but the seed also contains lectins, proteins that can bind cell surfaces, and protease inhibitors, proteins that block digestive enzymes such as trypsin and chymotrypsin, the pancreatic enzymes that normally cut dietary protein into smaller absorbable fragments. In red kidney beans the main acute lectin problem is phytohaemagglutinin, often shortened to PHA, a lectin concentrated strongly enough in raw or undercooked beans to provoke severe gastrointestinal symptoms. Food-safety sources and review literature describe these proteins as heat-labile, which means their biological activity depends on a folded structure that can be disrupted by enough heat and water.

Proper cooking changes that structure before the gut has to meet it. A folded lectin or protease inhibitor works because its shape still fits the surface or enzyme it is meant to bind. Once boiling or pressure cooking pushes enough heat into the hydrated seed, the protein begins to denature. Its folding loosens, its binding geometry is damaged, and the active defense starts losing function. That is why proper boiling matters so much with beans. The problem is not only that raw beans are harder to digest. The problem is that their active protein defenses are still close enough to the plant's original form to keep doing the job they were built to do. Review literature notes that boiling, autoclaving, and pressure cooking can irreversibly denature lectins, while cooking of presoaked seeds can reduce enzyme inhibitor activity very sharply, often into a range where the digestive sequence is dealing with ordinary protein much more than with active resistance.

The difference between proper heat and weak heat is not small. Undercooking can leave enough lectin activity behind that the bowel still receives a toxic contact event instead of a cooperative food. That is why guidance around kidney beans stays unusually blunt. Soaking helps shorten the time needed, but soaking does not finish the job on its own. FDA- and WHO-linked safety language reflected in review literature continues to emphasize vigorous boiling because low-temperature warming can leave phytohaemagglutinin active enough to remain dangerous. The seed may look softened. The chemistry can still be wrong. With protease inhibitors the pattern is similar but less dramatic. As heat treatment is done properly, trypsin inhibitor activity falls, protein digestibility rises, and the pancreas is no longer being forced to work against a seed still trying to block proteolysis in the lumen.

This is why proper heat changes the biological event instead of merely changing the recipe. A raw or undercooked legume asks the gut to negotiate with active protein defenses. A fully boiled or pressure-cooked legume reaches the stomach and small intestine after much of that defense has already been dismantled. The seed is still seed tissue. It may still carry phytate, fermentable carbohydrate, saponins, tannins, or residual resistance in the matrix. But the bowel is no longer meeting the same lectin burden or the same level of protease blockade. Heat does not make every bean low-burden. It does remove one of the harsher layers of plant logic before the intestine has to absorb the cost itself.

Phytate Reduction Through Fermentation and Sprouting

A dry seed is storing phosphorus in a locked form because the plant is not trying to feed the eater. It is trying to preserve mineral and phosphorus reserves for germination. Phytic acid, also called myo-inositol hexakisphosphate, holds that reserve tightly, often as mineral phytate salts. The burden is not only that the phosphorus is locked. Zinc, iron, calcium, and magnesium can be held in the same chemistry. A raw grain or legume therefore reaches the bowel as compact storage tissue still treating its minerals as future plant property. Fermentation and sprouting change that because both move the seed out of static storage and into breakdown. The seed is no longer only protecting its reserve. It has begun letting go of it. Review literature on phytic acid reduction describes both processes as effective because they increase phytase activity, the enzyme that cleaves phosphate groups off phytic acid and starts dismantling the storage form itself.

Sprouting does this from inside the seed. Water enters, metabolism wakes up, and the seed begins spending what it had previously locked away. Phytase activity rises because the young plant now needs access to the phosphorus and minerals it stored for itself. That is why germination is not a cosmetic preparation step. It changes the direction of the tissue. During germination, studies repeatedly show increasing phytase activity alongside falling phytate content, sometimes with substantial reductions depending on species, duration, and conditions. The seed is no longer a vault. It is a vault being opened from the inside. A person eating the sprouted grain or legume is meeting a storage tissue that has already begun digesting its own reserves instead of defending them in the original dry form.

Fermentation pushes on the same problem from another side. The tissue is broken, wetted, acidified, and handed over to microbial work before the human intestine has to do all the damage itself. Microbes can supply phytase of their own, and the falling pH during fermentation helps create conditions in which phytate breakdown becomes easier. That is why fermentation often reduces phytate more aggressively than soaking alone and in many comparisons more aggressively than germination. Liang and colleagues found fermentation to be the most effective of the common wet-processing methods they tested, with phytate reductions reported in the range of roughly 56% to 96%, while simple soaking often removed much less. The plant reserve is being chemically opened before the gut sees it. The bowel is no longer facing the same intact seed logic.

The reduction is real, but it is not a magic release of all value. Species differ, cultivars differ, and some of the same wet processes that lower phytate can also carry losses of dry mass or minerals into the soak water or fermenting medium. The seed may become easier. It does not become automatically low-burden. A sprouted or fermented grain can still carry resistant structure, residual phytate, fermentable carbohydrate, or other antinutrients that matter in the wrong host. What changes is the basic direction of the tissue. Dry storage resists surrender. Sprouting and fermentation begin forcing surrender before the first bite. The minerals are still not guaranteed. The lock is simply being broken open instead of arriving in the bowel untouched.

Why Preparation Can Improve a Food Without Turning It Into a Different Species

Preparation changes the biological event by changing what survives into the meal. It does not change what the plant is. A soaked bean is still a bean. A boiled spinach leaf is still spinach. A fermented grain is still grain. The species identity stays put while the chemistry and structure presented to the gut shift in important ways. Water enters where the tissue was dry. Heat denatures proteins that were still folded in their active defensive form. Soluble compounds move out into soak water or cooking water. Starch swells and loosens. Cell walls soften. Enzymes inside the plant are shut down or activated depending on the method. Microbes begin digesting part of the matrix before the human intestine has to do it. All of that can reduce burden. None of it turns the seed, leaf, tuber, or fruit into something biologically unrelated to the original plant.

That distinction matters because food language often swings between two bad extremes. One extreme pretends raw and cooked are basically the same. The other pretends a traditional preparation has somehow purified the food into a different category of substance. The body does not see either fantasy. It sees the same plant tissue under altered conditions. A pressure-cooked kidney bean reaches the bowel with far less active lectin and far less protease inhibitor activity than the undercooked bean, but it still arrives as legume storage tissue that may carry phytate, fermentable carbohydrate, and residual matrix resistance. Boiled spinach can lose part of its soluble oxalate into the water and still remain a high-oxalate leaf compared with low-oxalate greens. Fermented grain can surrender part of its phytate burden and still remain seed tissue whose minerals are not delivered with the ease of a food that never locked them away so tightly in the first place. Preparation improves the terms of contact. It does not erase the original design.

The reason is structural. The plant built a particular tissue for a particular job. A seed was built to preserve reserves. A peel was built to face the outside world. A tuber was built to store energy underground under chemical guard. A leaf was built to expose surface area while still defending itself from predation and mineral loss. Preparation can damage that design enough to make the tissue easier on the eater, but it cannot rewrite what kind of tissue it was. Sprouting can turn a seed from static storage into early growth and reduce part of the phytate burden because the seed has begun spending its own reserves. Fermentation can let microbes break down part of the matrix and acidify the tissue. Boiling can leach out mobile compounds and soften structure. Peeling can remove harder outer layers. But the food that reaches the mouth is still the descendant of the same plant logic. The defenses may be weaker. The storage chemistry may be partly opened. The tissue is still carrying the biological priorities it was built with.

This is why preparation has to be judged by net yield instead of by ritual status. The right question is never whether the food was prepared in a traditional, ancestral, artisanal, or wholesome way. The right question is what the preparation physically removed, what it denatured, what it dissolved out, what it opened up, and what still remained for the digestive tract, liver, thyroid, kidney, or colon to handle afterward. A soaked and pressure-cooked legume may be far easier than the raw or lightly cooked version and still produce heavy fermentation in an irritable bowel. A peeled fruit may reduce peel chemistry and still deliver enough fructose or sorbitol to overrun small-intestinal absorption. A fermented crucifer may alter one burden while still arriving as sulfur-rich plant tissue. Improvement is real. Rescue is conditional.

That is the useful middle ground. Preparation can make a food less chemically aggressive, less structurally resistant, and less demanding of the gut without turning it into a different organism or a different class of nourishment. The bean remains a bean. The leaf remains a leaf. The fruit remains fruit. The body simply receives less of the raw plant logic intact than it would have without the preparation. Sometimes that reduction is enough to make the food workable. Sometimes it is only enough to make the burden smaller.

The Limits of Processing as a Rescue Strategy

Processing can reduce burden because it can remove part of the chemistry before the body has to meet it. It can peel away outer tissues, leach out soluble compounds, denature active proteins, soften cell walls, gelatinize starch, acidify a matrix, or let microbes begin dismantling storage chemistry before the intestine has to do the same work alone. That improvement is real. It is also where people start lying to themselves about the food. A seed that needed soaking, fermenting, and pressure cooking before it became tolerable has already told you what kind of tissue it was. A leaf that has to be boiled to cut down soluble oxalate has already told you what chemistry the raw plant was carrying. A potato that needs aggressive peeling and trimming before it stops looking dangerous has already told you the outer tissue was not neutral. Processing can weaken the plant's grip. It does not prove the grip was never there.

The limit appears when the food's main problem is not only one removable fraction sitting at the surface. Some burdens are distributed through the tissue. Some are rebuilt as soon as the structure is broken. Some are reduced without disappearing. A boiled high-oxalate green can still remain a meaningful oxalate exposure because boiling removes more of the soluble fraction than the insoluble fraction and because the leaf is still the same mineral-binding plant tissue it was before the pot. A pressure-cooked bean can lose enough lectin activity to stop behaving like an acute gastrointestinal hazard and still arrive as fermentable legume storage tissue carrying phytate, residual inhibitor burden, and enough carbohydrate to overrun an irritable bowel later. A fermented grain can lower phytate substantially and still remain a grain whose minerals were stored under chemical guard strongly enough that the person needed fermentation in the first place. The food is easier. The food is not transformed into an unrelated species of nourishment.

Processing also forces tradeoffs the language of rescue usually hides. Water can leach out oxalate and at the same time pull out water-soluble vitamins and minerals. Fermentation can lower phytate and at the same time raise amine burden or acidity in a sensitive host. Peeling can remove protective outer chemistry and also remove fiber, pigments, and whatever nutrients were concentrated near the surface. Heat can denature lectins and protease inhibitors while also destroying heat-sensitive compounds. The change is not one-directional. The body does not receive a food that has simply been cleansed. It receives a food whose burdens and benefits were both rearranged. That is why processing has to be judged by net biological yield rather than by culinary virtue. The relevant question is not whether the preparation sounds traditional, careful, or health-conscious. The relevant question is what the preparation subtracted, what it degraded, what it concentrated, and what the gut, liver, thyroid, kidney, or colon still have to carry afterward.

The hardest limit is host context. Processing can move a food from impossible to tolerable in one body and from difficult to only slightly less difficult in another. A soaked and pressure-cooked bean may become workable in a person with broad digestive reserve and still remain a gas-producing, bowel-distending problem in a person with fermentation sensitivity. A boiled spinach serving may lower oxalate enough to matter for one host and still remain an unwise renal burden in a person with enteric hyperoxaluria or recurrent calcium oxalate stone formation. A peeled fruit may spare one person the peel chemistry and still deliver too much sorbitol, fructose, or acid for another. That is the real limit of rescue through processing. Preparation can reduce how much raw plant logic survives into the meal. It cannot guarantee that the remaining chemistry is worth the price of absorption, transformation, and clearance in the body eating it.

Chapter 29

Dose Makes the Burden Visible

A garnish can stay below consequence simply by staying below repetition. The chemistry is still there. The lectin is still a lectin. The oxalate is still oxalate. The glucosinolate still breaks toward thiocyanate and related sulfur compounds when the tissue is damaged. But a few leaves, a small spoonful, an occasional bitter note, or a rare condiment exposure may pass through the gut and liver without recruiting enough of the system often enough to make the cost visible. Toxicology has always had to distinguish acute exposure from chronic exposure for exactly this reason. One asks what happens after a single exposure or a short burst. The other asks what happens when the same chemistry keeps arriving over time. WHO's food-chemical risk guidance treats acute and chronic dietary exposure as different biological questions, not as the same question scaled up or down.

A staple is different because the body does not get to forget it between meals. The same tissue keeps being chewed, digested, absorbed, and cleared through the same surfaces and the same organs. The same bowel keeps seeing the same fermentable load. The same thyroid keeps seeing the same iodine competition. The same hepatocyte, the main working liver cell, keeps taking the same first pass at the same absorbed compounds in portal blood. The same nephron keeps concentrating the same dissolved remainder into urine. An occasional food and a foundational food are not the same physiological decision. The garnish can remain background chemistry. The staple becomes part of the organ's standing workload. WHO's exposure framework reflects that difference directly by separating short-term acute exposure from long-term chronic dietary exposure across the total diet.

This is where plant burden becomes easier to see than public nutrition language usually allows. A handful of spinach once in a while is not the same renal event as a daily high-oxalate smoothie habit. A side of sauerkraut is not the same histamine and amine exposure as building large amounts of fermented food into every day for a person with poor tolerance. A little cabbage in a soup is not the same thyroid problem as a repetitive raw-heavy Brassica pattern in a host already thin on iodine. The chemistry did not change. Dose pattern changed. Frequency changed. The host's ability to clear, compensate, and recover between exposures changed with it. Repeated-dose toxicology exists because organisms do not meet the fiftieth exposure with the same empty physiological slate they brought to the first one. EFSA's repeated-dose guidance is built on that same premise.

So dose makes the burden visible by turning a quiet chemical fact into recurring tissue work. The garnish may stay too small and too infrequent to recruit much consequence. The staple keeps returning until the subtraction stops looking theoretical. Mineral binding becomes lower mineral status. Fermentation becomes daily distension. Hepatic handling becomes standing liver workload. Urinary solute becomes supersaturation and crystal pressure. The body does not rank foods by image or category. It ranks them by how much of their chemistry arrives, how often it arrives, and whether the same membrane, gland, hepatocyte, or nephron still has enough reserve left to keep that chemistry quiet.

Daily Smoothie Exposure Versus Occasional Intake

A smoothie changes the food before the body ever sees it. The blade has already done much of the structural damage that chewing, gastric grinding, and slower release would have done more gradually with intact fruit or greens. Cell walls are ruptured, the water is no longer being held in the same tissue architecture, and the sugars, acids, polyols, pigments, oxalate, and smaller plant compounds are suspended in a fluid the stomach can move forward with much less resistance than a bowl of intact produce would impose. Solid foods generally slow gastric emptying and produce stronger satiety than liquid forms, while whole fruit tends to produce more fullness than fruit juice for the same broad category of food. The tissue still came from fruit or leaves. The digestive event is no longer the same.

That difference grows when the smoothie becomes daily instead of occasional. A handful of spinach once in a while is one oxalate exposure. A daily smoothie built from spinach, nut butters, cacao, berries, beets, or other favored "healthy" ingredients can become a repeated portal load and, in the wrong host, a repeated urinary load. Dietary oxalate intake is associated with urinary oxalate and kidney stone risk, and recent case literature has described oxalate nephropathy from smoothie-heavy or high-oxalate dietary patterns that looked health-conscious on the surface. The food keeps the wholesome reputation. The kidney still has to concentrate the dissolved remainder after absorption and hepatic handling are over.

The sugar side changes too. A whole fruit still imposes chewing time, gastric bulk, and a slower physical release of carbohydrate. A smoothie can deliver the equivalent of several pieces of fruit quickly, with much less stopping power from intact structure. The literature comparing whole fruit with juice and processed fruit keeps returning to the same point: the fruit matrix changes glycemic response, appetite, and fullness, even when the starting plant is the same. Some smoothie studies show nuances depending on the fruit and fiber still present, but the broader lesson holds. Once the tissue has been pulverized into a drinkable load, the small intestine and liver are no longer receiving the same paced carbohydrate event they would have received from intact fruit eaten piece by piece.

The bowel can read the same change from another angle. A smoothie makes it easier to combine large fructose loads, polyol-bearing fruits, and fibrous greens into one fast exposure that outruns the quieter limits of appetite and intestinal handling. A person who would never sit down and chew through three apples, a pear, a banana, a handful of greens, and a spoonful of nut butter can drink that combination quickly. If the small bowel does not absorb all of the fructose and polyols cleanly, the retained carbohydrate stays in the lumen, holds water there, and then reaches the colon as fermentation substrate. In a resilient host that may remain tolerable. In an irritable bowel, it becomes repeated luminal water retention, gas, stretch, and altered transit from a drink still wearing the identity of produce.

That is why daily smoothie exposure and occasional intake do not belong to the same physiological category. The occasional whole-food exposure still carries structure, friction, and natural stopping points. The daily smoothie removes much of that friction, makes large combined doses easier, and can keep returning the same sugars, oxalate, acids, and smaller plant compounds through the same bowel, the same portal route, and the same kidney day after day. A single smoothie may pass quietly. A daily smoothie habit can turn a reputation for health into repeated intestinal overrun, repeated hepatic sorting, or repeated urinary burden because the body is no longer judging one fruit or one leaf. It is judging a pulverized, concentrated, and easily repeated delivery system.

Repetition as the Bridge From Nuisance to Burden

A single exposure can stay small enough that the body absorbs the subtraction quietly. The bowel stretches a little, the liver oxidizes and conjugates a little, the kidney filters and concentrates a little, and the person calls the result annoyance, sensitivity, or just one of those things. Repetition changes the meaning of the same chemistry because the tissue receiving it does not reset to innocence between exposures. The same lumen sees the same fermentable residue again. The same intestinal membrane sees the same fructose, sorbitol, oxalate, amines, or sulfur breakdown products again. The same portal blood delivers the same compounds back to the same hepatocyte, the main working liver cell, again. A molecule that looked trivial in isolation can become a standing demand once it stops arriving as an exception and starts arriving as routine.

The gut usually reveals this first because repetition is easy to feel in a tube. One fruit-heavy meal that leaves fructose or polyols behind may produce a little gas and water retention. A daily pattern of smoothies, dried fruit, onions, garlic, legumes, or other poorly handled plant foods keeps returning unfinished carbohydrate to the same bowel until the residue stops looking episodic and starts becoming part of the bowel's normal workload. The lumen holds water again. The colon ferments again. The wall stretches again. Motility shifts again. At that point the person often thinks the symptoms appeared mysteriously or that their gut suddenly "got worse." More often the chemistry never stopped arriving long enough for the tissue to recover its margin. The nuisance became a pattern because the exposure became a pattern.

The same bridge exists in organs that do not speak as loudly. A single crucifer meal may not move the thyroid enough for anyone to notice. Repetitive raw-heavy Brassica intake in a host already thin on iodine is different because the gland has to trap iodide and build hormone under the same interference every day. A single oxalate-rich meal may pass without visible consequence. Repeated high-oxalate intake keeps returning soluble oxalate to the intestine, keeps sending part of it into blood, and keeps asking the kidney to filter and concentrate the same dissolved burden into urine. A single grapefruit exposure may not matter unless the wrong drug is on board. Repeated grapefruit intake in a person taking a CYP3A4-sensitive medicine keeps thinning the intestinal enzyme field that dose after dose depends on. The chemistry is not becoming more symbolic with repetition. It is becoming more continuous.

The liver sits in the middle of that continuity. One absorbed plant compound can be oxidized, conjugated, pushed into bile, and forgotten. Repetition is different because the cell does not experience those exposures as isolated tasks. The same chemistry keeps returning through the same portal route to the same cell. Phase I handling keeps generating reactive intermediates. Glutathione, the sulfur-rich antioxidant the liver uses to quench reactive chemistry, keeps being spent. Transporters keep loading altered compounds into bile or back into blood. Some of that chemistry returns again through enterohepatic circulation, meaning the liver secretes it into bile, the intestine receives it, part of it is reabsorbed, and portal blood brings it back for another pass. A mild burden can stay mild while it is occasional. Repetition is what teaches the organ to live inside the burden.

That is the bridge from nuisance to burden. Not drama. Not one spectacular poisoning. Frequency. The same food, the same tissue, the same chemistry, the same organ surface, repeated often enough that compensation becomes part of daily physiology instead of a brief repair job after a meal. A garnish can stay small. A staple keeps returning until the body has to organize itself around the cost. That is when the bowel stops feeling merely touchy, the thyroid stops feeling merely sluggish, the urine stops looking like a neutral waste stream, and the liver stops handling a passing compound and starts devoting real cellular work to it every day.

Why Concentrated "Health" Patterns Can Backfire

A concentrated health pattern usually begins by removing friction from the food and then removing doubt from the eater. The person stops eating one spinach salad and starts drinking spinach every morning. One handful of almonds becomes almond flour, almond butter, almond milk, and low-carbohydrate baking built around the same nut chemistry. Fruit stops arriving as a piece of intact tissue and starts arriving as juice, smoothies, dried fruit, bowls, snacks, and cleanses. Crucifers stop appearing as a side dish and become a daily raw habit because the vegetable has been assigned a cleaner moral status the more often it is repeated. The chemistry does not become safer when it is concentrated inside a health routine. It becomes easier to deliver in larger doses, easier to repeat without appetite pushing back hard enough, and easier to defend psychologically because the pattern now carries the identity of discipline, wellness, and self-care. The body does not see discipline. It sees more oxalate, more fructose, more sorbitol, more glucosinolate breakdown products, more fermentable residue, or more low-yield plant compounds crossing the same membranes more often.

That is where the backfire begins. Intact food usually comes with some natural brakes. Chewing slows the dose. Bulk stretches the stomach. Water and fiber occupy space. Variety interrupts repetition. Preparation changes some of the chemistry. Appetite tires of the texture before the load becomes extreme. Concentrated health patterns strip many of those brakes away. Blending breaks the tissue open before digestion begins. Juicing removes much of the structural resistance and leaves the sugars and acids moving through the gut as a fast fluid load. Drying compresses the same chemistry into a smaller volume that can be eaten absentmindedly. Powders and flours make it possible to build the same plant into every meal without the visual signal that intake has become excessive. Once that happens, a food that was tolerable as part of a varied diet can become a repeated high-dose exposure simply because the person found a more efficient delivery system and wrapped it in the language of health.

The organs then start reading the pattern more clearly than the person does. The bowel sees repeated fructose and polyol overrun, repeated fermentation, repeated luminal water retention, and repeated stretch. The thyroid sees repeated sulfur-rich crucifer chemistry landing on the same iodide-trapping sequence. The liver sees repeated portal delivery of plant compounds that may add little constructive value while still demanding oxidation, conjugation, and export. The kidney sees repeated oxalate or other dissolved burdens entering urine and being concentrated in a shrinking volume of water day after day. One spinach smoothie is one event. A daily smoothie habit built from spinach, almond butter, berries, cacao, and other chemically dense "superfoods" is another. One piece of fruit after a meal is one sugar exposure. Juices, bowls, and dried fruit layered across the day create a different portal load. Repetition turns the health pattern into an organ pattern. The food keeps the clean reputation while the same bowel, the same follicle, the same hepatocyte, and the same nephron keep paying for the chemistry.

That is why concentrated health patterns can backfire so badly in people who are trying hardest to eat well. The problem is rarely that one food was secretly poison. The problem is that a narrow set of praised foods is being delivered with too little structural resistance, too much repetition, and too much faith in the category label to notice when net biological yield has started falling. The person thinks they are increasing nourishment because the foods are socially approved. The body may be getting less mineral return, more fermentation, more endocrine friction, more liver sorting work, and more urinary burden than the reputation of the pattern would ever suggest. The cleaner the pattern sounds in public language, the easier it becomes to miss that the same chemistry is hitting the same tissue every day until the burden stops looking like a side effect and starts becoming the physiology of the person eating that way.

Juicing, Green Powders, Smoothies, Raw Food Habits, and Snack Frequency

These habits look clean because they remove so much of what normally makes a person stop. A whole fruit asks for chewing. A plate of greens occupies volume in the stomach. A cooked vegetable cools the appetite with bulk, heat, and finishing power. Juicing strips the tissue down to fluid and dissolved solids. Green powders remove water, freshness, and visible plant form, then compress the chemistry into a scoop. Smoothies break cell structure before the mouth ever touches it and turn several pieces of produce into one fast drink. Raw food habits keep more of the plant's original enzyme activity, sharper acids, harsher fibers, and unsoftened defense chemistry intact. Constant snacking removes the pause between exposures. The body is no longer meeting one meal at a time. It is meeting a stream.

That stream matters because plant burden is often limited by friction. Structure slows delivery. Chewing slows intake. Cooking denatures some proteins, softens cell walls, lowers some active compounds, and changes what the gut is forced to negotiate with. Time between meals allows gastric emptying to finish, the small intestine to clear, bile to cycle, the colon to calm, and the liver and kidney to finish handling what already crossed. Juicing, powders, and frequent snacking collapse those intervals. A fruit that would have been one piece of tissue becomes a glass. Greens that would have filled a bowl become a powder stirred into water. A handful of nuts becomes butter or flour and then disappears into a smoothie. The same chemistry is no longer arriving at the membrane in the same form or at the same pace. It is arriving faster, more repeatedly, and with less structural resistance.

The gut pays first. Fructose and polyols, sugar alcohols such as sorbitol, can be delivered in larger loads than the small intestine clears comfortably. Fiber that might have slowed intake in intact food is no longer playing the same mechanical role once the tissue has been pulverized or extracted. Raw crucifer tissue brings more active glucosinolate breakdown chemistry into the meal than cooked tissue does. Raw leafy greens can preserve more of the plant's original oxalate burden than boiling would have left behind. Frequent fruit and dried fruit snacking keeps acid and sugar contact returning to the teeth without much recovery time. A bowel that might have tolerated one apple after lunch may not tolerate an all-day pattern of smoothies, dried mango, dates, juice, and powdered greens because the same lumen, the hollow interior of the bowel where digestion is taking place, keeps receiving poorly cleared carbohydrate, acids, fibers, and plant compounds without enough pause for the previous burden to leave.

The liver and kidney read the same pattern differently but no less clearly. Portal blood keeps delivering the absorbed fraction to the hepatocyte, the main working liver cell, and repeated low-value plant chemistry still has to be oxidized, conjugated, and exported whether or not the person thinks they are eating lightly. A smoothie can feel easier than a meal and still deliver more sugar, more oxalate, more fruit acids, more supplement-like phytochemical density, and more repeated daily traffic than the intact foods would have imposed separately. The kidney inherits what the body did not turn into tissue. Oxalate-rich greens, cacao, nuts, beets, and powdered concentrates can all turn a health pattern into urinary chemistry if the habit becomes daily enough and dense enough. The danger is not always one spectacular poisoning. More often it is repetition without obvious stopping points.

Green powders are especially revealing because they expose the logic of concentration without the comfort of fresh produce. A powder is plant matter with the water removed and the tissue reduced to a transportable dose. The scoop looks small. The chemistry is not small. Minerals, oxalate, glucosinolates, polyphenols, fibers, dried fruit sugars, herbal extracts, and other compounds can be compressed into a form that bypasses appetite, chewing, cooking, and ordinary meal structure all at once. The person feels efficient. The body receives concentrated plant logic without much of the natural friction that might have kept dose lower or frequency less automatic.

That is why these habits can backfire so easily in people trying hardest to eat well. Juicing, green powders, smoothies, raw food habits, and constant snacking all move in the same direction. They reduce friction, increase repeat exposure, and make larger chemical loads easier to consume under the banner of health. The produce identity stays clean. The bowel still has to absorb it, the liver still has to sort it, and the kidney still has to clear what the body could not use. A habit built from approved foods can still become a daily delivery system for more burden than nourishment.

The Cumulative Effect of Chronic Plant Chemical Exposure

Chronic exposure changes the biology long before it produces a dramatic symptom. A single meal can pass as friction. The same chemistry repeated through the same tissues every day becomes architecture. The bowel keeps meeting the same fructose load, the same polyols, the same oxalate, the same phytate, the same sulfur compounds from damaged crucifer tissue, the same lectin fragments, the same peel acids, the same smaller plant molecules that were easy to dismiss when they arrived once. The lumen, the hollow interior of the gut where digestion is taking place, does not reset to theoretical neutrality between those exposures. It keeps absorbing what it can, fermenting what it cannot, stretching around retained water and gas, and handing the absorbed fraction forward in portal blood to the liver. A plant burden that stays below notice in one meal can become the background condition of the digestive tract when the same food pattern keeps returning before the tissues have recovered their margin.

The first cumulative cost is usually a loss of yield. Minerals keep arriving with binding partners that lower what the intestine can actually recover. Carbohydrate keeps arriving in forms that leave residue behind. Protein keeps arriving inside seed tissue that still resists cleavage more than animal tissue does. The body may not look acutely injured, but it is being underfed and overworked at the same time. Calcium is lost in the gut and then oxalate shows up later in urine. Zinc and iron stay bound often enough that the food keeps its nutrient reputation while the tissues receive a thinner return than the label implied. Fructose and sorbitol keep overrunning small-intestinal handling often enough that the colon inherits water and fermentation as part of ordinary life instead of as an occasional mistake. Chronic exposure turns a weak meal into a weak pattern, and weak patterns do not stay local to one bite.

Then the organs of handling begin living inside the repetition. The hepatocyte, the main working liver cell, keeps receiving the same absorbed chemistry in portal blood, the blood draining from the stomach and intestine into the liver first. It keeps oxidizing, conjugating, exporting into bile, and spending glutathione, the sulfur-rich antioxidant the liver uses to neutralize reactive chemistry before it binds proteins or injures membranes. The nephron, the kidney's microscopic filtering and reclamation unit, keeps concentrating the same dissolved remainder into urine. The thyroid keeps trying to trap iodide and build hormone while sulfur breakdown products keep pressing on the same sequence in a host with limited reserve. Chronic exposure does not need to look like poisoning to become expensive. It only needs to keep returning through the same route to the same cell until compensation stops being brief and starts becoming the organ's daily operating condition.

That is where people get misled by the absence of crisis. No collapse. No obvious intoxication. No single meal dramatic enough to blame. The chemistry still accumulates as work. The bowel keeps carrying residue. The liver keeps carrying clearance. The kidney keeps carrying concentrated solute. The gland keeps carrying interference. A person can therefore live inside the cumulative effect for years while describing the result with softer words such as bloating, sensitivity, fatigue, sluggishness, heaviness, food intolerance, irritability, or just getting older. The body is using harder language underneath. It is reallocating membrane transport, enzyme activity, antioxidant reserve, mineral balance, endocrine output, and excretory work around a food pattern that keeps arriving as more burden than nourishment.

This is the real danger of chronic plant chemical exposure. It does not need spectacular toxicity to matter. It only needs repetition strong enough that the same defended chemistry stops behaving like an occasional contact and starts behaving like a standing feature of the host's physiology. The meal is no longer one event. It is now the chemistry the bowel expects, the liver expects, the kidney expects, and the thyroid is forced to work around. Once exposure crosses that line, the food is no longer being judged by what it contained on paper. It is being judged by what the body had to keep doing with it day after day.

Chapter 30

Frequency, Variety, and the Illusion of Safety by Rotation

Rotation sounds safer because the plate keeps changing. The bowel, liver, thyroid, and kidney do not read the plate that way. They do not care that Monday was spinach, Tuesday was almonds, Wednesday was sweet potatoes, Thursday was beets, and Friday was Swiss chard. They care that oxalate kept returning to the same intestine, crossed into the same blood, and then reached the same nephron, the kidney's filtering unit, over and over again under different food names. The same thing happens with poorly absorbed sugars, FODMAPs, sulfur compounds from damaged crucifer tissue, salicylates, amines, and other plant burdens. Rotation changes the costume of the exposure. It does not always change the chemistry the organ has to handle. A person can therefore feel protected by variety while still delivering the same class of burden to the same membrane or gland often enough that the tissue never really gets a break.

Removing a burden is different. Removal gives the organ less of the same chemistry to process. Rotation often only changes where that chemistry came from. A bowel irritated by retained fructose and sorbitol may not care much whether the load came from apples one day, pears the next, dried fruit the day after, and a smoothie on the weekend. The lumen, the hollow interior of the bowel where digestion and absorption are taking place, still ends up carrying poorly absorbed carbohydrate, still pulls water in by osmosis, and still hands fermentable residue to the colon. A thyroid running on thin iodine reserve may not care much whether the raw Brassica burden came from kale, cabbage, Brussels sprouts, or collards across the week. The follicle still has to trap iodide and build hormone while sulfur breakdown products keep pressing on the same sequence. Rotation can lower the monotony of the menu and still preserve the workload of the organ.

Variety becomes especially deceptive when the burden is distributed across different foods that share the same destination. A person may stop eating spinach every day and replace it with almond flour, nut butter, dark chocolate, beets, and sweet potatoes, then believe they solved the oxalate problem because the diet looks more varied. The kidney sees something else. Urinary oxalate keeps arriving. Calcium oxalate supersaturation, the state in which urine holds more crystal-forming material than it can keep stably dissolved, still rises if the absorbed load remains high enough. The same illusion appears in the gut. One person rotates onions, apples, watermelon, legumes, mango, and stone fruit, all under the belief that no single food is being overused. The small intestine still fails to clear part of the fructose, polyol, or oligosaccharide burden, and the colon still receives repeated fermentation substrate. Different foods. Same bowel event.

Rotation can help under narrower conditions. If the burden is strongly dose-dependent and the tissue has time to recover between exposures, lowering the frequency of one specific chemical can reduce visible symptoms. A person may tolerate spinach once every few weeks better than daily. A person with bowel sensitivity may do better with occasional onion than with onion at every meal. That improvement is real. It is not the same as removal. The organ is still meeting the chemistry whenever it returns. Rotation is a spacing strategy. Removal is a subtraction strategy. In a sensitive host, spacing may not be enough because the threshold is low, the recovery is incomplete, or different foods are still converging on the same membrane, the same transporter, the same follicle, or the same urinary chemistry.

That is where the illusion of safety by rotation finally breaks. The eater sees different colors, different recipes, different produce, different labels. The tissues often see recurring classes of chemistry. A true reduction in burden means the bowel receives less retained fermentable residue, the thyroid receives less repeated interference with iodide handling, the liver receives less low-yield chemistry to transform, and the kidney receives less dissolved remainder to concentrate into urine. Rotation can disguise repetition when the chemistry is shared across many foods. The menu looks diverse. The organ workload stays familiar.

Why Many Moderate Irritants Can Still Add Up

A bowel surface does not need one spectacular insult to become a burdened surface. The mucosa, the living lining of the intestine, is built to face acid, enzymes, bile, food particles, microbes, and the smaller chemical debris released as plant tissue is broken down. It can tolerate contact. It cannot make contact meaningless. A moderately irritating fruit acid here, a fermentable carbohydrate there, a polyol load in one snack, a crucifer-heavy raw salad later, spices, coffee, alcohol, peel chemistry, emulsifiers, amines, poorly absorbed sugars, residual lectin activity, repeated rough fiber, and the day begins filling with small frictions that all land on the same tissue. None of them may be strong enough alone to look like poisoning. The intestine still has to secrete fluid around them, move them, buffer them, absorb what it can, ferment what it cannot, and then restore the surface afterward. The person sees many ordinary foods. The mucosa sees recurring contact and repeated recovery work.

Recovery is the part people miss because it is invisible when it is still working. After one irritating exposure, the bowel can dilute the contents, move them forward, replace mucus, restore ion balance, and quiet the local sensory nerves before the next challenge arrives. Repetition changes that sequence. The next meal lands before the previous chemical contact has fully cleared. The next snack reopens fluid shifts and stretch. The next "healthy" drink brings more acid, more sugar, more osmotic load, more plant residue, or more smaller compounds to a surface that is already a little more reactive than it was that morning. A membrane that keeps being asked to recover stays in recovery. At that point moderate irritants stop behaving like isolated events and start behaving like the day's operating conditions. The bowel is no longer responding to one food. It is living inside a pattern of repeated low-grade provocation.

Different irritants can also converge on the same physiological result even when they are chemically unrelated. One food may leave fructose behind and hold water in the lumen, the hollow interior of the bowel where absorption is taking place. Another may ferment heavily in the colon and raise gas pressure. Another may bring enough acidity to irritate the upper gut. Another may carry rough insoluble fiber that increases friction against a sensitive lining. Another may not be especially irritating in the gut at all but still alter bile flow, thyroid handling, histamine burden, or hepatic workload enough that the person becomes less tolerant of everything else layered on top. The body does not need the same molecule repeated to accumulate burden. It only needs several moderate exposures all leaning on the same weak points, fluid handling, permeability, motility, sensory threshold, enzyme reserve, clearance capacity, or inflammatory tone, until the total demand outruns what the tissue can neutralize quietly.

This is where a person can eat a diet full of foods that are each defensible in isolation and still feel chronically burdened. No single meal looks outrageous. No single fruit, vegetable, seed, grain, or condiment looks guilty enough to blame. But breakfast opens the day with a smoothie that delivers acid, fructose, polyols, oxalate, and fast plant chemistry in liquid form. Lunch adds raw crucifer tissue, nuts, seeds, and peel-heavy fruit. Afternoon snacking keeps the sugar and acid contact going in the mouth and keeps unfinished carbohydrate moving through the bowel. Dinner finishes with legumes, onions, garlic, and a dessert sold as light because it came from fruit. Every item can be described with a positive nutrient sentence. The bowel still received repeated osmotic pull, repeated fermentation substrate, repeated acid contact, repeated low-yield fiber, repeated small-molecule chemistry, and repeated clearance work. The labels stay moderate. The tissue sees the sum.

The same accumulation happens downstream. The hepatocyte, the main working liver cell, keeps receiving absorbed compounds in portal blood and keeps having to oxidize, conjugate, and export them. The kidney keeps filtering the dissolved remainder and concentrating it into urine. The thyroid keeps trying to hold hormone output while dietary interference and substrate weakness keep returning. A single moderate irritant can remain a nuisance. Many moderate irritants, repeated often enough, can become the background physiology of the host because the same liver, the same nephron, the same follicle, and the same bowel surface never get long enough between exposures to return fully to baseline. That is how people end up living inside symptoms that feel too vague to trace and too constant to ignore. The chemistry never needed to become dramatic. It only needed to keep arriving.

So many moderate irritants add up because tissues pay by frequency and overlap, not by drama alone. A membrane stretched three times, acid-bathed four times, fermented into pressure twice, and asked to absorb around all of it is carrying a real burden even if none of those exposures would have made a memorable story by itself. The body can hide that accumulation for a long time. It cannot make it cost-free.

The False Comfort of Variety When the Underlying Pattern Remains Plant-Heavy

Variety can hide repetition when the chemistry keeps changing names but not destination. A person stops eating spinach every day and feels safer because the plate now rotates through Swiss chard, beet greens, almonds, sweet potatoes, cacao, berries, and seeds. The menu looks broader. The bowel still receives oxalate-rich plant tissue again and again. Another person stops relying on apples and starts alternating pears, mango, watermelon, dried fruit, fruit bowls, smoothies, and honey-sweetened yogurt with granola. The colors change. The small intestine still keeps meeting fast sugar, fructose, polyols, acids, and fermentable residue. The eye sees diversity. The membrane sees recurring classes of chemistry.

A plant-heavy pattern can therefore stay chemically narrow while looking culinarily wide. One meal brings poorly absorbed carbohydrate that stays in the lumen, the hollow interior of the bowel where absorption is supposed to finish. Another brings seed chemistry that holds minerals in low-yield form. Another brings sulfur-rich crucifer tissue that pushes on the thyroid's iodide-handling sequence. Another brings fruit acids and sugars in liquid form. Another brings peel, seed, or skin compounds that make the mouth, stomach, or bowel do more work than the pleasant taste suggested. None of these foods needs to be repeated in identical form for the organs to feel the sameness. The colon still receives fermentation substrate. The hepatocyte, the main working liver cell, still receives low-yield plant chemistry in portal blood. The nephron, the kidney's filtering unit, still receives dissolved remainder it must concentrate into urine.

That is why variety can become a psychological anesthetic in plant-heavy eating. It lets the eater believe burden has been solved because boredom has been solved. The salad changes shape. The smoothie ingredients rotate. The fruit basket looks seasonal and colorful. The grain changes from oats to quinoa to brown rice to buckwheat. The legume changes from lentils to chickpeas to black beans. The chemistry remains recognizably similar at the level the body actually has to manage. Fermentable carbohydrate keeps returning. Phytate keeps returning. Oxalate keeps returning. Acids keep returning. Sugar delivered with too little structural resistance keeps returning. The pattern remains plant-heavy even while the menu keeps performing diversity.

A resilient host may absorb part of that quietly for a time. A vulnerable host loses margin much sooner. The irritable bowel does not care that the fermentable load came from different fruits and vegetables across the week. It still has to carry water and gas when absorption fails. The thyroid does not care that the raw crucifer rotated from kale to cabbage to Brussels sprouts. It still has to trap iodide and build hormone while sulfur breakdown products keep arriving. The kidney does not care that the oxalate came from greens one day and nuts the next. It still has to filter and concentrate the dissolved burden into a shrinking volume of urine. Rotation inside a plant-heavy framework can therefore preserve the same organ workload while giving the person the false feeling of having escaped repetition.

Real change begins when the underlying chemistry changes, not when the produce list becomes more interesting. A body burdened by fermentation needs less retained fermentable residue, not merely new sources of it. A body burdened by oxalate needs less absorbable oxalate, not a wider spectrum of oxalate-bearing foods. A thyroid running on thin iodine reserve needs less repeated interference, not a more imaginative rotation of interfering leaves. Variety can be useful when it truly lowers repeated exposure to the same burden. It becomes false comfort when it only changes the plant names while the same bowel, the same thyroid, the same liver, and the same kidney keep paying for the same kind of chemistry every day.

How Repeated Low-Grade Exposure Can Hide Inside Socially Approved Diets

A diet can look disciplined, colorful, plant-forward, and medically respectable while still delivering the same low-grade burdens to the same organs every day. That is what makes this pattern so easy to miss. No single food stands out as a villain. Breakfast is fruit and oats. Lunch is a large salad with nuts and seeds. Dinner is beans, whole grains, steamed vegetables, and maybe a green juice or fermented side dish. Each item arrives with a clean nutritional reputation. The bowel does not eat reputations. It receives fructose, polyols, rough fiber, oxalate, phytate, glucosinolate breakdown products, acids, polyphenols, and fermentable carbohydrate in repeated waves. None of these exposures has to be dramatic on its own. The problem is that the same classes of chemistry keep returning through the same lumen, the hollow interior of the bowel where digestion and absorption are taking place, often without enough interruption for the tissue to recover its margin.

This is how burden hides. A socially approved diet usually avoids the kinds of foods people are trained to distrust, so the symptoms that appear later are rarely blamed on the approved pattern itself. Gas is attributed to stress. Loose stool is blamed on sensitivity. Fatigue becomes aging. Slower thyroid function becomes bad luck. The kidney stone becomes a random event. Meanwhile the digestive sequence has been underpaid for months or years. The intestine keeps seeing carbohydrate it does not finish cleanly, so water stays in the bowel and bacteria inherit the residue. Minerals keep arriving inside storage tissues that bind part of their own value before absorption is complete. Sulfur-rich vegetables keep returning to the thyroid in a host whose iodine reserve may already be thin. Oxalate keeps crossing into blood and then into urine under the banner of vegetables and nuts that were never socially coded as renal burdens. The respectability of the diet becomes a shield that protects the pattern from scrutiny even while the body keeps absorbing the cost.

The low-grade nature of the exposure is exactly what lets it accumulate. Acute poisoning is easy to notice because the body is overwhelmed in one visible episode. Chronic plant burden usually works through repetition, not spectacle. A daily smoothie does not need to send a person to the hospital to matter. It only needs to keep delivering spinach, almond butter, berries, cacao, or other chemically dense plant tissue in a fluid form that removes chewing, reduces gastric friction, and makes larger intakes easy. A bowl of legumes every night does not need to cause violent illness to matter. It only needs to keep returning phytate, fermentable carbohydrate, and seed-storage chemistry to the same bowel often enough that lower mineral yield and heavier fermentation stop being occasional side effects and start becoming part of the host's normal physiology. Low-grade exposure hides best when the host can still function. The organs are compensating. The person confuses compensation with safety.

The liver and kidney make this easier to overlook because their work is quiet until the workload becomes too heavy to hide. Portal blood, the blood draining from the intestine into the liver first, keeps delivering the absorbed fraction to the hepatocyte, the main working liver cell. The hepatocyte keeps oxidizing, conjugating, and exporting chemistry that added little constructive value to the body in the first place. The nephron, the kidney's filtering unit, keeps taking the dissolved remainder, reclaiming water around it, and pushing the rejected solutes toward urine. A healthy-looking diet can therefore become a daily source of hepatic sorting work and urinary burden without ever feeling like intoxication. The person still believes they are eating clean because the foods remain approved. The liver still has to transform what crossed. The kidney still has to concentrate what the body could not use.

That is why socially approved diets can be some of the hardest diets to question honestly. The person is not eating recklessly. They are often trying hardest. That effort becomes the hiding place. Repeated low-grade exposure survives because the foods are morally protected, the symptoms are distributed across different organs, and the damage usually appears first as reduced margin rather than collapse. The bowel becomes easier to provoke. The thyroid has less room. The kidney chemistry shifts. The liver carries more routine sorting work. Nothing dramatic has happened, so the pattern keeps going. The chemistry stays low enough to avoid public alarm and frequent enough to keep shaping the host underneath it.

Why Symptom Fluctuation Can Confuse People Into Missing the Cause

Plant burden rarely behaves like a courtroom confession. The food is eaten, the symptom appears, and the body does not always draw a clean line between the two in a way the person can feel. One day the bowel bloats after fruit and legumes. Another day the same meal seems tolerable. One week the mouth stings after citrus. Another week it does not. Raw crucifers feel fine for a while, then a period of cold hands, slower bowels, and heaviness begins to build without any single meal dramatic enough to blame. Oxalate-heavy foods can accumulate into urinary chemistry long before a stone makes the sequence visible. The host is trying to read causation through fluctuating outputs, while the real biology is being shaped by thresholds, reserves, overlap, and timing. A symptom does not only depend on whether the food was eaten. It depends on what else was eaten with it, how much of it arrived, how the tissue was prepared, how much margin the bowel, thyroid, liver, or kidney had that day, how much of the same chemistry had already arrived earlier in the week, and whether the organ receiving it was still recovering from the previous round.

That makes fluctuation deeply misleading because people expect causes to behave consistently at the level of sensation. The body is often consistent at the level of mechanism and inconsistent at the level of symptoms. Fructose and polyols can remain in the lumen, the hollow interior of the bowel where absorption is supposed to finish, both times a person eats the fruit. One day the retained sugar load is small enough, transit is steady enough, and the colon quiet enough that little is felt. Another day the same fruit lands on top of prior fermentation, poor sleep, stress-mediated motility change, or a larger total carbohydrate burden and the bowel becomes visibly distended. The chemistry did not change sides. The threshold moved. Oxalate can bind calcium in the gut every time and still produce no immediate sensation at all, which makes the person think the food was harmless even while urinary oxalate shifts quietly downstream. Crucifer chemistry can press on iodide handling for months before the thyroid runs out of room and begins showing the slower, colder, more sluggish outputs that finally get noticed. The symptom is late and variable. The mechanism was early and repetitive.

Overlap makes the confusion worse because many foods can converge on the same tissue burden. A person may react to apples one day, onions another day, beans another day, and conclude that nothing makes sense because the foods seem unrelated. The bowel sees something simpler. Poorly absorbed carbohydrate, retained water, fermentation, pressure. Another person rotates spinach, almonds, dark chocolate, beets, and sweet potatoes and never notices the oxalate pattern because no one food is eaten in obvious excess on a single day. The kidney sees something simpler. Repeated oxalate delivery, repeated filtration, repeated concentration into urine. Symptom fluctuation then hides the pattern because the burden is being built by classes of chemistry rather than by one memorable food. The person keeps asking which item was guilty. The organ keeps paying for the sum.

There is also a delay problem. The food is eaten now. The consequence may declare itself later and somewhere else. Dental sensitivity may build after repeated fruit acid contact rather than after one orange. A kidney stone forms long after the meals that shaped the urine chemistry. Histamine-like or salicylate-like symptoms may flare only when the total chemical load crosses a threshold rather than after every isolated exposure. A hepatocyte, the main working liver cell, can spend months oxidizing, conjugating, and exporting low-yield plant chemistry before fatigue, heaviness, poor tolerance, or other softer outputs make the person suspect anything at all. Fluctuation then becomes false reassurance. Yesterday felt better, so the pattern must not matter. The organs are not reading yesterday alone. They are reading cumulative traffic.

That is why symptom fluctuation confuses people so effectively. It teaches them to trust the dramatic day and ignore the repeated day. It makes the cause look inconsistent when the host reserve was what changed. It makes the pattern look random when the chemistry kept returning through the same route to the same tissue. The bowel, thyroid, liver, and kidney do not need a symptom every time to prove the burden is real. They only need the same low-yield chemistry to keep arriving often enough that margin thins, thresholds drop, and one day the person finally feels what the organ had been compensating for all along.

Part IX

How to Judge a Food Correctly

Chapter 31

A Better Standard Than "Contains Nutrients"

"Contains nutrients" is the weakest possible defense of a food. It says the laboratory found minerals, vitamins, amino acids, fatty acids, or phytochemicals inside the sample after the tissue was broken apart hard enough to measure them. The body does not eat laboratory ash, solvent extracts, or nutrient tables. It eats plant and animal tissues that still have to be torn open, acidified, emulsified, cleaved by enzymes, moved across membranes, circulated through blood, and either retained or excreted. A food can test rich and still nourish poorly. It can carry impressive chemistry and still lower net yield. It can give the label something to praise while giving the bowel, liver, thyroid, and kidney more work than the tissues received in return. So the first real question is not what the food contains. The first real question is whether you can digest it. Can the stomach acidify it properly. Can the pancreas and brush border enzymes, the enzyme-rich surface of the small intestine, actually break it down. Can the matrix be opened without excessive fermentation, irritation, or incomplete cleavage. A food that resists digestion keeps much of its value trapped behind its own structure.

The second question follows immediately. Even if the tissue is broken down, can you absorb what it contains. Presence inside the food is not the same thing as membrane crossing. Calcium inside a high-oxalate leaf is not the same as calcium entering blood. Iron inside a phytate-rich seed is not the same as iron reaching the absorptive surface in usable form. Fructose inside fruit is not the same as fructose clearing the small intestine without residue. Absorption is the point where the body decides whether the food was generous or merely dense on paper. A nutrient that remains bound, precipitated, encapsulated, or left behind in the lumen is not yet nourishment. It is only inventory the intestine failed to recover.

The third question is harsher because a food can underperform and still do collateral damage at the same time. Does it block other nutrients. A plant can carry magnesium, calcium, zinc, iron, and phosphorus and still arrive with oxalate, phytate, tannins, or other binding chemistry that lowers the yield of those same minerals or of minerals elsewhere in the meal. That is where many "healthy foods" fail the body while keeping their reputation. They are not only low-yield. They are antagonistic. They alter the mineral environment of the meal. They tie up calcium before calcium can be absorbed. They hold zinc and iron in complexes the intestine does not reclaim well. They bind proteins or interfere with digestive enzymes and reduce what another part of the plate might have delivered cleanly on its own. A food that blocks other nutrients is not merely disappointing. It changes the whole arithmetic of the meal around it.

The fourth question moves from yield into tolerance. Does it irritate or destabilize the gut. The intestine is not only a site of absorption. It is also a living surface that has to tolerate contact, stretch, acidity, osmotic load, fermentation, and microbial traffic without losing coordination. A food can fail here without ever becoming an acute toxin. Poorly absorbed carbohydrates can hold water in the bowel and feed gas production later. Rough fibers can increase friction against a bowel that is already easy to provoke. Fruit acids can irritate oral and upper-gut surfaces. Lectins, saponins, peel chemistry, sulfur breakdown products, and other plant compounds can make the digestive sequence less stable even if the person never uses the word poison. The gut does not need to collapse for the food to be biologically expensive. It only needs to keep receiving residue, water, pressure, and chemical contact it cannot clear quietly.

The fifth question finishes the sequence where many nutrition discussions never bother to look. Does the food leave the liver, thyroid, or kidney with avoidable work. Once a compound crosses the intestine, the argument is not over. Portal blood, the blood draining from the intestine into the liver first, brings the absorbed fraction to the hepatocyte, the main working liver cell, which now has to oxidize, conjugate, export, or otherwise sort chemistry the body may never have wanted in the first place. The thyroid has to trap iodide and build hormone while certain plant sulfur compounds crowd the same sequence. The kidney has to filter and concentrate dissolved remainder into urine, sometimes pushing oxalate, uric acid, drug metabolites, and other low-value compounds toward crystal formation or tubular irritation. A food that adds little nourishment and still recruits hepatic sorting, thyroid interference, or renal excretion has failed at the level that matters most. It entered as food and left as organ workload.

Those are the real questions because they follow the actual path of the meal. Can you digest it. Can you absorb what it contains. Does it block other nutrients. Does it irritate or destabilize the gut. Does it leave the liver, thyroid, or kidney with avoidable work. A food that answers those questions badly is not redeemed by a nutrient label. A food that answers them well does not need much marketing. The body judges by digestion, absorption, interference, tolerance, and downstream burden. Everything else is reputation.

Net Biological Value as the True Measure

The body does not live on what a food contains. It lives on what it can actually take from that food without paying too much for the privilege. That is the standard the whole book has been working toward. A nutrient chart can show calcium, magnesium, iron, folate, carotenoids, polyphenols, fiber, and protein, and still tell you almost nothing about what the meal accomplished in a human body. Digestion has to fracture the tissue first. Acid has to unfold what can be unfolded. Enzymes have to cleave what can be cleaved. Bile has to emulsify what can only move in fat-handling pathways. Minerals have to remain soluble long enough to reach the absorptive membrane. Sugars have to clear the small intestine without being left behind as osmotic load and fermentation substrate. The liver has to sort what crossed. The kidney has to clear what the body could not use. A food can look dense at the level of composition and still come out weak once the full sequence is finished.

Net biological value is the measure taken after the body has done all the work. Everything before that is only promise.

That is why the right question is never whether the food is rich. The right question is whether the food yields. A high-oxalate leaf can carry calcium and still deliver very little usable calcium because the same leaf releases the mineral and its binding partner into the same intestinal field. A phytate-rich seed can test dense in zinc and iron while holding those minerals in chemistry the intestine reclaims poorly. A fruit can look light and hydrating while leaving behind fructose or polyols that hold water in the lumen, the hollow interior of the bowel where absorption is supposed to finish, and then feed fermentation in the colon. A crucifer can look virtuous while still asking a thyroid with thin iodine reserve to complete hormone assembly under added interference. None of those foods becomes innocent because the chart admired them. The body is harsher than that. It counts what crossed, what was blocked, what irritated tissue, and what had to be excreted afterward.

Net biological value also forces the question of cost back into the same frame as nourishment. A food is not high value merely because some useful molecules entered the body. A food can nourish and burden at the same time, and that second half is where most nutrition language becomes evasive. The intestine may absorb part of the sugar while the bowel still pays in water retention and gas. The liver may take in plant compounds that add little constructive value and still has to oxidize, conjugate, and export them. The kidney may receive oxalate, uric acid, or other dissolved remainder and still has to concentrate that chemistry into urine without letting it precipitate into crystals. The thyroid may keep pace for a while and still do so under rising strain. Net biological value has to include that downstream work or it is not measuring the food honestly. A food that gives little and costs much is biologically poor even if the ingredient list sounds pure and the nutrient panel looks impressive.

This is where socially protected foods often fail most clearly. Fruit keeps its reputation through sweetness and freshness. Greens keep theirs through color and vitamin language. Seeds and nuts keep theirs through density and mineral numbers. Legumes keep theirs through fiber and plant protein language. Those reputations are not the same as net biological value. A smoothie built from spinach, almond butter, berries, and cacao can sound exemplary and still become a low-yield, high-oxalate, fast-delivery burden in the wrong host. A bowl of beans and grains can sound balanced and still leave the intestine with fermentable residue, the meal with lower mineral yield, and the liver with more handling work than the tissues received in return. Net biological value strips away the social protection and asks what the body was left with after digestion, absorption, interference, and clearance were over.

That is the true measure because it is the only one the organs actually recognize. The bowel does not care how a food was marketed. The liver does not care how natural it sounded. The kidney does not care how colorful the plate looked. Each organ reads the chemistry it actually received. A high-value food digests well, yields what it carries, blocks little else, irritates little, and leaves the organs of clearance with work proportionate to its return. A low-value food may still contain impressive compounds, but it gives back less than it costs. The body never confuses those two states. Only food language does.

Why the Body Cares About Usable Yield, Not Public Reputation

Public reputation is built from words the body never sees. Fresh. Natural. Whole. Plant-based. Nutrient-dense. Antioxidant-rich. Clean. Those labels are attached to foods before chewing begins, before the stomach acidifies anything, before enzymes cut into the structure, before the intestine decides what can cross, and long before the liver and kidney are forced to finish handling what the meal left behind. The body does not absorb reputation. It absorbs dissolved compounds that survived digestion, reached the membrane in a usable form, and crossed into blood. That is why a food can keep a clean public identity and still perform badly in human physiology. The reputation belongs to the plate. The value belongs to what the tissues actually receive.

Usable yield is a harsher standard because it begins after the food has already been broken open. A mineral only counts if it remains soluble long enough to reach the absorptive surface and cross it. Protein only counts if it is unfolded, cleaved, and reduced into amino acids or small peptides the intestine can take up. Carbohydrate only counts as a low-friction fuel if it clears the small bowel instead of remaining in the lumen, the hollow interior of the intestine, where it can hold water and feed fermentation later. A food can therefore contain calcium and still nourish poorly if oxalate traps it in the gut. It can contain zinc and iron and still underdeliver if phytate keeps them bound. It can carry fruit sugar and still become bowel burden if fructose or polyols outrun absorptive capacity. The body does not grade the intention of the food. It grades the fraction it could actually extract and use.

That is why defended plant foods are so often overrated by nutrient language. The laboratory can grind the tissue to dust, dissolve it aggressively, and report everything that was there. The intestine does not receive the food under those conditions. It receives leaf, seed, peel, flesh, tuber, kernel, and hull still wrapped in the plant's own logic. Some tissues were built to invite contact. Others were built to survive it. Some carry sugar in soft flesh while keeping a harder chemistry in the skin or seed. Some store minerals in the same structure that also keeps those minerals difficult to recover. Some release acids, sulfur compounds, alkaloids, tannins, or poorly absorbed carbohydrates into the same meal that was praised for vitamins and fiber. Public reputation flattens those contradictions because it speaks at the level of category. The body restores them because it has to handle the full tissue, not the marketing summary.

The downstream organs make the same judgment more brutally. The liver does not ask whether a fruit, seed, or vegetable was socially approved. It receives the absorbed fraction in portal blood and decides what has to be oxidized, conjugated, exported into bile, or sent back into blood for renal clearance. The kidney does not ask whether the food was colorful or clean. It filters the dissolved remainder and concentrates it into urine until what could not be used has to leave without damaging the tubule or precipitating into crystals. A food with low usable yield can therefore fail twice. It can undernourish on the way in and still impose clearance work on the way out. That is a poor bargain no matter how attractive the food looked in public language.

The body cares about usable yield because tissue is built from what was retained, not from what was admired. A good food is not the one that wins the nutrient argument in theory. It is the one that digests cleanly, gives up what it carries, blocks little else, destabilizes the gut as little as possible, and leaves the liver, thyroid, and kidney with work proportionate to its return. That is why public reputation and biological value so often separate. Reputation is assigned before the meal. Usable yield is the verdict after the body is done with it.

Chapter 32

How to Think About Fruits and Vegetables Without Ideology

The body does not sort food into moral camps. It does not eat a slogan, a tribe, a documentary, or a backlash. It eats tissue. It meets structure, chemistry, digestibility, residue, and clearance. That is where the argument has to begin again. Fruits and vegetables are neither redeemed by color and public praise nor condemned automatically because they are plants. They are plant tissues built for plant purposes. Some are soft and easy enough that the human digestive tract can take useful value from them with little friction. Some arrive carrying sugars that overrun absorption, acids that irritate, oxalate that binds minerals and later burdens urine, glucosinolates that matter to a thin-margin thyroid, polyols that stay in the bowel, peels and seeds that carry harder chemistry than the flesh around them, or fibers and storage compounds that reduce yield more than the reputation of the food would suggest. The useful question is not whether plants are good or bad. The useful question is what kind of tissue this is, what chemistry it is carrying, what digestion has to do to it, what the intestine can actually recover from it, and what the body is left clearing afterward.

That is why pro-plant language fails as badly as anti-plant language. The first hides the burden behind nutrient content and symbolic purity. The second hides real variation behind anger and simplification. Both stop looking too early. A watermelon wedge, a grapefruit, a glass of orange juice, raw kale, boiled spinach, pressure-cooked lentils, almonds, avocado, pickles, onions, and blueberries do not belong to one physiological category merely because they came from plants. They differ in water content, sugar form, acid load, fiber structure, mineral-binding compounds, peel chemistry, fermentation burden, and downstream organ cost. One may be easy in a resilient host and expensive in a sensitive one. One may be tolerable when occasional and biologically costly when it becomes a daily concentrate in smoothies, powders, juices, bowls, or snack habits. One may be improved meaningfully by peeling, boiling, fermenting, or pressure cooking. Another may remain low-yield even after preparation has done what it can. A serious standard has to be specific enough to see those differences. Ideology blurs them because it wants the category to carry the verdict before the tissue has been examined.

A better way to think begins with friction. How much force does the body have to spend to get the useful part. Does the food digest cleanly. Does it release what it contains in a form the intestine can absorb. Does it bind or block other nutrients in the same meal. Does it leave behind water-retaining sugar, fermentable residue, crystal-forming solute, gland-interfering chemistry, or hepatic sorting work that exceeds its return. That line of thought is less emotionally satisfying because it does not let the eater join a side. It does something better. It puts the stomach, the small intestine, the colon, the thyroid follicle, the hepatocyte, and the nephron back at the center of the judgment. A food can contain useful compounds and still fail that standard. A food can sound chemically unimpressive and still pass it well because the body extracts it cleanly and is left with little damage control afterward. Once that becomes the frame, slogans begin to look childish. The body was never debating plants. It was measuring yield against burden all along.

This is also the only frame that leaves room for host reality without collapsing into relativism. The same food is not the same event in every body because bodies do not begin from the same margin. An intact bowel with steady transit and broad reserve can tolerate chemistry that a fermentation-sensitive bowel cannot carry quietly. A thyroid with ample iodine reserve can absorb small amounts of interference that a strained gland cannot. A kidney with strong clearance can move solutes out that a reduced-clearance kidney cannot handle safely. None of that means the chemistry is imaginary. It means physiology decides how expensive the chemistry becomes. That is the part ideology hates because it refuses simple universal heroes and villains. The food can be acceptable in one context, costly in another, improved by preparation in a third, and still not worth forcing in a fourth. A person thinking clearly about fruits and vegetables has to be willing to hold all of that at once.

So moving beyond slogans does not mean becoming neutral in the weak sense. It means becoming exact. Stop asking whether plants are virtuous. Start asking which fruits and vegetables digest with low friction, which ones underdeliver, which ones create more fermentation or clearance work than they justify, which ones become worse when concentrated, juiced, dried, or repeated, and which ones change sharply with host vulnerability. A person thinking this way can keep what yields, reduce what merely irritates, prepare what can be improved, and stop romanticizing foods that keep costing more than they return. That is not anti-plant. It is anti-confusion. The plate stops being a moral stage and becomes what it always was: a set of tissues the body has to turn either into nourishment or into work.

Foods as Chemical Structures with Tradeoffs

A food is never just a nutrient list. It is a physical structure carrying chemistry in a particular arrangement, and that arrangement decides what the body actually has to face. A fruit carries sugars inside water-rich flesh, acids in solution, polyols in some species, peel compounds at the surface, and reproductive chemistry in the seed or pit. A leaf carries minerals inside a photosynthetic tissue that may also hold oxalate, nitrate, salicylate-like compounds, or sulfur-rich precursors that change once the tissue is cut and chewed. A seed carries protein, fat, phosphorus, and minerals inside a storage organ built to preserve those reserves, not to hand them over cheaply to the eater. That is why tradeoffs are built into the food before the first bite. The useful fraction is real. The resistance is real. Digestion has to take both at once.

The body experiences those tradeoffs as competing events inside the same meal. A food can carry calcium and the chemistry that lowers calcium yield. It can carry iron and the chemistry that keeps iron bound. It can carry carbohydrate and still leave part of that carbohydrate behind as osmotic load and fermentation substrate. It can carry polyphenols that sound attractive in public language and still bind proteins or minerals in the gut. It can carry water, potassium, and vitamin C and still deliver acid to the mouth, fructose to the small intestine, and drug-interacting compounds to the intestinal wall if the tissue happens to be grapefruit. The question is never whether one side of the tradeoff exists. The question is which side dominates after chewing, stomach acid, pancreatic enzymes, bile, absorption, liver handling, and urinary clearance are finished. A food that gives something useful and costs little is a different biological event from a food that gives something useful and still drags three other burdens behind it.

This is why processing, host context, and dose keep changing the verdict without changing the species. Boiling a high-oxalate leaf can lower part of the soluble oxalate burden and still leave the leaf as a mineral-poor bargain compared with a lower-oxalate green. Pressure cooking a bean can strip away much of the active lectin burden and still leave fermentable carbohydrate, phytate, and storage-tissue resistance for the gut to negotiate. Peeling a fruit can reduce part of the peel chemistry while leaving the fructose, polyols, and acids in the flesh unchanged. The food remains the same food. The tradeoff profile shifts because the structure the body receives has shifted. A resilient host may absorb that tradeoff quietly. A sensitive host may expose it immediately because the bowel, thyroid, liver, or kidney has less margin left to hide the cost.

Good food judgment therefore starts where ideology ends. Instead of asking whether the food is natural, colorful, traditional, plant-based, anti-inflammatory, antioxidant-rich, or nutrient-dense, the better question is what kind of exchange this tissue is offering. What does it release easily. What does it hold back. What does it block. What does it irritate. What does it leave for the liver to transform or the kidney to excrete after the useful fraction has already been taken. Foods are chemical structures with tradeoffs. The body does not object to that fact. It lives by it. The mistake is pretending the tradeoff disappears because one side of the structure sounds healthier than the other.

Why Some People Can Tolerate Certain Plants and Others Cannot

The plant does not change from person to person. The host does. A spinach leaf still carries oxalate. A bean still carries storage chemistry that asks for real digestive work. A cabbage leaf still releases sulfur compounds when the tissue is damaged. A peach still delivers fructose, acids, and in some cases polyols into the bowel. The difference begins in the body receiving that chemistry. One person has stronger stomach acid, steadier pancreatic output, broader bile flow, more calcium available in the gut to trap oxalate, better small-intestinal transport capacity for sugars, calmer motility, less visceral hypersensitivity, more resilient mucosa, broader thyroid reserve, stronger liver clearance, and kidneys that still have room to concentrate and excrete dissolved burden without losing control of the urine chemistry. Another person meets the same food with less margin at one or several of those steps. The food keeps the same chemistry. The sequence inside the body changes.

The intestine is often where that difference becomes visible first. A person with good fat absorption keeps more calcium free in the bowel and may trap more oxalate before it ever crosses into blood. A person with fat malabsorption ties that calcium up in fatty acid soaps, leaves more soluble oxalate free in the lumen, the hollow interior of the bowel where digestion is taking place, and absorbs more of the burden into the body. A person with broad fructose tolerance can clear a piece of fruit quietly. Another reaches the limit of transport more quickly, leaves fructose or sorbitol behind, pulls water into the bowel by osmosis, and then hands that residue to the colon for fermentation. A person with a calm colon may barely notice the gas. A person with an irritable bowel state feels pressure, stretch, urgency, or pain from the same intraluminal chemistry because the bowel wall is more reactive to the same load.

The same host difference appears in organs that do not announce themselves as quickly. A cruciferous vegetable can remain a modest exposure in a person with strong iodine intake and a thyroid gland that still has room to compensate. In a person with thin iodine reserve, rising thyroid-stimulating hormone, or already narrowed thyroid margin, the same damaged Brassica tissue lands as repeated interference in iodide trapping and hormone assembly. Grapefruit can behave like an ordinary fruit in someone not taking a susceptible medication and become a pharmacologic exposure in someone whose oral drug depends on intestinal cytochrome P450 3A4 for first-pass metabolism. Star fruit can remain uneventful in one person and become retained neurotoxin plus oxalate burden in a person with reduced kidney clearance. The produce identity stays constant. The organ reserve does not.

Microbial variation widens the difference further because the bowel is not a sterile tube. Some people carry microbial communities that degrade more oxalate or handle carbohydrate residue with less symptom intensity. Others lose that margin through antibiotics, bowel disease, inflammation, surgical alteration, or long-standing dietary patterns that changed the ecology of the colon. The same food then enters a different fermentative system and leaves behind a different set of gases, acids, and microbial byproducts. A person can believe they suddenly became sensitive to a food when the deeper change was that the host environment stopped neutralizing the same chemistry quietly. The plant did not become more aggressive. The internal buffer thinned.

Tolerance is therefore not a moral certificate proving the food is benign. It is a sign that the body still has enough reserve to carry the burden without making the cost obvious. Intolerance is not always a mysterious overreaction either. It is often the point where the same defended plant chemistry finally meets a membrane, gland, hepatocyte, or nephron with too little room left to hide the price. One person still has margin. Another has already started spending it.

Why the Question Is Burden-to-Return Ratio

A food does not earn its place by carrying attractive chemistry. It earns it by what the body is left with after the full encounter is over. That is why the right question is burden-to-return ratio. The return is what digestion actually liberates, what remains available in the lumen, the hollow interior of the bowel where digestion is taking place, what crosses the absorptive membrane, what reaches blood in a form the tissues can use, and what is retained as structure, energy, enzyme substrate, mineral value, or signaling material. The burden is everything the body had to spend or suffer to get that return. Mineral binding in the gut. Enzyme inhibition. Osmotic pull. Fermentation. Acid contact. Sulfur compounds pressing on thyroid iodine handling. Hepatic transformation of low-yield chemistry. Renal excretion of dissolved remainder. A food can therefore look rich and still score badly if the body had to fight through too much interference to get too little back. The nutrient list is only the offer. The burden-to-return ratio is the settlement.

This is why foods with strong reputations so often underperform once the physiology is followed all the way through. A leaf can carry calcium and still deliver little calcium because oxalate traps part of the mineral before absorption and later burdens urine if enough soluble oxalate crosses into blood. A seed can carry zinc, iron, protein, and phosphorus and still return them weakly because phytate keeps minerals bound and the storage matrix keeps the tissue from surrendering its contents cheaply. A fruit can carry water, potassium, vitamin C, and attractive sweetness and still leave behind fructose or polyols that hold water in the bowel and feed fermentation, or acids that irritate the mouth, or furanocoumarins that change drug handling at the intestinal wall. The return may be real in each case. The ratio still fails if the organ cost remains too high relative to what the body actually kept.

The ratio also changes with dose, preparation, and host reserve. A garnish can have a low enough burden that the return still wins. A staple can keep returning the same chemistry to the same membrane, gland, hepatocyte, or nephron until the burden side of the equation grows larger than the eater realizes. Preparation can improve the ratio by peeling away outer chemistry, denaturing active proteins, leaching out soluble oxalate, reducing phytate through fermentation or sprouting, or softening cell walls enough that digestion can extract more value with less friction. But preparation does not erase the equation. It only moves the numbers. Host context moves them too. The same fruit, bean, green, or grain can remain acceptable in a person with broad digestive and clearance reserve and become expensive in a person with fat malabsorption, bowel hypersensitivity, thin iodine supply, or reduced kidney function. The tissue stayed the same. The ratio changed because the host changed.

That is the standard the body has been using all along. Not whether the food was natural. Not whether it was colorful. Not whether it was praised. Not whether it contained something beneficial in isolation. The body keeps asking one harder question. After digestion, absorption, interference, and clearance were finished, was there enough usable return to justify the burden required to get it. A food with a good burden-to-return ratio can be plain and still valuable because the body extracts it cleanly and is left with little repair or disposal work afterward. A food with a bad ratio can sound chemically impressive and still be biologically poor because too much of the interaction was spent on surviving the food instead of building from it.

Judging by Tissue Consequence Instead of Cultural Prestige

Cultural prestige attaches to foods long before the body has done anything with them. A food becomes clean, vibrant, ancestral, medicinal, anti-inflammatory, plant-based, or nutrient-dense in language before the stomach has acidified it, before enzymes have cut into it, before the intestine has decided what can cross, and before the liver and kidney have finished handling what the meal left behind. Tissue consequence begins later and speaks more bluntly. Did the food release usable mineral or trap it in the lumen, the hollow interior of the bowel where digestion is taking place. Did the carbohydrate clear the small intestine or stay behind as osmotic load and fermentation substrate. Did the leaf, fruit, seed, or tuber nourish cleanly, or did it leave the thyroid with interference, the liver with sorting work, and the kidney with dissolved burden to concentrate into urine. Prestige is assigned from outside. Consequence is assigned by organs that have to survive the chemistry.

This is why prestige is such a poor guide. A spinach smoothie can carry more cultural approval than a plate of simpler food and still give the body a worse bargain if the oxalate load strips calcium value in the gut and then reappears as urinary work later. A bowl of beans, grains, nuts, seeds, and greens can sound disciplined and complete while the intestine is still fighting through phytate, fermentable carbohydrate, storage-tissue resistance, and mineral binding strong enough to lower net yield. A fruit bowl can look light and restorative while fructose, sorbitol, acids, and peel chemistry are producing a very different event in the bowel, teeth, or intestinal wall. None of that requires the food to lose its public reputation. The body does not need the reputation revoked before it starts paying the cost.

Tissue consequence forces the judgment back into anatomy. The bowel wall cares about pressure, water retention, incomplete absorption, acid contact, and chemical irritation. The thyroid follicle cares about iodide reaching the cell, being oxidized, and being fixed onto thyroglobulin without too much interference from sulfur-rich plant breakdown products. The hepatocyte, the main working liver cell, cares about what crossed into portal blood and now has to be oxidized, conjugated, exported into bile, or returned to blood for renal clearance. The nephron, the kidney's filtering unit, cares about what remained dissolved, what has to be concentrated into a shrinking volume of urine, and whether the rejected chemistry can leave without crystallizing or irritating the tubule. Those organs do not ask whether the food was fashionable, traditional, or socially protected. They ask whether the chemistry arriving there was worth what it cost to handle.

Judging by tissue consequence also strips away a common confusion. A food can be culturally high-status because it symbolizes restraint, purity, color, freshness, or botanical virtue and still be biologically expensive when it becomes a staple, a concentrate, a juice, a powder, or a daily exposure in a vulnerable host. Prestige can even make the burden harder to see because the person keeps explaining symptoms around the food instead of through it. The bowel is called sensitive. The thyroid is called sluggish. The kidney stone is called unfortunate. The fatigue is called stress. Tissue consequence asks the harder question first. What did this food become after digestion. What did it leave behind. Which organ had to carry the remainder.

That is the better standard because it is the one the body has been using all along. Not whether the food looked virtuous on the plate. Not whether it won a cultural argument. Not whether it contained nutrients in theory. The real verdict is written later, in absorbed yield, in bowel stability, in gland function, in hepatic workload, in urinary chemistry, and in whether the tissues were strengthened or merely burdened. Cultural prestige can protect a food from criticism. It cannot protect the body from the consequence of what the food actually does.

Chapter 33

The Foods Most Likely to Burden the Body

High-oxalate greens and roots belong near the top of the burden list because they can fail the body in two directions at once. The first failure happens in the gut. The leaf or root enters the meal carrying calcium, magnesium, potassium, folate, carotenoids, and whatever other nutrients made the food look attractive on paper, but it is carrying oxalate in the same tissue. Oxalate is an organic acid the plant uses and stores in forms that can bind calcium and other minerals. When the tissue is broken open in the stomach and small intestine, the mineral and the binding chemistry are released into the same intestinal field. A high-oxalate food can therefore test dense and still underdeliver because part of the calcium is no longer reaching the absorptive surface in a freely usable form. Reviews of dietary oxalate and stone disease keep coming back to this exact contradiction, and current kidney guidance still treats oxalate-rich foods as a meaningful issue for calcium oxalate stone risk because dietary oxalate can raise urinary oxalate later as well.

The second failure happens after absorption. If enough soluble oxalate remains free in the gut, crosses the intestinal wall, and enters blood, the kidney inherits the burden. The nephron filters it, may secrete more of it into tubular fluid, and then pulls water back around it as urine is concentrated. At that point the question is no longer whether the food was rich in minerals or "full of greens." The question is whether the urine can keep calcium and oxalate dissolved at the same time. Once that chemistry becomes too crowded, supersaturation develops and calcium oxalate crystal formation becomes more likely. That is why spinach is such a hard model case. It can already lower calcium yield in the gut and still become a urinary oxalate problem downstream. The same molecule underperforms on the way in and burdens the kidney on the way out.

The foods that keep appearing here are not obscure. Spinach, Swiss chard, beet greens, beets, rhubarb, sweet potatoes, and some potato preparations show up again and again on high-oxalate food lists used in stone prevention because the burden is built into the tissue strongly enough to remain relevant in real diets, not just in chemistry textbooks. Harvard's updated oxalate table and kidney-stone diet resources continue to place spinach and Swiss chard near the high end, and clinical stone-prevention materials continue to list beets, sweet potatoes, and related foods among the items that matter when oxalate is already a problem in the host. The plate may still look respectable, colorful, and mineral-rich. The body is reading the same foods as repeated oxalate delivery.

This is why high-oxalate greens and roots deserve special suspicion in a book like this. They are not necessarily dramatic toxins in the acute sense. They are often worse than that because they hide inside the language of health while steadily lowering mineral yield, raising urinary oxalate, and teaching the kidney to live inside a repeated crystal-forming chemistry. A serving once in a while is one event. A daily spinach smoothie, almond-heavy snack pattern, beet habit, or sweet potato staple is another. The food keeps the prestige of vegetables and roots. The bowel and kidney keep paying for the oxalate.

Undercooked or Heavily Relied-On Legumes

A legume is a storage organ first and a human food second. The seed is holding starch, protein, minerals, and phosphorus for the young plant, and it protects that reserve with folded protein defenses and mineral-binding chemistry that make cheap predation harder. In the raw or undercooked state, that protection remains close enough to the original plant design that the bowel still has to face it directly. Lectins remain active enough in some beans, especially red kidney beans, to bind gut surfaces and produce abrupt nausea, vomiting, abdominal pain, and diarrhea within hours when the cooking was inadequate. Protease inhibitors remain active enough to interfere with trypsin and chymotrypsin, the pancreatic enzymes that normally cut dietary protein into smaller absorbable fragments. The eater sees beans. The small intestine receives a defended seed that has not yet been opened enough to behave like generous food.

Proper heat changes the event because these defenses depend on shape. A lectin or protease inhibitor works only while its folded protein structure is still intact enough to fit the surface or enzyme it was built to bind. Boiling and pressure cooking push water and heat through the hydrated seed and denature those proteins, meaning the folded structure loosens and the active defense loses much of its function. The change is real and large. Reviews of legumes and antinutritional factors report that proper boiling can eliminate lectin activity in kidney beans and sharply reduce protease inhibitor activity, while at the same time softening the matrix and improving protein digestibility. Weak heat is a worse bargain because the seed may look softened while still carrying too much active protein defense into the bowel.

Heavy reliance creates a different problem because full cooking does not remove the storage logic of the seed. The acute lectin hazard may be largely dismantled, but the legume still arrives as phytate-rich storage tissue with fermentable carbohydrate and a protein matrix that remains less cooperative than animal tissue. Protein digestibility in legumes is influenced not only by cooking but by intrinsic structure and by residual antinutrients such as phytate, tannins, saponins, and remaining protease inhibitor activity. Build the diet heavily around beans, lentils, chickpeas, peas, and their flours or processed forms, and the same bowel keeps receiving the same seed chemistry meal after meal. Mineral yield can stay lower than the label implied. Fermentation can stay higher than the eater expected. The food does not need to be undercooked to become biologically expensive. It only needs to remain a staple while still behaving like storage tissue under partial surrender.

This is what makes legumes such a clear burden food when they are either underprepared or overrelied on. Undercooking leaves too much of the active defense intact and turns the meal into a more immediate gut problem. Heavy reliance lowers the drama and raises the repetition. The same seed chemistry keeps returning through the same lumen, the hollow interior of the bowel where digestion is taking place, keeps asking for enzymatic work, keeps contributing fermentable residue, and keeps presenting minerals and protein in a form that often yields less generously than the numbers on the package suggest. A side dish of properly cooked beans is one physiological event. A diet structurally built from legumes is another. The seed may have been softened enough to stop punishing the gut acutely. It can still keep the body working harder than the return justifies.

Greening or Sprouting Potatoes

A potato is easiest to misread when it still looks familiar. The tuber is sold as starch, comfort, and ordinary food, so people keep treating greening or sprouting as a cosmetic defect that can be cut around casually. The chemistry is harsher than that. In potatoes, the main glycoalkaloids, steroidal defense compounds called alpha-solanine and alpha-chaconine, are not distributed evenly through the tuber. They are concentrated more heavily in the peel and just beneath it, and they rise further in the eyes, sprouts, and stressed outer tissues. EFSA's risk assessment notes that glycoalkaloid levels are substantially higher in the peel than in the flesh and that light exposure, storage conditions, and damage can all alter those levels. The potato still looks like a starch food. The plant is tightening its chemical guard around stored carbohydrate.

Greening confuses people because the green color itself is chlorophyll, not the toxin. Chlorophyll is only the visible sign that the tuber has been exposed to the same conditions that often raise glycoalkaloids as well. USDA materials make that distinction directly. Greening by itself does not perfectly predict how high the glycoalkaloids are, but light exposure, age, and physical damage are all associated with elevated glycoalkaloid levels, which is why green tissue is treated as a warning rather than as harmless discoloration. The plant has shifted away from quiet storage and back toward active defense. The color is only the readable part of that shift.

Sprouting is a harder warning because a sprout is not passive damage. It is active growth. The tuber is mobilizing reserve material into a vulnerable new shoot, and vulnerable new growth needs protection. USDA and other technical sources note that sprouts, green parts, and the skin of sprouted potatoes contain higher glycoalkaloid levels than the inner flesh. A sprouting potato is therefore no longer just a potato that has been stored too long. It is a storage organ that has begun behaving like growing plant tissue again, and the chemistry moves with that change. The starch is still there. The biological posture of the tuber has changed.

This is why greening or sprouting potatoes belong in a chapter on burden rather than in a kitchen note about quality. The food does not need to become inedible in the theatrical sense to become biologically worse. It only needs to move back toward the chemistry it uses to make feeding less profitable. Peel it deeply and some of that burden can be cut away. Trim the sprouts and some of it can be reduced. The underlying fact remains the same. A greened or sprouting potato is no longer quiet starch reserve. It is a defended tuber whose outer tissues are carrying more of the very chemistry the body did not need in the first place.

Raw-Heavy Crucifer Patterns in Vulnerable Hosts

A raw-heavy crucifer pattern becomes a different biological event the moment the leaf is damaged and swallowed without much chemical softening beforehand. Kale, cabbage, Brussels sprouts, collards, arugula, broccoli, cauliflower, and related Brassica tissues do not enter the meal as blank vegetables. They carry glucosinolates, sulfur-containing plant compounds held in intact cells until cutting, chewing, shredding, juicing, or blending ruptures the tissue and lets those compounds meet myrosinase, the plant enzyme that begins breaking them down. When crucifer tissue is chopped and eaten raw, more glucosinolate breakdown products survive into the meal than after cooking. The bowel is not receiving a generic green food at that point. It is receiving damaged sulfur-rich plant tissue whose chemistry has already started changing before the first part of the meal has even cleared the stomach.

A resilient host can absorb some of that friction quietly because the gland still has room. The thyrocyte, the hormone-producing thyroid cell, pulls iodide, the charged form of iodine, out of blood through the sodium-iodide symporter, or NIS. It then has to move that iodide toward the follicular lumen, oxidize it through thyroid peroxidase, or TPO, and attach it to thyroglobulin, the large protein scaffold on which thyroid hormone is built. A person with good iodine supply, broad thyroid reserve, and ordinary cooked crucifer intake may never notice much cost from this sequence. A vulnerable host is different. If iodine intake is thin, if the gland is already compensating hard, or if the person keeps sending raw crucifer chemistry into the same pathway day after day, the margin narrows quickly. The issue is not that the vegetable became poison. The issue is that the gland has to keep building hormone while more of the plant's sulfur chemistry is still alive in the meal.

The raw pattern matters because it removes some of the buffering that cooking would have imposed. Heat does not erase Brassica chemistry, but it does change the terms of contact by reducing plant enzyme activity and shifting how much of the original breakdown sequence happens before the food reaches the gut. Raw-heavy intake leaves more of that work active and more of the sulfur burden closer to the original damaged-tissue state. A kale salad once in a while is one event. A daily pattern of shredded raw cabbage, green smoothies, kale slaws, crucifer juices, and large uncooked portions is another. The same gland keeps seeing the same class of interference. Thiocyanate crowds iodide uptake. Goitrin and related compounds press further into hormone synthesis. The food keeps the public reputation of greens. The follicle keeps absorbing the subtraction.

Vulnerable hosts usually have more than one weakness at the same time, which is why the pattern becomes easy to miss. Low iodine is one weakness. Low total protein is another because thyroid hormone is built and transported inside a protein-dependent system. Slower digestion, chronic underfeeding, bowel disease, heavy endurance stress, calorie restriction, postpartum strain, and long periods of plant-heavy low-animal-food eating can all reduce the room the gland has to work with before the first raw leaf hits the plate. A person living inside that physiology may still tolerate cooked broccoli with dinner and then run into trouble when the diet shifts toward daily raw crucifer concentration under the banner of health. The raw pattern did not create the vulnerable host from nothing. It found the host where the reserve was already narrowing and kept pressing on the same sequence until the cost stopped being invisible.

That is the real shape of the problem. Raw-heavy crucifer patterns do not prove that all crucifers are dangerous and they do not deserve the sentimental protection people give them either. They are damaged sulfur-rich plant tissues delivering chemistry that can be modest in one body and expensive in another. In a strong host with adequate iodine and enough reserve, the gland may hold the line. In a vulnerable host, the same chopped raw leaf keeps returning through the same meal pattern, landing on the same iodide-trapping machinery, and asking a narrow-margin thyroid to do the same work with less room every day.

High-FODMAP Produce in Gut-Sensitive People

A gut-sensitive person does not meet an onion, apple, mango, watermelon, cauliflower, or asparagus as a list of vitamins and plant pigments. The bowel meets the part that escaped absorption. That is the real event. FODMAPs, fermentable oligosaccharides, disaccharides, monosaccharides, and polyols, are small carbohydrates that either cross the small-intestinal membrane poorly, arrive in excess of transport capacity, or move slowly enough that too much of them remains in the lumen, the hollow interior of the bowel where absorption is supposed to finish the meal. Onions and garlic carry fructans. Many fruits carry excess fructose relative to glucose. Apples, pears, peaches, cherries, and related fruits can add sorbitol, a sugar alcohol absorbed incompletely enough to leave a residue behind. A resilient bowel can sometimes carry part of that residue without much protest. A gut-sensitive person cannot hide the same chemistry as easily.

The first problem is mechanical, not mysterious. When these carbohydrates stay in the small intestine, they hold water there by osmosis, which means dissolved particles pull and retain water around themselves. The bowel is now carrying a wetter, heavier, more distending column of contents than the eater expected from produce that looked light and wholesome on the plate. Then the same residue moves into the colon, where bacteria inherit what the small intestine failed to clear. Gas begins to rise. Pressure begins to rise with it. The wall stretches. The tube fills. In a person with good reserve, that may remain background physiology. In a person with a gut already prone to visceral hypersensitivity, meaning the bowel senses pressure and stretch too strongly, or altered motility, meaning the bowel does not move its contents with steady timing, the same retained carbohydrate becomes bloating, cramping, urgency, diarrhea, constipation, or an unstable mix of all of them.

This is why high-FODMAP produce can look innocent while behaving badly in the wrong host. The problem is not that the produce stopped being natural. The problem is that the small intestine did not finish the meal cleanly enough to spare the colon from inheriting the residue. A mango can still carry carotenoids and vitamin C and still overrun fructose handling. An apple can still look like one of the safest foods in the room and still deliver both fructose and sorbitol to a bowel that clears neither very gracefully. Cauliflower can still sit under the banner of healthy vegetables while the colon reads it as fermentable load. The produce keeps the public reputation. The bowel reads the osmotic burden first and the fermentation burden second.

The sensitive host changes the event even when the food does not change at all. One person eats onions or stone fruit and barely notices. Another carries the same meal into an intestine already easy to provoke, already too aware of pressure, already unstable in its transit pattern, and the same FODMAP load becomes visible almost immediately. This is why so many people get confused by these foods. They expect a food problem to act like a poison, clear and consistent, the same every time. FODMAP burden is more conditional than that. It depends on total dose, what other foods arrived with it, how fast the meal was eaten, how much residue was left from earlier in the day, and how much margin the bowel had left before that meal even began. The chemistry is still real. The threshold moves.

A gut-sensitive person therefore does not need ideology about produce. They need a clearer read on which plant foods leave too much unfinished carbohydrate behind. High-FODMAP produce matters because it is easy to praise, easy to repeat, and easy to misread as harmless when the symptoms fluctuate. But the bowel does not care that the food was colorful, fresh, or socially protected. It cares whether the carbohydrates crossed the membrane or stayed in the tube long enough to become water, gas, pressure, and unstable transit. That is the actual burden.

Grapefruit With Medications

Grapefruit becomes dangerous at the intestinal wall, not because the fruit suddenly stops being fruit, but because the bowel is doing pharmacology while the person thinks they are eating breakfast. A swallowed drug dissolves into the fluid inside the small intestine and then has to cross the intestinal epithelium, the absorptive cell layer lining the bowel. Those cells are not passive. They carry cytochrome P450 3A4, abbreviated CYP3A4, one of the main enzyme systems that metabolizes many oral drugs during first-pass metabolism, the early metabolic loss that happens before the full dose reaches the wider circulation. FDA warns that grapefruit and grapefruit juice can block this intestinal CYP3A4 step for certain medicines, which means less of the drug is broken down in the bowel wall and more unchanged parent compound reaches blood than the dose was designed to deliver.

The fruit does this through furanocoumarins, citrus defense compounds stored strongly enough in grapefruit tissue that they reach the enterocyte, the absorptive intestinal cell, in active form. Bergamottin and 6',7'-dihydroxybergamottin are two of the best known examples. They do not merely sit beside the drug in the stomach. They interfere with the enzyme field the drug is supposed to meet on its way through the gut wall. The result is simple and severe. The prescription still says the same milligrams. The intestinal filter has thinned, so the body absorbs a larger effective dose than the label assumed under ordinary conditions.

This is why grapefruit belongs in a different category from fruits that are only sugar, acid, or fermentation problems. Grapefruit can become a pharmacologic fruit, a fruit whose plant chemistry changes drug handling directly. FDA's consumer guidance says the practical consequence plainly: instead of being metabolized in the small intestine, more drug may enter the bloodstream and stay in the body longer. That does not happen with every medicine. It matters most when the oral drug depends heavily on intestinal CYP3A4 to limit how much parent compound survives the crossing from bowel to blood. That is also why so many drug labels tell patients to avoid grapefruit or grapefruit juice entirely rather than simply "be careful" with it.

The danger is easy to underestimate because the fruit keeps all the ordinary signals of innocence. It is wet, bright, acidic, sweet, and sold as produce. The bowel still meets a defense chemistry strong enough to alter the dose of certain medications before the rest of the body ever sees them. The fruit did not add more medicine to the tablet. It reduced how much medicine the gut wall destroyed. That is enough.

Cassava Without Proper Processing

Cassava looks like simple starch until the root is broken open and the plant's defense chemistry starts moving. The tissue carries cyanogenic glycosides, mainly linamarin and a smaller amount of lotaustralin, compounds that remain comparatively quiet while the root is intact and become dangerous once peeling, grating, pounding, or chewing collapse the plant's internal compartments. WHO identifies cassava as one of the important food plants containing cyanogenic glycosides, and cassava reviews describe the same basic structure: the root stores carbohydrate for the plant while keeping a cyanide-releasing system in reserve. The sweetness of the starch never cancelled the chemistry wrapped around it.

The danger begins when the tissue is damaged without being processed far enough to carry the chemistry out. Once the cells rupture, endogenous enzymes gain access to the glycosides and begin converting them toward hydrogen cyanide, the small rapidly acting toxin the body then has to neutralize or suffer from. Cassava therefore does not become safer simply because it was cut, mashed, or milled. Those steps can make it more dangerous if they activate the release sequence and stop before enough cyanide and cyanogenic intermediates have been removed. Food Standards Australia New Zealand notes that disruption of the plant cells is what allows the chemistry to break down toward hydrogen cyanide, and the CDC outbreak report states bluntly that cassava can cause fatal cyanide poisoning if it is not properly detoxified.

Proper processing works because it does more than soften the root. Peeling removes outer tissues that often carry higher cyanogenic content than the inner pulp. Soaking, grating, fermenting, drying, and boiling then give the released chemistry somewhere to go other than the body. FAO notes that the peel contains higher cyanide content than the pulp and that removal of the peel lowers the burden immediately. Older cassava detoxification work and food-safety guidance keep returning to the same practical conclusion: combined methods work better than partial ones, with soaking plus boiling, or broader traditional sequences such as soaking, fermenting, and drying, reducing cyanide far more effectively than casual preparation or single weak steps alone.

That is what makes improperly processed cassava such a useful food in this book. It shows the full plant bargain without much camouflage. A root can look like neutral starch and still carry chemistry strong enough to produce acute poisoning or chronic neurologic damage if the tissue is opened and the burden is not driven out far enough before eating. The CDC described an outbreak from inadequately processed cassava flour in Uganda, and WHO continues to treat cassava as a major cyanogenic food precisely because safe use depends on adequate preparation, not on the public reputation of the root itself. Cassava does not become a better food because the eater wants to believe the starch is the whole story. The root is only as safe as the processing that dismantled its chemistry before the meal began.

Bitter Cucurbits

A bitter cucurbit is the plant dropping the mask. Zucchini, squash, cucumbers, pumpkins, bottle gourds, and related fruits are usually eaten only because generations of selection drove the flesh away from the harder chemistry still common in the family. The fruit keeps the soft texture, pale water-rich flesh, and easy kitchen identity, but the plant never abandoned its deterrent system entirely. Cucurbitacins are the main compounds behind that system, bitter triterpenoids, meaning thirty-carbon terpene-derived molecules built strongly enough to make feeding costly when their levels rise. In ordinary edible fruit the burden is usually low. When the chemistry reasserts itself, the bitterness stops being a flavor note and becomes the readable surface of defense.

That return can happen without the fruit looking suspicious. The skin may still look normal. The flesh may still slice and cook like a vegetable. The problem sits in the chemistry, not in dramatic spoilage. Pacific Northwest Extension notes that modern zucchini and squash should generally be low in these bitter compounds, but fruit from inadvertent cross-pollination with higher-cucurbitacin lines, along with abiotic or biotic stress such as water stress, can produce fruit with elevated cucurbitacin levels. The eater sees zucchini. The bowel receives a fruit that has shifted back toward defended cucurbit tissue.

Once enough of that chemistry is swallowed, the burden declares itself quickly because cucurbitacins are not passive plant decorations. They are directly irritating compounds. Extension and review sources describe severe gastrointestinal effects after surprisingly small exposures, with drooling, vomiting, diarrhea, headaches, severe abdominal cramping, collapse, and broader organ effects reported when the dose is high enough. Older literature cited in review work notes that severe symptoms have followed only one or two bites of contaminated squash, which shows how little the public reputation of the fruit matters once the deterrent chemistry rises far enough. The meal is no longer a vegetable side dish. It is an acute chemical insult moving through the gut.

Cooking does not rescue that event reliably. The fruit may soften, the seasonings may cover the bitterness, and the preparation may make the person more willing to keep eating it, but at least some forms of cucurbitacin appear heat-stable enough to persist through processing. The danger then becomes easier to miss because the tissue still looks edible while the warning signal is being masked. Bitter cucurbits belong in this book for that reason. They show the principle in a clean brutal form. A familiar fruit can still carry a deterrent chemistry strong enough to make the bowel pay quickly, and the bitterness was the plant's attempt to tell the eater that the fruit had stopped behaving like selected food and started behaving like defended tissue again.

High-Frequency Juice and Smoothie Patterns

A juice or smoothie habit changes the food before the body ever has a chance to slow it down. The blade, press, and filter have already done much of the mechanical damage that chewing, salivary mixing, gastric grinding, and slower release would otherwise have spread across time. Cell walls are ruptured. Sugars are loosened from the tissue that once held them. Fruit acids are dispersed through fluid instead of being met gradually inside intact flesh. Greens that would have occupied chewing time and stomach volume arrive as suspended particles or liquid. A person who would never sit down and chew through several apples, a pear, a banana, a handful of spinach, berries, almond butter, cacao, and a scoop of green powder can drink that chemistry in minutes. The produce identity stays intact in the mind. The structure that once put brakes on delivery is already gone.

Frequency is what turns that altered delivery into burden. One smoothie can be a meal. A daily smoothie, an afternoon juice, a fruit-and-greens drink after training, a powdered greens drink at night, and the body is no longer dealing with occasional produce. It is dealing with repeated fluid delivery of sugar, acids, polyols, oxalate, peel chemistry, seed-adjacent chemistry, and smaller plant compounds through the same bowel and into the same portal circulation. The stomach empties liquid more easily than intact food. The small intestine sees a faster carbohydrate wave. Fructose and sorbitol have less structural resistance slowing their arrival at the absorptive surface. If the transport capacity is exceeded, the retained sugar stays in the lumen, holds water there by osmosis, and moves into the colon as fermentation substrate. If the chemistry crosses, the liver receives a larger and more repetitive portal sugar load than the same plants would have delivered in slower intact form. The body is no longer reading fruit and greens as separate tissues. It is reading a concentrated daily infusion.

Greens make the same pattern harder in another direction. A handful of spinach in a salad is one oxalate exposure. Spinach pulverized into a daily smoothie with almond butter, cacao, beet powder, or sweet potato is another. The person feels virtuous because the ingredients are all culturally protected. The intestine still has to decide how much soluble oxalate stays free, how much calcium is available in the gut to trap it, and how much of that burden crosses into blood. The kidney then inherits whatever the bowel failed to leave behind. What looked like a clean habit can become repeated urinary oxalate delivery under the banner of health. The same distortion can happen with raw-heavy crucifer smoothies. The glass is carrying damaged sulfur-rich plant tissue with far less of the slowing and softening that cooking would have imposed. A person can therefore build fructose load, fermentable residue, oxalate burden, thyroid interference, fruit-acid exposure, and hepatic sorting work into one visually simple routine and then repeat it often enough that the organs stop experiencing it as food variety and start experiencing it as daily traffic.

The attraction of these patterns is exactly what makes them risky. They feel efficient. They compress time, chewing, meal preparation, and appetite signals into one approved ritual. They also compress chemistry. A whole-food meal usually pushes back through bulk, texture, satiety, and boredom before the dose becomes extreme. Juice and smoothies make overdelivery easier while keeping the health halo intact. The bowel still has to clear what stayed behind. The liver still has to sort what crossed. The kidney still has to excrete what the body could not use. High-frequency juice and smoothie patterns do not fail because blending is morally wrong or because every drink is a poison. They fail when repeated processing removes enough structural resistance that the body keeps receiving more plant chemistry, more sugar, and more low-yield burden than the pleasant ease of drinking ever warned the person was there.

A Practical Ranking System From Low Concern to High Concern

The safest way to rank plant foods is not by moral language and not by nutrient density on paper. Rank them by what the tissue does in the body and how often ordinary eating turns that chemistry into real organ work. At the low-concern end sit foods that still behave like food after digestion begins. The structure softens easily, the sugars or starches clear the small intestine without much residue, the minerals are not tightly trapped behind binding chemistry, and the liver and kidney are left with little cleanup after absorption is over. The return is clear and the burden stays modest. A fresh whole fruit with low polyol burden, eaten occasionally and tolerated well by the host, can belong here. So can lower-oxalate vegetables that do not arrive with much mineral-binding chemistry and do not demand unusual preparation before the gut can handle them. The point is not that these foods are chemically blank. The point is that the body extracts what it needs with relatively little friction and relatively little downstream waste handling.

The next level is moderate concern. These foods can work in some hosts, in some doses, and in some preparations, but the tradeoffs are real enough that they should never be judged by reputation alone. This is where many common fruits and vegetables belong. A fruit may still carry fructose or sorbitol in amounts that leave residue behind if the serving grows too large or the host has less absorptive room. A crucifer may be uneventful when cooked and eaten occasionally, then become a thyroid problem when eaten raw, concentrated, and repeated in a host with thin iodine reserve. A legume may be acceptable when soaked, thoroughly cooked, and used as one food among many, while still remaining a lower-yield protein and mineral source than its public image suggests. These foods are not automatically harmful. They are conditional foods. Dose, preparation, host reserve, and frequency decide whether they stay tolerable or start taking more than they give back.

High concern begins when the food carries chemistry that predictably lowers yield and predictably creates organ burden in ordinary use. High-oxalate greens and roots sit here because they can reduce calcium value in the gut and then shift the same burden into urine if enough soluble oxalate is absorbed. Heavy reliance on legumes can sit here too, especially when they become structural staples rather than occasional foods, because the person keeps receiving fermentable carbohydrate, phytate, and seed-storage resistance meal after meal even if the beans are properly cooked. Juice and smoothie patterns also climb into this range quickly because processing strips away much of the natural braking system and makes repeated delivery of sugar, acids, oxalate, and smaller plant compounds far easier than intact food would have allowed. These are not usually acute poison foods. They are burden foods. They become expensive through repetition, concentration, and underwhelming net yield.

Very high concern belongs to foods or conditions where the chemistry becomes hard to defend even before host sensitivity is added. Greening or sprouting potatoes belong here because the tuber has shifted back toward active glycoalkaloid defense. Bitter cucurbits belong here because the bitterness is the plant making cucurbitacin burden visible before the bowel is forced to absorb the lesson more violently. Cassava without proper processing belongs here because the tissue still carries a cyanide-releasing system that preparation must dismantle before eating. Raw or undercooked kidney beans belong here because the lectin burden can still act as an acute gastrointestinal toxin when proper heat has not denatured it. These foods do not merely ask for more digestion. They can punish the host quickly if the plant chemistry is allowed through intact enough.

The highest-consequence tier is narrower but more severe. This is where the food becomes dangerous because a specific host weakness turns ordinary-looking produce into a direct toxic event. Grapefruit with susceptible medications belongs here because the fruit changes drug exposure at the gut wall by thinning intestinal CYP3A4 handling. Star fruit in reduced kidney function belongs here because the host may no longer clear oxalate and caramboxin safely. High-oxalate foods in enteric hyperoxaluria, raw-heavy crucifer patterns in a thyroid already short on iodine reserve, or dense fruit and polyol exposure in a severely fermentation-sensitive bowel can enter the same practical zone for the person living in that physiology. The food may still be praised publicly. The host has lost enough margin that the chemistry no longer stays modest.

So the ranking system is simple in use even though the biology underneath it is not. Low concern means the body digests it easily, absorbs a meaningful return, and is left with little residue and little organ work. Moderate concern means the food can be workable but only under the right dose, preparation, and host conditions. High concern means the burden is built into ordinary use strongly enough that repetition commonly turns it into gut, hepatic, thyroid, or urinary work. Very high concern means the plant's own defense chemistry is still active enough that the food can become an acute problem if handled badly. Highest consequence means host vulnerability and plant chemistry have lined up cleanly enough that the food stops behaving like ordinary food at all. That is the ranking worth using because it follows tissue consequence, not prestige.

Conclusion

The Reputation of the Food Is Not the Same as Its Biological Result

The reputation of a food is assigned before digestion. It is built from color, freshness, sweetness, fiber language, vitamin language, cultural prestige, epidemiologic shorthand, and the emotional comfort of calling a tissue natural. The biological result is assigned later. It is assigned in the stomach that had to acidify the meal, in the small intestine that had to break it down and move its dissolved chemistry across a membrane, in the colon that inherited whatever residue absorption did not finish, in the liver that received the absorbed fraction in portal blood and had to transform it, in the thyroid that had to keep building hormone while certain plant compounds pressed on the same sequence, and in the kidney that had to concentrate the dissolved remainder into urine without letting it crystallize or injure the tubule. That is the principle this book has been following from the first chapter forward. A food can keep a clean public identity and still produce a poor biological result. A food can look chemically impressive on paper and still undernourish, destabilize digestion, interfere with endocrine function, or increase the burden of clearance once the full sequence is made visible.

The body experiences chemistry, not marketing. It does not absorb a halo. It does not absorb the phrase plant-based, antioxidant-rich, anti-inflammatory, heart-healthy, or nutrient-dense. It absorbs what digestion released and what the intestine allowed into blood. It carries what survived the gut into tissues that then have to decide whether the compound can be used, stored, transformed, buffered, filtered, or excreted. That is why a fruit can still become a bowel problem, a liver problem, a dental problem, or a pharmacologic problem. That is why a green can still become a mineral problem in the gut and a crystal problem in the kidney. That is why a crucifer can still become a thyroid problem in the wrong host. The market sees categories. The body sees molecules meeting membranes, enzymes, transporters, colloids, tubules, and glandular tissue under conditions that either favor use or favor burden.

The modern conversation about plants fails because it stays too abstract to explain real symptoms. It speaks in categories broad enough to flatter and too broad to diagnose. Vegetables are healthy. Fruit is natural sugar. Fiber is good for the gut. Antioxidants are protective. Diversity is beneficial. The problem is not that these phrases are always false. The problem is that they are too weak to explain why one person bloats after fruit, why another forms stones on a plant-heavy smoothie pattern, why another slows metabolically while building the diet around raw crucifers, why another feels chronically burdened on a socially approved high-legume, high-seed, high-green diet, and why these symptoms often fluctuate enough to hide the mechanism from the person living inside them. A bowel does not respond to abstraction. It responds to retained fructose, sorbitol, water, gas, acids, and rough or irritating residue. A kidney does not respond to vegetable virtue. It responds to oxalate, urine volume, pH, calcium, and supersaturation. A thyroid does not respond to kale's public status. It responds to iodide delivery, transport, oxidation, organification, and interference. The abstract plant conversation fails because it never enters the tissue where the event is actually happening.

A better standard is now simple enough to carry forward without ideology. What does the meal yield. What does it block. What does it burden. What does it cost to clear. Those are the four questions that survive contact with physiology. Yield asks what the body actually extracted and retained after digestion and absorption were finished. Block asks whether the same food tied up minerals, slowed enzymes, trapped nutrients, or reduced the value of the rest of the meal. Burden asks what the food left behind in the gut, what it asked the liver to transform, what it asked the thyroid to work around, and what it sent to the kidney as dissolved remainder. Cost to clear asks what the body had to spend in bile flow, enzyme activity, glutathione, urinary concentration, and organ reserve just to get rid of chemistry it never meaningfully turned into tissue. A food that answers those questions badly is biologically poor no matter how strong its reputation remains. A food that answers them well does not need much praise because the tissues already showed the result.

That is the closing argument of this book. Common fruits and vegetables can carry real toxic, antinutritive, endocrine, digestive, and renal consequences, not because every plant is secretly poison and not because the answer is to react with a new ideology, but because plant tissues are chemical structures with tradeoffs that simplistic nutrition language has flattened almost beyond recognition. Some plants are low burden and worth keeping. Some are improved meaningfully by peeling, boiling, fermenting, sprouting, or pressure cooking. Some are tolerable only in modest amounts or in hosts with broad reserve. Some are structurally poor bargains that keep returning more interference than nourishment. The body has never been confused about this. It has been measuring the difference between reputation and result all along. The confusion lived in the language. The chemistry was always there.

Made in the USA
Monee, IL
05 November 2026

67914358R00226